Applied Health Fitness Psychology

Mark H. Anshel, PhD

Middle Tennessee State University

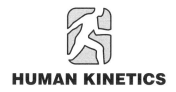

HUMAN KINETICS

Library of Congress Cataloging-in-Publication Data

Anshel, Mark H. (Mark Howard)
    Applied health fitness psychology / Mark Anshel.
        p. ; cm.
    Includes bibliographical references and index.
    I. Title.
    [DNLM: 1. Exercise--psychology. 2. Physical Fitness--psychology. 3. Health Behavior. QT 255]
    RC482
    616.89'13--dc23

                                    2013015458

ISBN-10: 1-4504-0062-0 (print)
ISBN-13: 978-1-4504-0062-6 (print)

The web addresses cited in this text were current as of August 6, 2013, unless otherwise noted.

Acquisitions Editor: Myles Schrag; **Developmental Editor:** Judy Park; **Managing Editor:** Katherine Maurer; **Assistant Editor:** Casey A. Gentis; **Copyeditor:** Alisha Jeddeloh; **Indexer:** Andrea J. Hepner; **Permissions Manager:** Dalene Reeder; **Graphic Designer:** Joe Buck; **Graphic Artist:** Yvonne Griffith; **Cover Designer:** Keith Blomberg; **Photograph (cover):** © Hakan Hjort/ Johner Images RF/age fotostock; **Photographs (interior):** © Human Kinetics, unless otherwise noted. Photos p. 1 and 215 © Bananastock, photo p. 67 © Blend Images, photo p. 74 courtesy of the author, photo p. 143 © Flashon Studio/fotolia.com, photo p. 217 © BOLD STOCK/age fotostock; **Photo Production Manager:** Jason Allen; **Visual Production Assistant:** Joyce Brumfield; **Art Manager:** Kelly Hendren; **Associate Art Manager:** Alan L. Wilborn; **Printer:** Sheridan Books

Printed in the United States of America   10 9 8 7 6 5 4 3 2 1

The paper in this book is certified under a sustainable forestry program.

Human Kinetics
Website: www.HumanKinetics.com

United States: Human Kinetics
P.O. Box 5076
Champaign, IL 61825-5076
800-747-4457
e-mail: humank@hkusa.com

Canada: Human Kinetics
475 Devonshire Road Unit 100
Windsor, ON N8Y 2L5
800-465-7301 (in Canada only)
e-mail: info@hkcanada.com

Europe: Human Kinetics
107 Bradford Road
Stanningley
Leeds LS28 6AT, United Kingdom
+44 (0) 113 255 5665
e-mail: hk@hkeurope.com

Australia: Human Kinetics
57A Price Avenue
Lower Mitcham, South Australia 5062
08 8372 0999
e-mail: info@hkaustralia.com

New Zealand: Human Kinetics
P.O. Box 80
Torrens Park, South Australia 5062
0800 222 062
e-mail: info@hknewzealand.com

E5270

This book is dedicated to the memory of my parents, Bernard and Rochelle Anshel, who gave me the opportunity to learn, to grow, to mature, and to feel compassion in helping others through my teaching and writing. My parents taught me to embrace the values of health, education, performance excellence, family, and faith that served me well on my journey through life. I also am very grateful for their patience during my childhood, which allowed me the chance to mature and to explore my independence in a safe and secure environment. Thanks, Mom and Dad, for providing me with a roof over my head, food on the table, and the opportunity to learn and to make a difference in the lives of others.

I can relate to the following quotation by former world heavyweight boxing champion, Mohammad Ali: "Champions aren't made in the gyms. Champions are made from something they have deep inside them—a desire, a dream, a vision." Amen!

Contents

9 Cognitive and Behavioral Strategies 169

10 Fitness Goal Setting and Leadership. 199

Part IV Professional Considerations   215

11 Fitness Consulting With Special Populations. 217

12 Dysfunctional Eating Behaviors 237

13 Professional Organizations and Ethics 255

Preface

This book addresses the need to assist a group of professionals who are devoted to changing the health behavior of clients and patients. A book about changing health behavior is a book about making a difference in peoples' lives. There is no greater source of satisfaction. The information contained in this book will empower health professionals to fulfill their ambition to help others create lifelong habits and make long-term changes in their lives. Though modifying a person's—or a culture's—disdain for exercise will not happen quickly, we can mobilize a group of educated and trained professionals to change the culture of inactivity and overeating to becoming more aware and fully engaged in the many benefits of a more active lifestyle. Lifestyle change cannot be forced, but juxtaposing the benefits of a healthier lifestyle with the many short-term costs and long-term consequences of a sedentary lifestyle and linking people to a vast network of social support, particularly with the involvement of health professionals, will help change the way we live.

The motivation to write this book was based on three factors:

1. As a society, we engage in unhealthy habits every single day.
2. These unhealthy habits are misaligned (i.e., disconnected) from our values—what we cherish and what matters most to us (e.g., health, happiness, family, faith, energy, character).
3. This disconnect between our unhealthy habits and values results in serious short-term costs and long-term consequences to our health and quality of life.

The results of our unhealthy habits are increased rates of obesity and obesity-related diseases, especially type 2 diabetes, heart disease, hypertension, and various cancers. A new professional industry is blossoming whose mission is to support people on their journey to a better life, providing physical, mental, emotional, and often spiritual support to help them reach their destination of better health and happiness. This book provides one source of information in support of this mission. *Applied Health Fitness Psychology* represents a new area of practice and research, and it addresses ways in which professionals who attempt to improve physical and mental health can help others take control of their lives and overcome obstacles in their journey to become healthy members of society.

FITNESS AND HEALTH ATTITUDES

Once upon a time, we loved physical activity. As children, we played, competed, and had fun in our quest to remain active. We didn't call it exercise, but our activity level was persistent, gratifying, and made us feel good. So what happened? At some point we stopped finding the time to be active, and our attitudes toward exercise and other forms of physical activity turned increasingly negative. Computers, demands of the academic world and work, television, and an array of electronic devices have worked jointly toward creating a society that has increasingly rejected opportunities to be physically active. As a result, our weight has increased while our health has decreased. Our sedentary lifestyle is killing us, and the data supporting this contention are current and compelling. This is the primary rationale for writing this book and helping health professionals to deliver a much-needed service to those who desperately need to change their lives.

The time is ripe to create an educational program that helps professionals in the health industry to help others replace their negative, unhealthy habits with better, healthier rituals that improve energy and quality of life. It is this new professional for whom this book was written. The primary purpose of this book is to understand, explain, and achieve one of the most challenging goals confronted by health and fitness professionals—replacing a person's negative habits with ones that are healthier. The causes of human behavior, particularly the self-destructive choices we make, are complex. The book reflects an evidence-based approach in which the research literature forms the foundation for using techniques and interventions that foster the motivation for people to improve their health and quality of life.

HOW THIS BOOK IS ORGANIZED

Applied Health Fitness Psychology is divided into four parts. Part I, Theoretical Foundations of Health Fitness Psychology, includes chapters 1 through 3, which address the scientific basis on which the book was conceived and developed. This section recognizes the contributions of multiple disciplines that can make a difference in changing unhealthy habits. These disciplines include sport and exercise psychology, counseling and clinical psychology, exercise science, sports medicine, nutrition, and behavioral medicine.

Part II, Factors That Influence Health Behavior, includes chapters 4 through 7. These chapters ask and attempt to answer profound questions about the primary objective of health professionals. Why do people engage in self-destructive behavior? Why are we our own worst enemy when it comes to unhealthy habits? Not surprisingly, there are many obstacles to adopting a healthy lifestyle.

In part III, Strategies for Health Behavior Interventions, chapters 8 through 10 discuss the use of cognitive and behavioral strategies and interventions for changing health behavior. This section addresses ways to promote exercise adherence, the use of cognitive and behavioral strategies to improve exercise performance and fitness, and the proper way to set goals.

Part IV, Professional Considerations, includes chapters 11 through 13, which address issues related to being a professional in health fitness psychology. These considerations include working with special populations and dysfunctional eating. They also include learning about professional organizations, their codes of ethics, and the criteria required to join them in order to attend their conferences, obtain their professional journals, and acquire other publications regarding the requisite skills for professional practice. Professional organizations help their members to remain current with new advances in professional practice and to acknowledge areas for needed future research and advancement.

SPECIAL FEATURES OF THIS BOOK

Each chapter begins with a set of chapter objectives that reflect what the reader should know after finishing the chapter. Chapter objectives help learners to focus on the most relevant features of the chapter so that key concepts can be applied.

Tables, figures, and highlight boxes help readers focus on relevant features of material explained more fully in the text. Learning is more efficient when we reduce the amount of information we are exposed to at one time; avoiding information overload is a teaching technique that promotes retention. Highlight boxes, tables, and figures perform this function.

The *From Research to Real World* section concerns the application of research findings, theories, models, and general literature concepts. The key word in writing this book was *applied*. An extensive effort was made to bridge research to the application of key concepts, which reflects an evidence-based approach.

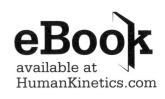

Each chapter ends with a summary of content, student activity, and key concepts. Summary material is intended to improve the learner's retention of chapter information. Each *Student Activity* has been developed to practice and apply a concept presented in the chapter in a meaningful way. Finally, references for each chapter reflect the most important research findings, theories, and other concepts that give credibility to the application of book material.

NOTE TO INSTRUCTORS

The primary goal of this book is to provide the tools for health and fitness professionals—both current (professionals) and future (students)—to help others lead healthier and more productive lives. Current and future professionals will be challenged by what familial and cultural norms view as typical or even healthy. For example, because obesity is ubiquitous, it is therefore considered acceptable and normal.

As instructors, we teach our students—our future health and fitness professionals—how to help clients acknowledge that there will be consequences for their unhealthy habits, and we promote the process of helping clients acknowledge the need for a "new normal" of desirable lifestyle choices. Instructors need to challenge students to think about their mission in helping others make better decisions that are consistent with their values.

Consider using current events and recent research reported in the media that reflect why we should be concerned about our health and what we should do about it. For example, one of the consequences of a sedentary lifestyle is financial, as health care is becoming more and more expensive. Who pays for these consequences?

Ancillary resources for each chapter include PowerPoint slides (which the instructor may alter). I have found that students will benefit from class lectures if they have access to

PowerPoint slides that are saved in handout format as a PDF, which allows for three slides per page with room for taking notes adjacent to each slide. The book is also accompanied by a test package of objective (i.e., multiple choice, true–false) and essay examination questions that instructors may use to assess student learning.

NOTE TO STUDENTS

A final word about the writing style of this book. Because this book is intended for university students and practitioners, I purposely avoided extensive use of references and the so-called scholarly prose that is more common in research journals. I wanted readers to be able to understand and apply the information clearly with minimal distractions from extensive reviews of research literature and accompanying references. The narrative style should make it easier to apply concepts. In addition, it was important for me to provide information that reflects my background as an educator, researcher, and practitioner. My initial career was as a fitness director in community recreation, and I have directed several wellness programs on campus, in the community, and in law enforcement. The application of literature required a less formal, more hands-on writing style.

Here's wishing you—current and future health and fitness professionals—success and pleasure in the power you have in making a difference in the lives of others.

Mark H. Anshel, PhD
Mark.Anshel@mtsu.edu

Acknowledgments

Many thanks to my Middle Tennessee State University librarian Sharon Parente for her assistance with this book. Thank you also to the Human Kinetics team of Myles Schrag, Judy Park, Kate Maurer, Casey Gentis, and their crew for their hard work and diligence in getting this book to press.

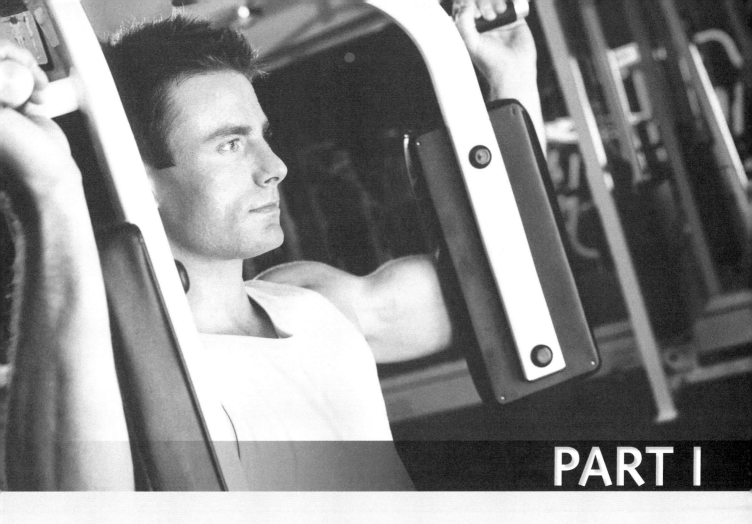

PART I

THEORETICAL FOUNDATIONS OF HEALTH FITNESS PSYCHOLOGY

Introducing a new area of study and practice, particularly one that connects disparate academic disciplines such as health fitness psychology, must begin with a strong theoretical foundation. Theoretical foundations provide a basis on which to describe, explain, and predict human behavior and determine how professionals can favorably change it. There is a great need to bring together multiple disciplines that can make a difference in changing unhealthy habits, including sport and exercise psychology, counseling and clinical psychology, exercise science, sports medicine, nutrition, and behavioral medicine.

Chapter 1 concerns the advantages of exercise. It describes explanations and theories of the mental and physical benefits of exercise,

explains exercise motives, and defines and clarifies terms and concepts. Chapter 2 discusses the various motivation theories and addresses what fitness coaches, mental health professionals, and health care workers can do to improve exercise motivation. Finally, chapter 3 includes the definitions and clarification of theories and models. It maintains the momentum from chapter 2 by focusing more exclusively on health-related theories to explain and predict exercise behavior. This area is especially important because researchers and practitioners are interested in determining which interventions are most effective at improving health behavior and replacing unhealthy habits with more desirable ones.

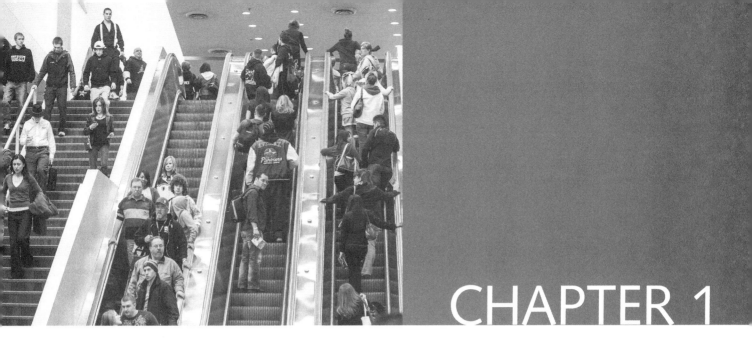

Introduction to Applied Health Fitness Psychology

66 *People are always blaming their circumstances for what they are. I don't believe in* 99 *circumstances. The people who get on in this world are the people who get up and look for the circumstances they want, and if they can't find them, make them.*

George Bernard Shaw (1856-1950), playwright and philosopher

CHAPTER OBJECTIVES

After reading this chapter, you should be able to:

- define and differentiate among the concepts of applied health psychology, fitness psychology, and exercise psychology;

- list and describe the reasons people maintain unhealthy habits, many of which are self-destructive and long-term;

- explain the process of replacing these negative habits with healthier routines; and

- identify the types of credentialing and ethical issues in applied health fitness psychology.

At no time in our history has it been more important to help others rid themselves of unhealthy behavior patterns. We live in a culture of self-destructive habits, and the cost of our poor lifestyle is staggering. Obesity in particular, often the consequence of poor eating habits combined with a sedentary lifestyle, has reached epidemic proportions in the United States and many other countries. The economic costs of obesity are extensive, and adult obesity is the second leading cause of death in the United States (U.S. Department of Health and Human Services [HHS], 2006). In addition, childhood obesity is soaring. For the first time in U.S. history, children today will live shorter lives than their parents, mainly due to obesity and the resultant type 2 diabetes, which shortens the life span (National Center for Health Statistics, 2010). Obese people are far more likely to suffer from diabetes and resultant conditions such as kidney failure, leg amputations, stroke, various types of cancer, and blindness (Jebb, 2004). Only 1% to 3% of obesity can be explained by heredity; its main causes are environmental and due to human behavior (Bauman et al., 2012).

An extensive review of related research indicates that "physical inactivity accounts for more than 3 million deaths per year" (Pratt et al., 2012, p. 282). In an analysis of 100 physical activity interventions, researchers examined the effects of various interventions on increasing the frequency and duration of physical activity (Pratt et al., 2012). Types included web-based, Internet-based, mobile phone (including texting), and transportation-related interventions. The researchers found that the use of electronic communication, particularly if the messages were "personally tailored behavioral and cognitive tips for increasing activity" (p. 290), significantly increased the number of minutes per week of physical activity, particularly in high-income countries. Thus, conscious attempts at cognitive and behavioral interventions can increase physical activity levels if the activity becomes habitual and part of the person's lifestyle. Nevertheless, in another review, Bauman et al. (2012) concluded that more effective interventions are needed to improve physical activity rates, especially exercise participation and long-term adherence.

It is important to understand the known causes of unhealthy behavior patterns and to institute interventions that prevent and treat changes in health behavior. The psychology of health behavior change has received surprisingly little attention in the education and training of health care professionals to influence client behavior. Increasing people's physical activity, particularly exercise, is a primary aim of this book, which focuses on assisting health professionals, including exercise trainers, dietitians, medical practitioners, rehabilitation specialists, and mental health professionals, to develop and maintain client attitudes and emotions for improving energy and promoting a healthy lifestyle. Students who plan to enter the health care industry or professionals who are currently providing services to improve clients' physical or mental health will be provided with strategies and interventions to help others develop and maintain healthy habits to improve their quality of life.

Changing the thoughts, emotions, and behaviors of others is a challenging, often impossible task. This is especially true when it comes to replacing an unhealthy habit with a healthier one. Coaches, for example, try to influence an athlete's psychological readiness to compete before a competitive event and transfer those feelings (e.g., self-confidence, concentration, motivation) and emotions (e.g., managing anxiety and arousal level) to the contest for optimal performance. Personal trainers and fitness coaches attempt to do the same thing with respect to completing exercise routines and meeting performance goals. Most of us need a coach—a person who will guide us to perform optimally and consistently—to help us replace our unhealthy habits with more desirable ones. We need to change our self-destructive behaviors and lifestyle choices.

The purpose of this book is to help the helper, that is, to assist the person whose professional mission is to provide a service that enables clients to acknowledge their unhealthy habits and to replace them with more desirable routines. Health behavior change is the responsibility of educators, medical practitioners, mental health professionals, dietitians, and fitness coaches, among others, who provide clients with the incentive to lead a more productive and happy life.

PSYCHOLOGICAL BENEFITS OF EXERCISE

Results of scientific research have been clear and consistent for many years regarding the benefits of exercise and other forms of physical activity on an array of physiological processes. In addition to the physical health benefits, it is important to recognize the strong influence of regular exercise on mental health and numerous psychological factors, particularly the aging process and quality of life. Personality traits, such as trait anxiety and perfectionism, are stable across situations and permanent; they are not susceptible to exercise effects and other short-term treatments. Other mental states, however, are clearly influenced by both short-term (often called *acute*) and long-term (often called *chronic*) exercise behavior. The focus of this section is to examine how exercise influences a person's mental health and certain psychological characteristics. Perhaps the most notable changes in psychological functioning concern stress, state anxiety, mood, self-esteem, cognitive functioning, and depression.

Reduced Stress

Results of several studies have confirmed that both short-term (a single exercise bout) and long-term (over a period of weeks, months, or years) exercise markedly reduce both acute and chronic forms of stress (Dishman and Jackson, 2000). The mechanisms of this positive effect are explained by the distraction, or time-out, hypothesis (Bahrke and Morgan, 1978) in which the exerciser is concentrating on the exercise activity and avoiding or minimizing stressful thoughts. The pleasant thoughts that distract the person by attending

to the task at hand—exercise—also increase feelings of self-control. This is beneficial because the lack of self-control is a source of acute and chronic stress. Stress-reducing properties are more likely if each exercise session lasts for at least 30 minutes. In their review of literature, Buckworth and Dishman (2002) concluded that "aerobic exercise programs lasting at least a few months seem best for reducing reports of chronic stress" (p. 79). However, exercising will not reduce stress and may actually increase stress if the person is required or coerced to exercise.

Reduced State Anxiety

Anxiety differs from stress. Stress reflects a sense of immediate danger or a physiological response related to confrontation or escape, often termed *fight-or-flight response*. Anxiety, on the other hand, consists of feelings of worry or threat regarding future harm. For instance, a person who has been injured might feel threatened by reinjury when engaging in physical activity after rehabilitation. This is one reason why athletes commonly do not perform as well when they return to competition after rehabilitating an injury.

Anxiety has two forms, trait and state. Trait anxiety is, as the name implies, a personality trait and therefore is stable across situations and not amenable to change. People with high trait anxiety (which can be measured with a written inventory) are predisposed to perceive apparently harmless situations as threatening. Exercise will not change their level of trait anxiety, but it can alter their disposition to feel anxiety in a certain situation. A low trait-anxious individual is less susceptible to situational anxiety compared with a high trait-anxious person. State anxiety, on the other hand, refers to an emotional state of worry in which the person interprets a particular future situation as threatening. Examples of self-talk of an anxious person might include "I hope I don't reinjure my arm" or "What if I cannot finish the race?"

What is important to remember about anxiety is that the person's feelings reflect the anticipation or prediction of a *future* event or condition that causes psychological discomfort. If the threatening anticipated event is *currently* being experienced, the feeling is categorized as perceived stress.

Hackfort and Spielberger (1989) state that anxiety "is an emotional state that consist of a unique combination of feelings of tension, apprehension and nervousness, unpleasant thoughts (worries), and physiological changes" (p. 5). The experience of threat, they explain, is a state of mind that has two main characteristics:

1. It is oriented toward the future, generally involving the anticipation of a potentially harmful event that has not yet happened (e.g., "Will others look and laugh at me when I am trying to work out at the fitness club?").

2. It is mediated, or influenced, by complex mental processes that are involved in appraising, interpreting, and perceiving the situation (e.g., "Just perform your routines and stop looking around the weight room; focus on the next task").

Differences between stress and anxiety are important with respect to their treatment and interventions, which are discussed later in this chapter and in chapter 5.

Another area of clarification includes knowing the difference between acute (short-term) and chronic (long-term) anxiety and how exercise, particularly aerobic exercise, helps reduce both types of anxiety. Exercise benefits only state, not trait, anxiety, however. The findings from numerous research studies is that even a single bout of aerobic exercise, as well as involvement in a longer-term aerobic exercise program, markedly reduces state anxiety. Aerobic exercise has also benefited patients with various anxiety disorders (e.g., panic disorder, post-traumatic stress disorder) and clinical depression (Petruzzello, Landers, Hatfield, Kubitz, and Salazar). These findings were similar for people with varying levels of initial fitness. Exercise of any type, however, is not likely to influence trait anxiety because of its long-term, unchanging nature.

How does exercise help manage anxiety? Although trait anxiety is not altered by exercise or any other behavior pattern because, like any other trait, it is stable and intrinsic to an individual's personality, there are valid explanations of the mechanisms that help reduce state (i.e., situational) anxiety. As briefly discussed earlier in this chapter, the primary theory is the distraction or time-out hypothesis, which posits that exercise reduces stress and anxiety because exercisers take a time-out by focusing on the exercise experience instead of reflecting on unpleasant thoughts. This is one reason it is important to disconnect from the real world and stop thinking and talking about stressful topics while engaged in exercise and other forms of pleasant physical activity. This is also why it is important that exercisers perceive their form of physical activity as pleasant and desirable. If people feel negative about jogging, for example, they should try to achieve aerobic fitness through another type of aerobic exercise that they find less unpleasant, such as using elliptical equipment or a stationary bicycle, perhaps while listening to music.

Improved Mood

Mood, often called *mood state*, is a situational characteristic ranging from the immediate present to one week in duration. Moods are subjective states and consist of a person's thoughts. Because mood is usually measured as a state (situational) rather than trait characteristic, research on the effects of exercise on mood have focused on immediate rather than long-term effects.

Berger and Motl (2000) conducted a comprehensive review of the research literature related to the effects of exercise on mood. The authors examined studies over the past 25 years in which mood was measured specifically by the Profile of Mood States (POMS). They concluded that there is unequivocal support for the mood-enhancing effects of exercise, specifically on improved vigor and reduced tension, depression, anger, confusion, and fatigue. The authors attributed changes in mood following exercise to psychological mechanisms, including "enhanced self-concept, feelings of self-efficacy, enjoyment, expectancy of psychological benefits, 'time out' from one's routine and daily hassles, and an increased sense of control" (p. 84). Physiological mechanisms (e.g., cortisol, endorphins, monoamines) reflecting biochemical changes may also partly explain mood alteration during and after exercise. With respect to exercise intensity, the authors recommend that unless a participant prefers low or high exercise intensity, moderate-intensity exercise creates optimal conditions for mood changes.

Lox, Martin Ginis, and Petruzzello (2010) identify three ways in which moods differ from emotions. First, moods last longer than emotions; emotions are usually short-lived. Second, the causes of emotions can usually be explained, whereas moods often cannot.

People who say, for instance, "I'm in a bad mood," often cannot identify the cause of these feelings. Third, emotions are usually more intense and variable than moods.

Research on the effects of exercise on mood state has focused on immediate rather than long-term effects. Results of these studies indicate that exercise generally improves mood. As mentioned earlier, the POMS instrument shows that exercise increases vigor while reducing tension, depression, anger, and mental fatigue. In other words, positive mood tends to increase after an exercise bout and negative mood tends to decrease.

There are several possible explanations for an elevated positive mood state following exercise or, for that matter, following most forms of physical activity. As mentioned earlier, optimal conditions for mood changes for

EMOTIONAL SUPPORT FOR NOVICE EXERCISERS

If exercise reduces stress and anxiety and improves mood state, why do so many people find exercise unpleasant and quickly drop out of programs? Practitioners such as fitness leaders, personal trainers, physical education teachers, and others in the business of promoting healthy habits must remember that most exercise novices will find the road to improved fitness challenging and threatening. Usually, they have not engaged in formal exercise for many years, are currently unfit and overweight, and feel self-conscious about their appearance compared with other exercisers in the facility who might be fitter, younger, and thinner. Follow these procedures when working with such clients:

1. Be sensitive to their mind-set upon entering an exercise facility. They will be nervous and self-conscious about their appearance.

2. Novices require instruction on proper exercise techniques (e.g., how to lift weights to avoid injury and to improve muscular strength, how to stretch correctly). Their lack of understanding of how to use equipment increases their self-consciousness and discomfort in the fitness facility. Teach them proper exercise movements and praise high-quality performance and, especially, performance improvement.

3. Attempt to greet clients near the entrance of the facility so that they see a friendly face upon entering, and take the time to provide exercise instruction. (Client interaction is discussed in greater detail later in the book.)

4. Always pay attention to clients when providing instruction or giving performance feedback; they can spot a consultant who is going through the motions and does not really care about their well-being. Observe them while they lift weights, for instance, and jog or walk with them at least part of the way.

5. Provide clients with positive feedback during and at the end of the exercise session so that they feel competent, feel they are learning and improving exercise techniques, and start to feel comfortable. It is imperative to slowly introduce novice clients to the unfamiliar world of exercise. The combination of feeling comfortable and successfully completing the workout will provide the incentive to return and build an exercise routine. Taken together, these early steps will help clients feel less threatened (i.e., anxious) and more confident and secure in pursuing a regular exercise habit.

all of these possible explanations occur at a moderate intensity of exercise.

- *Endorphin hypothesis.* One possible cause of mood change following exercise is a function of biochemical changes via endorphins, hormones known to create a state of euphoria during physical activity. This process is thought to at least partially explain exercise dependence in which the person is addicted to exercise, especially cardiorespiratory exercise (see Hoffmann, 1997, for a review).

- *Distraction hypothesis.* Exercise has stress-reducing properties by distracting the person from stressful and unpleasant thoughts and feelings, thereby improving mood (Bahrke and Morgan, 1978). Stress, anxiety, and unpleasant feelings are either forgotten or ignored while the person's focus is on the exercise task, the environment in which exercise is performed, or other people who form an integral part of the exercise experience. Exercise is an excellent time-out strategy from the day's demands.

- *Thermogenic hypothesis.* Another explanation for a positive mood following exercise is that the elevation of body temperature caused by exercise has a relaxing effect. Researchers have found that elevated body temperature produces therapeutic benefits, such as muscle relaxation and reduced anxiety (Koltyn and Morgan, 1992). The thermogenic hypothesis holds that a similar reaction follows exercise, which causes an elevated internal body temperature (see Koltyn, 1997, for a review). A similar change in psychological factors may occur, such as reduced anxiety and other negative feelings.

- *Social interaction hypothesis.* Exercise may improve mood state if the person exercises in the company of others and enjoys this type of environment. This is especially true in special programs that improve health, fitness, or rehabilitation where a group of individuals meet regularly to experience therapy, such as patients who attend postcoronary exercise programs (Burke, Carron, and Shapcott, 2008). The social interaction hypothesis also explains the value of a related concept called *social support.* Numerous studies clearly indicate that people who exercise with others, a form of direct social support, or receive verbal encouragement from others, a form of indirect social support, are more likely to have positive feelings about their exercise program and maintain their participation than people who want to exercise with others but instead do so alone (Watson, Martin Ginis, and Spink, 2004).

Increased Self-Esteem

Self-esteem, also referred to as *self-worth,* concerns the degree to which people value or approve of their personal identity (i.e., how you feel about who you are). Positive self-esteem is associated with good mental health.

Self-esteem is a multidimensional concept, meaning that it has a variety of sources. It includes knowledge (academic), physical (also called *somatic*), sport, social, religious, family, and work dimensions. Exercise is more likely to improve self-esteem if people (a) consider exercise a source of enjoyment, (b) feel a sense of achievement due to improving their exercise performance and fitness, and (c) believe that exercise is related to good health and, in many cases, improved physical appearance (e.g., maintaining healthy body weight).

The influence of exercise on self-esteem is related to the exerciser's initial level of self-esteem. For example, Buckworth and Dishman (2002) concluded that "positive associations between exercise and self-esteem have been found, but effects are stronger for individuals initially lower in self-esteem," and "exercise has more potent effects on physical self-concept and self-esteem than on general self-perceptions" (p. 168). The authors also found that, among females, exercise especially improves self-esteem if they have a particularly strong body or physique self-esteem (i.e., if they link their self-worth—their sense of value and competence—to their physical attributes). Concomitant changes in other forms of self-esteem (e.g., family, academic, sport) were not noted.

Improved Cognitive Functioning

Cognitive functioning describes the entire process of how we take in, use, and respond to information. Processing information begins with detecting an environmental stimulus, followed by perceiving and interpreting the stimulus to make sense out of it, then often thinking about the perceived information, sometimes storing it in memory for later use, making a decision that determines what happens next (react versus don't react), and often executing a coordinated action. *Cognitive functioning*, then, is defined as the process of detecting, interpreting, storing, determining, and acting at the proper speed, accuracy, and efficiency.

The important point about cognitive functioning in the present context is that exercise, especially aerobic exercise, improves the speed, efficiency, and accuracy of cognitive functioning (Etnier and Chang, 2009). Several studies on various age groups have confirmed that exercise benefits cognitive functioning by improving attentional focus, concentration, monitoring of one's thought processes and emotions, information storage and retrieval from short-term and long-term memory, and execution of motor skills in children (Davis et al., 2007) and older adults (Larson et al., 2006).

The aging process normally slows and reduces the capability of the brain and nervous system to function at optimal levels. The brain structure and function deteriorate with advanced age, and cognitive functioning is inhibited as a result. The combination of aging and a sedentary lifestyle hastens the effects of aging on cognitive functioning.

Can exercise reverse the effects of aging on cognitive functioning? In their extensive review of this literature, Lox and colleagues (2010) concluded that "we can expect a program of regular exercise results in improvements in cognitive function and even reverses the loss of function seen with aging" (p. 390). Does a single exercise bout, however, benefit cognitive functioning? Using laboratory tasks, such as reaction time (i.e., the time interval between detecting a stimulus and initiating a response), decision-making speed, and visual tracking, the authors determined that "it appears that single bouts of activity may have utility in the short term, in terms of enhancing the processing of information" (p. 391). It seems, therefore, that exercise has both

short-term and long-term benefits for cognitive functioning.

Depression Prevention

The *Diagnostic and Statistical Manual of Mental Disorders (DSM)* classifies depression as a mood disturbance that includes disorders that influence mood regulation. Exercise has been shown to reduce symptoms of depression. The characteristics of depression include sustained feelings of sadness, feelings of guilt or worthlessness, disturbances in appetite, disturbances in sleep patterns, lack of energy, difficulty concentrating, loss of interest in all or most activities, problems with memory, thoughts of suicide, and hallucinations.

The research has focused primarily on exercise as a preventive measure of depression and effects of exercise on existing depression. Extensive reviews of literature by Lox et al. (2010) and Biddle and Mutrie (2001) have reported extensive benefits of exercise on both depression prevention and remedy. For instance, several studies have shown depression prevention effects. Their reviews indicated that women who are sedentary or engaged in little physical activity are twice as likely to develop depression compared with women who are at least moderately active. In addition, there is an association between inactivity and incidence of depression. The risk of developing depression is significantly greater for both men and women if they are inactive. Further, physical activity at baseline is negatively associated with depression in later life, whereas more physical activity predicts lower depression.

Can exercise serve as a treatment for depression? In a meta-analysis of 80 studies, North, McCullagh, and Tran (1990) found that exercise resulted in decreased depression, and it was as effective as or more effective than traditional therapies. They also found that all types of exercise similarly reduced depression—weight training, aerobic activity, and walking all had similar effects on depression. Exercise helped decrease depression for all age groups and genders, and people who trained harder experienced a greater reduction in depression than people who trained at moderate or low intensity. Finally, the optimal conditions under which exercise improved clinical depression were when exercise training

- occurred over at least five weeks,
- was performed at least three times per week,
- was of low to moderate intensity (50% of predicted maximum heart rate), and
- occurred over 20 to 60 minutes per session.

PHYSICAL BENEFITS OF EXERCISE

An extensive number of studies for over 50 years have examined the extent to which various forms of exercise improve structural and physiological processes of the human body. The evidence of physical benefits of a regular exercise program on normal physical functioning is overwhelming. These benefits are particularly evident with respect to cardiorespiratory exercise.

Cardiorespiratory Benefits

Cardiorespiratory exercise is used interchangeably with *aerobic exercise*. The term *aerobic*, which means "with oxygen," refers to a form of physical activity (or work) in which the amount of oxygen taken in and used by the body is sufficient to provide the energy necessary for performing the task (Greenberg, Dintiman, and Myers Oakes, 2004). The terms *aerobic* and *cardiorespiratory* are used interchangeably because they both represent a type of exercise that results in a significant increase in heart rate, such as jogging or any rapid movement of the legs or arms.

The importance of this type of exercise cannot be overstated. The heart is a muscle, and similar to improving muscular strength by resistance training (weightlifting), increasing the heart rate makes the heart stronger, increasing the ability to pump blood throughout the body. This results in two physical benefits:

1. More blood is pumped with each beat (this is called *cardiac output*).
2. A person with high aerobic fitness is more likely to survive a heart attack (called a *myocardial infarction*).

The other important benefit of aerobic fitness is the foundation of this book—the mental benefit.

It is essential that clients engage in aerobic exercise because it is directly responsible for most of the health benefits associated with exercise in general. This includes weight control, reduced levels of bad cholesterol (low-density lipoprotein, or LDL), improved levels of good cholesterol (high-density lipoprotein, or HDL), lower triglycerides (fat cells in the blood), reduced blood pressure, increased metabolism (the number of calories burned per minute to sustain life), and a stronger cardiac muscle, making the heart more likely to withstand the effects of a heart attack. Techniques to achieve aerobic fitness are beyond the scope of this chapter; however, the psychological benefits are well established, as discussed earlier.

Strength Gains

Resistance training and strength fitness are essential components of long-term good health (e.g., prevention of osteoporosis) and high quality of life (e.g., greater mobility, resistance to injury and pain, physical stability). According to the American College of Sports Medicine (ACSM, 2010), muscular fitness is important for overall physical health for the following reasons:

- Improved bone health and stronger bones
- Increased muscle mass, which raises resting metabolic rate (i.e., the number of calories burned per minute to sustain life), which improves weight control
- Increased glucose tolerance, which reduces the chance of having type 2 diabetes
- Reduced risk of injury and low back pain
- Improved ability to carry out activities of daily living

- Improved balance and decreased risk of falls in older adults
- Improved self-esteem and general mood

Improved Flexibility

Improving flexibility decreases the chance of injury and allows a greater range of motion—that is, mobility. Stretching is the best way to improve flexibility. ACSM (2010) defines *stretching* as "the systematic elongation of musculotendinous units to create a persistent length of the muscle and a decrease in passive tension. . . . The application of stretching can result in a continued deformation (longer length) of the muscle at a lower tension, which is commonly known as improved flexibility" (p. 159).

According to ACSM (2010) guidelines, stretching is sometimes performed incorrectly. There are two primary types of stretching techniques, *static* and *ballistic* (also called *dynamic*). The latter—ballistic or dynamic—should be avoided. Here's why.

ACSM (2010) recommends static stretching to reduce muscle soreness, which involves slowly stretching a muscle to the point of mild tension and then holding the position for 10 to 30 seconds. Ballistic stretching, on the other hand, involves using momentum in repetitive bouncing movements. According to the ACSM (2010), there is a greater risk of muscle strain injury due to dynamic stretching if the person exerts too much force during dynamic ("bouncing") movements.

Thus, the problem with ballistic stretching is that your tendons react to the bouncing—which is an attempt to maximize the stretch effect—by protecting the muscle. The automatic response is to tighten, not loosen, the muscle and the tendon that attaches it to the bone. Therefore, ballistic stretching is counterproductive.

ACSM (2010) offers nine general guidelines for stretching:

1. Stretch to the point of mild tension or discomfort.
2. Hold each stretch for 15 to 30 seconds.
3. To avoid back strain, keep your back in its natural alignment.
4. Do not lock your joints.
5. Do not hold your breath while stretching.
6. Do not bounce or use momentum.
7. Do not allow the weight-bearing knee to flex more than 90°.
8. Do not hyperextend (i.e., move backward) the neck or lower back.
9. Complete two to four repetitions of each stretch.

MOTIVES FOR EXERCISING

In my former career as a fitness director in the community recreation field, I used to ask club members why they thought other people did not like to exercise or tended to begin an exercise program and then quit within a few months. This section is about describing those reasons. One of them told me, "Every time I feel like exercising I lie down until the feeling passes." No doubt there are personal and situational factors that promote exercise behavior—and statistically predict it. When exercise leaders and program administrators know the motives of their clients for engaging in exercise, they can develop programs that meet those needs. They are as follows:

- *Social physique anxiety and physical self-esteem.* There are personal dispositions—ways of thinking that are consistent across different situations—that often lead to certain behavior patterns related to exercise. *Physique anxiety* is a condition in which people feel self-conscious and worried about their physical features and body appearance. People with high physique anxiety are less likely to exercise in public settings than people who feel relatively secure and satisfied with their physical features. The results of two studies, for instance (Martin Ginis, Jung, and Gauvin, 2003; Martin Ginis, Burke, and Gauvin, 2007), indicated that exercise novices should not exercise in front of a mirror, because it exacerbates feelings of worry, threat, and discomfort about their physical appearance. Self-esteem reflects the extent to which people value themselves. There are several dimensions and sources of self-esteem, one of which is called *physique* or *physical self-esteem*. People who value their health, feel satisfied with their physique, and wish to improve and maintain their physical appearance usually have relatively high physique self-esteem. They are more likely to exercise, especially in a public setting, than people who have low physique self-esteem.

- *Weight control.* As is well known, most Western countries suffer from an epidemic of overweight and obesity. Not surprisingly, this is due to the combination of overeating and maintaining a sedentary lifestyle. Though losing weight is a primary motivation to begin and maintain an exercise program, weight loss happens slowly for many reasons. It is also important to remember that exercise, especially resistance training, builds muscle, and muscle weighs more than fat. Therefore, the scale will not necessarily reflect improved fitness and less fat. If the person maintains a regular exercise schedule and does not indulge in overeating (see a registered dietitian for dietary guidelines), body weight will come off.

- *Social affiliation.* Social affiliation is a strong predictor of exercise motivation and persistence, as Markland and Ingledew (1997) found in their development of the Exercise Motivation Inventory. Fitness classes, weight training, yoga, running clubs, or simply attending a fitness center or health club are examples of programs in which the primary motive for attending includes a strong social component.

- *Improved health.* Naturally, many people are motivated to exercise in order to improve physical health, reduce stress, and improve mood and energy. One technique that meets this need to improve health is to provide health-related data to exercisers. As Loehr and Schwartz (2003) have found from their clinical work, people are motivated to change health behavior based on numerical information, such as test scores and other forms of assessment. If those numbers indicate that one's health is at risk due to a current habit or behavior pattern, it is likely the person will feel more motivated to change the behaviors that are responsible for those undesirable numbers than she would if she were merely asked to change her behaviors. For instance,

an unhealthy lipids profile, which lists the person's cholesterol data, is a strong motivator to change eating habits and increase physical activity output given the relatively high prediction of heart disease or a fatal medical event (e.g., myocardial infarction, stroke). This information must come from a credible source, however, such as the person's medical care provider or a registered dietitian, nurse, or mental health professional.

- *Ill-health avoidance.* For many people, the desire to improve health is less motivating than the desire to avoid poor health and disease. Because clients tend to strongly value their family and work, developing an illness or disease would be devastating. Few people would continue to act in a way that would lead to ill health or premature death, considering the importance of their family and other aspects of their lives. Guilt, fear of being a burden to family and caregivers, and pain are related motivators to avoid ill health. Exercise thus becomes more desirable.

- *Competitiveness.* For people who have a strong competitive orientation, exercise can be a form of competition, whether against one's own past performance, called *intraindividual competition*, or against the performance of others, called *interindividual competition*. Running speed or endurance, number of repetitions of an exercise, and fitness test scores are all sources of competition that may increase motivation to exceed current fitness level.

WHY WE KEEP OUR UNHEALTHY HABITS

Humans are the only species on earth who consciously engage in behavior that they acknowledge are unhealthy and can have serious health consequences. For example, humans often eat for emotional rather than for biological reasons, and they may refuse to engage in physical activity unless absolutely necessary (Winett et al., 2007). Habits such as emotional eating and a sedentary lifestyle based on conscious choice are antithetical to good physical, mental, and emotional health and quality of life. We eat to satisfy hunger and our bodies are stronger and more efficient when we engage in physical activity. So why do so many of us eat when we are not hungry and move as little as possible? This book will address this question. Chapter 4 in particular provides a more in-depth discussion of the barriers to exercise and other forms of physical activity.

What is apparent is that many of us depend on others to motivate us to do the right thing. We need experts to tell us what to eat, how and when to exercise, and how to develop routines that give us daily structure and proper habits to maintain our energy and good health. Many of us also need companions to share our health-related routines and to remind us to do the right thing, such as an exercise partner, a personal trainer, or a dietitian. Collectively, these individuals provide a role called *social support*. Coaching, sometimes conducted by a personal trainer, registered dietitian, or mental health professional, enables a person to self-regulate, that is, to carry out an array of routines on one's own volition. How to get someone to stop engaging in self-destructive behaviors and to make lifestyle changes, however, is a psychological issue—the main focus of this book.

Perhaps one of the most perplexing questions about human behavior is, why do we behave in a manner every day that we know is unhealthy and not in our best interests? For instance, we do not get adequate sleep, we often go nonstop all day without taking a rest or what is known as a recovery break, we eat high-fat foods on the run, we often feel stressed and rushed, and we are controlled by the demands and requirements of others. Is it a lack of self-awareness of our self-destructive ways? Why do we make conscious decisions about our thoughts, feelings, and actions that run counter to our best interests? The reasons we maintain bad habits and make poor choices about unhealthy behavior patterns—why we persist in a self-destructive lifestyle—have been studied by many researchers.

Peter Hall and Jeffrey Fong (2007) from the University of Waterloo in Ontario have developed a model that explains individual health behavior. They have concluded that our self-destructive nature is based primarily on two factors. First, we acknowledge that the benefits of a given action outweigh the costs and consequences. Eating that pizza before bedtime, for instance, has the benefit of satisfying hunger and, besides, most people enjoy the taste of pizza when they are hungry, even late at night. Second, the benefits of an unhealthy habit are experienced quickly, sometimes even immediately, while the short-term costs (e.g., indigestion, weight gain) and long-term consequences (e.g., heart disease, obesity, type 2 diabetes) are farther down the road and sometimes are not experienced for many years. Because our culture demands immediate rather than delayed gratification, we opt for outcomes that are quickly satisfying.

In summary, perhaps the best explanation of self-defeating behavior patterns is about the short-term versus long-term costs and benefits of a particular habit. Hall and Fong (2007) explain:

> Behaviors judged to be maladaptive in the long run are usually driven by a strongly favorable balance of immediate costs and benefits. That is, many "maladaptive" behaviors are associated with substantial long-term costs and few (if any) long-term benefits; however, these same behaviors are frequently associated with many benefits and few costs for the individual at the time of action. In contrast, many avoided behaviors that seem "adaptive" to the outside observer (e.g., consuming raw vegetables) are, in fact, associated with substantial costs (and few benefits) at the time of actions, leading to the perplexing but common state of affairs where individuals know "what is good for them," but do not do it. (p. 6)

This book addresses the ways that health care providers can overcome resistance to doing the right thing and combat the cultural addiction of immediate gratification. Most health-protective behaviors such as maintaining proper eating habits, applying sunscreen, driving within the speed limit (or slower in inclement weather), exercising regularly, not smoking, and many others involve inconvenience and sometimes discomfort, embarrassment, and additional expense.

How many of us refuse to take an umbrella or any other rain gear with us upon leaving home, even when we see storm clouds and the weather forecast predicts rain? Most of the benefits of using the umbrella are well down the road. Eventually, we pay a price for leaving our umbrella home—we get wet from the rain. Along these lines, the most compelling reason why we might want to perform health-protective behaviors would be in response to these longer-term considerations (Hall and Fong, 2003). One day it's going to rain and we'd better have an umbrella with us; one day our health will suffer. To use another cliché, eventually we have to pay the piper.

CHALLENGES OF CHANGING HEALTH BEHAVIOR

Simply informing people about the ill effects of their unhealthy habits (e.g., eating late at night, smoking, eating high-fat foods, experiencing chronic stress, ingesting mind-altering drugs) will not necessarily result in behavior change. Numerous studies on the effects of educational programs on changing behaviors that are unhealthy (e.g., smoking, drinking alcohol, using anabolic steroids) or illegal (e.g., manufacturing or ingesting mind-altering drugs, committing crimes, texting while driving) have shown that providing educational information by itself does not result in long-term changes in attitudes or behaviors regarding the negative habit. Other forces, such as the influence of a peer group, self-esteem, chronic depression, and other social and psychological factors are far stronger predictors of these actions. Thus, merely increasing a person's knowledge about the negative consequences of a certain habit will not necessarily result in long-term change of that habit.

What will influence behavior change and get people to stop self-destructive actions? One approach is to stay positive. Instead of associating maladaptive behaviors with poor health, Loehr and Schwartz (2003) take a more positive approach. They associate healthy habits with improved energy and superior performance. These are outcomes with which most people can identify. According to the authors, "To be fully engaged we must be physically energized, emotionally connected, mentally focused and spiritually aligned with a purpose beyond our immediate self-interest" (p. 5).

The challenge of health care professionals, then, is to create two contrasting scenarios. The first is to help the person experience continued *short-term benefits* of a specific behavior pattern (e.g., favorable scores on a medical or fitness test, encouraging words from a fitness coach, dietitian, or medical practitioner), which will lead over time to a new habit of the desirable behavior. The second is to provide extensive and meaningful evidence of the eventual *long-term consequences* of the unhealthy habit (e.g., testimony of a cancer-stricken person who smoked for many years, an athlete whose health suffered from prolonged use of steroids, or a chronic

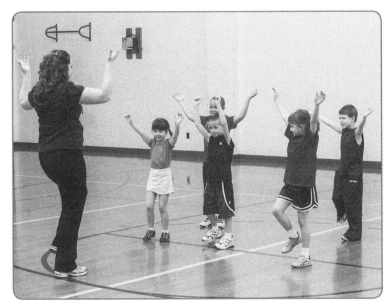

Positive health care professionals, such as PE teachers, should associate healthy habits with fun, improved energy, and superior performance.

smoker suffering from emphysema; photos and stories of drivers killed due to drinking alcohol or speeding).

How does a health care professional successfully prevent, stop, initiate, or maintain specific behavior patterns to improve a client's health and quality of life? How do we overcome the propensity toward careless and toxic behaviors, especially by younger people, who often do not identify with long-term consequences of their actions and therefore do not tend to take responsibility for them? What about people who suffer from mental illness, such as clinical depression, chronic anxiety, or irrational thinking, whose self-destructive behavior patterns are intrinsic to their survival and therefore the long-term consequences are irrelevant? These are just some of the challenges that health care professionals face that require more than sponsored educational programs, TV commercials, and most other external strategies to maintain an optimistic future.

DEFINING APPLIED HEALTH FITNESS PSYCHOLOGY

This book introduces an emerging area of study and practice called *applied health fitness psychology*. It is important to define each of these areas of study, research, and practice—applied psychology of health and fitness—in real-life settings in order to determine the parameters and framework of a given discipline and to identify the concepts that define it. Applied health psychology remains a relatively new area of study and practice, and the inclusion of fitness in this area has not been previously explained.

Health

Health is a positive state of physical, mental, and social well-being, not simply the absence of injury or disease, that varies over time along a continuum from wellness to illness or injury (Sarafino and Smith, 2011). To Sarafino and Smith, *health psychology* is a field of study and practice concerned with understanding the psychological, behavioral,

and social factors that predict, describe, and determine a person's health status, which can range from good physical and mental health to illness. For example, researchers know that prolonged psychosocial stress may result in heart disease, compromise the immune system, and promote the onset of disease. Severe clinical depression reduces energy and promotes thoughts of suicide. And a child's diet influences attention-deficit/hyperactivity disorder (ADHD), among other mental disorders.

Applied health psychology is defined, first, by understanding the concept of health, then by reviewing the concept of psychology, and finally by determining how the psychological factors that affect health have implications in real-world settings (Abraham, Conner, Jones, and O'Connor, 2008). These implications include examining how environmental and situational factors influence a person's mental and physical well-being and how practitioners (e.g., mental health professionals, fitness coaches, dietitians) can influence the individual's health, well-being, and quality of life. At the core of applied health psychology is the attempt to understand, prevent, manage, and, if possible, eradicate the onset of mental and physical disease.

Health psychologists attempt to promote a person's mental and physical health by

1. understanding the personal and situational factors that explain a person's health or illness;
2. favorably influencing the person's mental state by understanding the causes of dysfunctional or maladaptive behavioral patterns (i.e., bad habits that negatively influence health and well-being);
3. preventing or treating illness with various forms of therapy and interventions;
4. identifying the psychological, behavioral, and situational factors that explain a person's illness or dysfunction; and
5. determining the effects of cognitive and behavioral strategies on improving mental and physical health and quality of life (Abraham et al., 2008; Sarafino and Smith, 2011).

Use of the title (and credential) *health psychologist* implies that the person is a licensed mental health professional with a specialization in understanding the personal (e.g., thoughts, emotions, personality traits) and environmental (e.g., psychosocial stress, relationships) factors that may explain a person's physical and mental condition. In addition, health psychologists interact with medical practitioners, rehabilitation and physical therapists, dietitians, personal trainers and exercise coaches, and other specialists whose expertise will provide the array of services needed to provide proper counsel and intervention strategies.

Wellness and Fitness

Changing a person's well-learned habits is among the most challenging objectives in the health care industry. It is apparent that the science and practice of using programs that effectively replace unhealthy habits with more desirable ones and that improve a person's mental and physical well-being and quality of life come from various fields of study. One objective of this chapter is to illustrate how these fields converge to become the emerging field reflected in this book, called *applied health fitness psychology*. It is not an entirely new field of study and practice but rather an extension of an existing field called *exercise psychology*.

Exercise psychology is defined and discussed later in greater depth, but to briefly explain, it addresses the psychological factors that explain participation and adherence in physical activity programs. Applied health fitness psychology expands our current understanding of exercise psychology, integrating it into the more expansive area of health psychology. It contributes to the value of exercise psychology research and practice by expanding the mission of helping sedentary people change their health behavior, with a focus on increased physical activity.

More and more studies tell us about the undesirable long-term effects of an unhealthy lifestyle and the many health benefits of regular physical activity, particularly exercise. The lack of a daily exercise habit in particular contributes to heart disease (Liu et al., 2012) and poor mental health (Stathopoulou et al., 2006), among other maladies. Consequently, there is an emerging need to provide educational opportunities, expertise, and professional services to meet the needs of a public that is becoming less and less healthy due to following a lifestyle that is counterproductive to proper fitness, nutrition, energy, and health.

As described in this chapter, applied health fitness psychology is a new multidimensional field of study (e.g., research, formal instruction in educational institutions) and practice (e.g., consultancies, coaching, licensed mental health professionals). The various dimensions of applied health fitness psychology explained in this chapter converge seamlessly because they reflect the evolving needs of our society. New and creative professional expertise is required to address the expanded psychological and physical needs of people who are aging and becoming less and less healthy.

Concepts related to fitness psychology that need to be clearly defined include *wellness*, *physical wellness*, *physical fitness*, and *exercise psychology*, including the differences between fitness psychology and exercise psychology. The highlight box Fitness Psychology Terminology illustrates these dimensions and subdimensions.

Wellness, the most global concept, is usually defined as a generalized state of good health, the optimal soundness of body and mind. More specifically, wellness is "the achievement of the highest level of health possible in physical, social, intellectual, emotional, environmental, and spiritual dimensions" (Hopson, Donatelle, and Littrell, 2009, p. 2). *Wellness* and *health* are often used interchangeably. Wellness has several dimensions, and the dimension that is most closely allied with this book is *physical wellness*. To Hopson and colleagues, physical wellness consists of "all aspects of a sound body, including body size and shape, sensory sharpness and responsiveness, body functioning, physical strength, flexibility and endurance, resistance to diseases and disorders, and recuperative abilities" (p. 4).

One subdimension of physical wellness is a concept called *physical fitness*, which is the ability of the human organism to function efficiently and effectively (ACSM, 2010). Researchers have designated five subdimensions, or measures, of physical fitness. These are *cardiorespiratory endurance* (also called *aerobic fitness*), which focuses on improved function of the heart and lungs; *muscular strength*; *muscular endurance*; *flexibility*; and *body composition* (also referred to as *percent body fat*). Hopson et al. (2009) further define *health-related components of physical fitness* as "components of physical fitness that have a relationship with good health" (p. 31).

One method of achieving better physical fitness is physical activity, and exercise is the type of physical activity that is the focus of this book. Various forms of exercise achieve each of the five types of physical fitness. Why some people choose to exercise while others do not and how practitioners can improve exercise participation and maintenance are just a small part of a field that deals with the mental and emotional factors that explain exercise behavior. This field is called *exercise psychology*.

Exercise psychology is defined in *Dictionary of the Sport and Exercise Sciences* (Anshel et al., 1991) as "the study of psychological factors underlying participation and adherence in physical activity programs" (p. 56). Lox et al. (2010) define it as "the application of psychological principles to the promotion and maintenance of leisure physical activity (exercise), and the psychological and emotional consequences of leisure physical activity" (p. 4).

Researchers in exercise psychology study how exercise alters mood, reduces stress, reduces the effects of mental disorders such as depression and anxiety, improves self-confidence and self-esteem, increases energy, improves tolerance to acute and chronic pain, and enhances quality of life. Less well known is the extent to which these outcomes are influenced by some types of exercise (e.g., aerobic exercise) but not others (e.g., strength or flexibility training).

Fitness psychology is operationally defined in this book as the attempt to understand the manner in which personal factors (e.g., mental and emotional processes) and situational or environmental factors (e.g., exercise facilities, social support, exercise leadership and coaching, use of technology) interact to influence exercise performance and improve fitness. It also attempts to apply these factors in promoting exercise participation and long-term adherence.

To understand how exercise psychology differs from fitness psychology, we need to repeat an earlier statement, that one method of achieving better physical fitness is through physical activity, and the type of physical activity that best achieves fitness is exercise. Fitness psychology differs from exercise psychology, then, in that the psychological factors that influence exercise participation will eventually improve physical fitness. For example, a person will enter an exercise facility with one of two mind-sets, positive or negative. The person who enters the facility with enthusiasm and anticipates an enjoyable experience (fitness psychology) is more likely to demonstrate better exercise performance due to her heightened confidence and more energy and self-determination (exercise psychology). Another person, however, who shows up feeling self-doubt about his exercise skills and fitness level, worried about his appearance, or intimidated by the physical discomfort generated from muscular exertion is less likely to enjoy the experience and become fitter. In fact, the latter individual is far more likely to drop out of the exercise program. In other words, a person can view the exercise venue as an opportunity to get fitter and become healthier or as an unpleasant environment that should be avoided.

Fitness psychology is the more global concept; it is the goal, or eventual outcome, of maintaining an exercise habit. We improve physical fitness through exercise, and both concepts are described, explained, and predicted by psychological (e.g., confidence, positive self-talk, motivation, mental preparation) and emotional (e.g., anxiety, arousal) factors. Applied fitness psychology is the primary focus of this book in dealing with the ways we apply research findings and concepts in improving health and fitness.

Fitness psychology researchers also want to know the personal and situational factors that explain and predict the reasons some people initiate and maintain an exercise habit (or any other form of regular physical activity) while others do not and perhaps even have an aversion to physical activity. Are attitudes toward exercise related to childhood experiences in physical education classes or coaches who burned out their former athletes with excessive physical training and conditioning? In one rare study in this area, O'Rourke (2011) examined the relationship between perceived experiences in physical education in secondary school and current attitudes about physical activity among 700 middle-aged male and female adults. She found that attitudes toward experiences in secondary school physical education predicted exercise behavior. In particular, unpleasant experiences in physical education classes were significantly and positively related to negative attitudes toward physical activity. She concluded that current physical education programs in secondary schools are not promoting positive attitudes toward physical activity.

Attitudes toward exercise and other forms of physical activity, discussed at length in chapter 5, also partly explain why some people adhere to an exercise program, sometimes as a permanent lifestyle change, while others quit, often within the first three months after starting a new program. Researchers and practitioners have attempted to understand how psychological issues relate to a person's decision to begin and maintain an exercise program.

One factor that clearly influences exercise participation is mental health. Mental health professionals need to become aware of the importance of a client's mental well-being as one predictor of exercise participation, enjoyment, and adherence. It is well known that the presence of mental illness, or *psychopathology*, can strongly influence a person's energy and willingness to exercise regularly (Pinquart, Duberstein, and Lyness, 2007; Williams, 2008).

FITNESS PSYCHOLOGY TERMINOLOGY

- **health**—A positive state of physical, mental, and social well-being.
- **health psychology**—A field of study and practice concerned with understanding the psychological, behavioral, and social factors that predict, describe, and determine a person's health status.
- **applied health psychology**—A field of study and practice concerned with examining how environmental and situational factors influence a person's mental and physical well-being and how practitioners (e.g., mental health professionals, fitness and nutrition coaches) influence the person's health, well-being, and quality of life.
- **health psychologist**—A licensed clinical psychologist with a specialization in understanding the personal and environmental factors that may explain a person's physical and mental condition.
- **wellness**—A generalized state of good health; the optimal soundness of body and mind.

- **physical wellness**—All aspects of a sound body, including body size and shape, sensory sharpness and responsiveness, body functioning, physical strength, flexibility, endurance, resistance to diseases and disorders, and recuperative abilities.
- **physical fitness**—The ability of the human organism to function efficiently and effectively. Includes cardiorespiratory endurance (aerobic fitness), muscular strength, muscular endurance, flexibility, and body composition.
- **exercise psychology**—The study of psychological factors underlying participation and adherence in physical activity programs.
- **fitness psychology**—Understanding the manner in which personal (e.g., mental and emotional processes) and situational or environmental factors interact to influence exercise performance and improve fitness and applying these factors in promoting exercise participation and long-term adherence.

Examples include chronic stress, depression, anxiety, irrational thinking (e.g., "I don't deserve to be fit"), emotional eating, low self-esteem, low confidence, fear of failure, and somatic anxiety (i.e., worry about one's physical appearance). These examples will receive more attention in chapters 5 and 6 in examining the personal and situational factors that influence exercise participation and adherence. See Stathopoulou et al. (2006) for an in-depth review of the mental health literature related to exercise.

HISTORY OF APPLIED HEALTH FITNESS PSYCHOLOGY

All areas of practice have a beginning. How do the areas of health, fitness, and psychology come together to form this emerging field? In addition, under whose umbrella does this field of study and practice fall? Is it a branch of psychology, similar to health psychology?

Do academics, researchers, and practitioners and coaches who represent exercise science and sports medicine form the primary disciplines that govern this field? Or do all of these areas own a part of this field but are separated by their training, academic preparation, and practice?

Acknowledging the relatively brief history of applied health fitness psychology probably begins with the serious health crisis facing most Western countries, especially the United States. The Healthy People 2010 report, published by the U.S. Department of Health and Human Services (HHS, 2004), indicated that only 22% of American adults engage in moderate- to light-intensity physical activity for 30 minutes five or more times a week. Almost 25% of the population is completely sedentary. For those who begin a regular exercise program, up to 50% drop out within the first six months. Americans are eating more, exercising less, and getting fatter—about two-thirds of the U.S. population is overweight or obese. Thus, there is what's commonly

FROM RESEARCH TO REAL WORLD

Physique self-esteem has been studied as a factor that influences exercising in front of a mirror, which is common in many fitness facilities. Martin Ginis et al. (2003) wanted to know if one's level of physique anxiety while looking into a mirror would influence aerobic exercise performance among 58 sedentary (low-fit) women, average age 20.7 years. They found that exercising in front of a mirror increased negative mood significantly more than exercising with no mirror. The researchers speculated that negative body image and physical self-awareness may increase discomfort among unfit women, whereas fit women might find that the mirror sends a more positive, uplifting message.

In a follow-up study, Martin Ginis et al. (2007) examined the effects of a mirrored exercise environment and the presence of other exercisers on sedentary women's feeling states. Unfit (sedentary) participants (n = 92, mean age 20.2 years) performed 20 minutes of exercise at moderate intensity with or without a mirror and alone or with a coexerciser. They found that women who exercised with another person in the mirrored environment experienced greater physical exhaustion and did not recover from the exercise as well as the women who exercised alone and did not face a mirror. The mirror also increased the women's self-consciousness and elicited more social comparisons. These findings suggest that group exercise, particularly in front of mirrors, is not conducive to psychological well-being among unfit women. This is at least partially due to high physique anxiety.

referred to as an *obesity epidemic*, and the current state of the nation's health is costing 17% of the national budget at several billion dollars a year. An overweight employee costs the employer $5,000 more a year in health costs than an employee at a healthy weight, according to a survey by the National Business Group on Health (National Business Group on Health, 2011).

There is plenty of blame to go around for this sad state of affairs. Physical education in schools is a mess. Most courses focus on learning and performing sport skills and are almost void of fitness improvement. To make matters worse, students are often criticized for less-than-stellar performance during sport competition, teachers use exercise as a form of punishment, and coaches tend to overtrain their athletes, resulting in exercise burnout and negative attitudes toward exercise. The result is that athletes stop being physically active when they retire from sport.

From a cultural perspective, we are obsessed with food and disdain physical activity. Thus, weight gain as we age is not surprising. The rate of type 2 diabetes, which is usually attributed to obesity, is increasing annually.

Applied health fitness psychology, of which exercise psychology is one component, is particularly important in creating a field of research and practice that promotes a healthy lifestyle. It complements exercise science, the area that is devoted to understanding the physiological and psychological effects of exercise, because it addresses the effects of interventions that influence exercise participation and adherence.

SUMMARY

We live in a society in which lifelong unhealthy habits are resulting in poor health and enormous health care costs. Poor eating habits and lack of physical activity in particular are leading to obesity at a higher rate than ever before. There are many antecedents and known causes of unhealthy behavior patterns, and one focus of this chapter was a review of the antecedents that have implications for interventions to overcome self-destructive habits. Increasing physical activity, particularly exercise, and engaging in a healthier lifestyle are the primary aims of this book. Changing unhealthy habits, particularly helping people adopt exercise as a lifestyle habit, includes a strong psychological component called *fitness psychology*. Fitness psychology concerns understanding the manner in which personal and environmental factors interact to influence exercise performance and improve fitness and applying these factors in promoting exercise participation and long-term adherence. The purpose of this book is to provide information on ways students and professionals in health care can accomplish this objective.

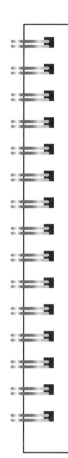

STUDENT ACTIVITY

Costs and Benefits of Habits

Think about one of your bad habits, something you do regularly that you know is not good for you. Perhaps the bad habit is unhealthy, or takes up too much of your time, or increases your stress, or prevents you from reaching short-term (daily or weekly) or long-term (end of the month or longer) goals.

1. Write down this negative habit and list at least two benefits of it. Why do you maintain this behavior? What is in it for you?

2. Write down two or three short-term costs (e.g., weight gain, lack of concentration and energy, headaches) and long-term consequences (e.g., heart disease, diabetes, pain) of this negative habit for your health and well-being.

3. Now, compare your lists and see if the benefits are more important than the costs and consequences. If the benefits are more important and immediate (experienced sooner) than the costs and consequences, you can now see the reason you continue to engage in this self-destructive behavior pattern.

4. Finally, discuss with your group or partner what will it take for you to give up this unhealthy habit and replace it with a more desirable one.

REFERENCES

Abraham, C., Conner, M., Jones, F., and O'Connor, D. (2008). *Health psychology topics in applied psychology.* London: Hodder Education.

American College of Sports Medicine (ACSM). (2010). *ACSM's guidelines for exercise testing and prescription* (8th ed.). Philadelphia: Lippincott, Williams and Wilkins.

Anshel, M.H., Freedson, P., Hamill, J., Haywood, K., Horvat, M., and Plowman, S.A. (1991). *Dictionary of the sport and exercise sciences.* Champaign, IL: Human Kinetics.

Bahrke, M.S., and Morgan, W.P. (1978). Anxiety reduction following exercise and meditation. *Cognitive Therapy and Research, 4,* 323-333.

Bauman, A.E., Reis, R.S., Sallis, J.F., Wells, J.C., Loos, R.J.F., and Martin, B.W. (2012). Correlates of physical activity: Why are some people physically active and others not? *Lancet, 380,* 258-271.

Berger, B.G., and Motl, R.W. (2000). Exercise and mood: A selective review and synthesis of research employing the Profile of Mood States. *Journal of Applied Sport Psychology, 12,* 69-92.

Biddle, S.J.H., and Mutrie, N. (2001). *Psychology of physical activity: Determinants, well-being and interventions.* New York: Routledge.

Buckworth, J., and Dishman, R.K. (2002). *Exercise psychology.* Champaign, IL: Human Kinetics.

Burke, S.M., Carron, A.V., and Shapcott, K.M. (2008). Cohesion in exercise groups: An overview. *International Review of Sport and Exercise Psychology, 1,* 107-123.

Davis, C.L., Tomporowski, P.D., Boyle, C.A., Waller, J.L., Miller, P.H., Naglieri, J.A., et al. (2007). Effects of aerobic exercise on overweight children's cognitive functioning: A randomized control trial. *Research Quarterly for Exercise and Sport, 78,* 510-519.

Dishman, R.K., and Jackson, E.M. (2000). Exercise, fitness, and stress. *International Journal of Sport Psychology, 31,* 175-203.

Etnier, J.L., and Chang, Y.K. (2009). The effect of physical activity on executive function: A brief commentary on definitions, measurement issues, and the current state of the literature. *Journal of Sport and Exercise Psychology, 31*, 469-483.

Greenberg, J.S., Dintiman, G.B., and Myers Oakes, B. (2004). *Physical fitness and wellness: Changing the way you look, feel, and perform.* Champaign, IL: Human Kinetics.

Hackfort, D., and Spielberger, C.D. (1989). *Anxiety in sports: An international perspective.* New York: Hemisphere Publishing Corp.

Hall, P.A., and Fong, G.T. (2003). The effects of a brief time perspective intervention for increasing physical activity among young adults. *Psychology and Health, 18*, 685-706.

Hall, P.A., and Fong, G.T. (2007). Temporal self-regulation theory: A model for individual health behavior. *Health Psychology Review, 1*, 6-52.

Hoffmann, P. (1997). The endorphin hypothesis. In W.P. Morgan (Ed.), *Physical activity and mental health* (pp. 163-177). New York: Taylor & Francis.

Hopson, J.L., Donatelle, R.J., and Littrell, T.R. (2009). *Get fit, stay well.* San Francisco: Benjamin-Cummings.

Jebb, S. (2004). Obesity: Causes and consequences. *Women's Health Medicine, 1*, 38-41.

Koltyn, K.F. (1997). The thermogenic hypothesis. In W. P. Morgan (Ed.), *Physical activity and mental health* (pp. 213-226). New York: Taylor & Francis.

Koltyn, K.F., and Morgan, W.P. (1992). Influence of underwater exercise on anxiety and body temperature. *Scandinavian Journal of Medicine and Science in Sports, 2*, 249-253.

Larson, E.B., Wang, L., Bowen, J.D., McCormick, W.C., Teri, L., Crane, P., and Kukull, W. (2006). Exercise is associated with reduced risk for incident dementia among persons 65 years of age and older. *Annals of Internal Medicine, 144*, 73-81.

Liu, K., Daviglus, M.L., Loria, C., Colangelo, L.A., Spring, B., Moller, A.C., and Lloyd-Jones, D.M. (2012). Healthy lifestyle through young adulthood and the presence of low cardiovascular disease risk profile in middle age. *Circulation, 125*, 996-1004.

Loehr, J., and Schwartz, T. (2003). *The power of full engagement: Managing energy, not time, is the key to high performance and personal renewal.* New York: The Free Press.

Lox, C.L., Martin Ginis, K.A. and Petruzzello, S.J. (2010). *The psychology of exercise: Integrating theory and practice.* Scottsdale, AZ: Holcomb Hathaway.

Markland, D. and Ingledew, D.K. (1997). The measurement of exercise motives: Factorial validity and invariance across gender of a revised Exercise Motivations Inventory. *British Journal of Health Psychology, 2*, 361-376.

Martin Ginis, K.A., Burke, S.M., and Gauvin, L. (2007). Exercising with others exacerbates the negative effects of mirrored environments on sedentary women's feeling states. *Psychology and Health, 22*, 945-962.

Martin Ginis, K.A., Jung, M.E., and Gauvin, L. (2003). To see or not to see: The effects of exercising in mirrored and unmirrored environments on women's mood states. *Health Psychology, 22*, 354-361.

National Business Group on Health (2011). *USA Today*, November 25, 2011, p. 2A.

National Center for Health Statistics. (2010). *Health, United States, 2010.* Washington, DC: U.S. Government Printing Office.

North, T.C., McCullagh, P., and Tran, Z.V. (1990). Effect of exercise on depression. *Exercise & Sport Sciences Reviews, 18*, 379-415.

O'Rourke, M. (2011). *Predictors of attitudes toward physical activity as a function of secondary school physical education experiences among adults.* (Unpublished doctoral dissertation). Middle Tennessee State University, Murfreesboro, TN.

Petruzzello, S.J., Landers, D.M., Hatfield, B.D., Kubitz, K.A., and Salazar, W. (1991). A meta-analysis on the anxiety-reducing effects of acute and chronic exercise: Outcomes and mechanisms. *Sports Medicine, 11*, 143-182.

Pinquart, M., Duberstein, P.R., and Lyness, M.M. (2007). Effects of psychotherapy and other behavioral interventions on clinically depressed older adults: A meta-analysis. *Aging and Mental Health, 11*, 645-657.

Pratt, M., Sarmiento, O.L., Montes, F., Ogilvie, D., Marcus, B.H., Perez, L.G., and Brownson, R.C. (2012). The implications of megatrends in information and communication technology and transportation for changes in global physical activity. *Lancet, 380*, 282-293.

Sarafino, E.P., and Smith, T.W. (2011). *Health psychology: Biopsychosocial interactions* (7th ed.). Hoboken, NJ: Wiley.

Stathopoulou, G., Powers, M.B., Berry, A.C., Smits, J.A., and Otto, M.W. (2006). Exercise interventions for mental health: A qualitative and quantitative review. *Clinical Psychology and Practice, 13*, 179-193.

U.S. Department of Health and Human Services (HHS). (2004). *Healthy People 2010.* Washington, DC: U.S. Government Printing Office.

U.S. Department of Health and Human Services (HHS). (2006). *Healthy People 2010 Midcourse Review.* Washington, DC: U.S. Government Printing Office.

Watson, J., Martin Ginis, K.A., and Spink, K.S. (2004). Team building in an exercise class for the elderly. *Activities Adaptation and Aging, 28,* 35-47.

Williams, D.M. (2008). Exercise, affect, and adherence: An integrated model and a case for self-paced exercise. *Journal of Sport and Exercise Psychology, 30,* 471-496.

Winett, R.A., Anderson, E.S., Wojcik, J.R., Winett, S.G., and Bowden, T. (2007). Guide to health: Nutrition and physical activity outcomes of a group-randomized trial of an Internet-based intervention in churches. *Annals of Behavioral Medicine, 33,* 251-261.

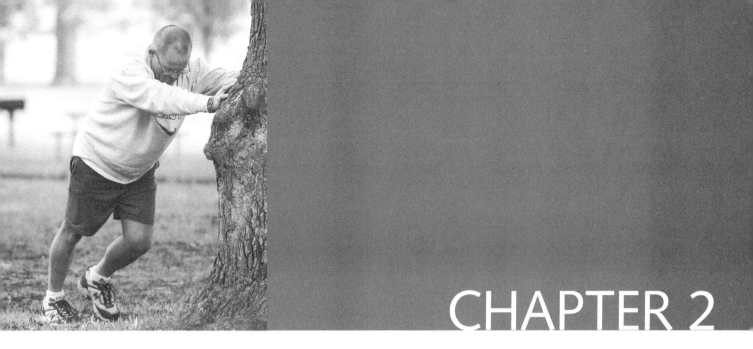

CHAPTER 2

Psychological Motivation Theories

" If I accept you as you are, I will make you worse; however, if I treat you as though you are what you are capable of becoming, I help you become that."

Johann Wolfgang von Goethe (1749-1832), author and philosopher

CHAPTER OBJECTIVES

After reading this chapter, you should be able to:

- discuss the various definitions of motivation,
- understand the theories that describe and predict health and fitness motivation, and
- list the factors that reduce and improve an exerciser's motivation.

There is no greater challenge in changing health behavior than feeling the need for change. Unless people feel that beginning a new habit or stopping an old one is in their best interests, change will not occur. They have to feel that their current level of fitness, body weight, medical condition, or appearance warrants a lifestyle change that will remedy the situation. Feeling the incentive to change is the ignition, or starting point, to motivate people to change or improve their current situation. This incentive cannot be externally imposed—at least not for long. Health behavior change is an active, not passive, process that requires energy. The primary source of energy is derived internally, and it's called *motivation*.

Motivating people to perform an activity they already enjoy doing, such as playing a sport, weight training, or jogging, may seem to be relatively easy. But improving people's motivation to engage in an activity that they do not enjoy or find beneficial is a far more sophisticated challenge for fitness leaders. The foundation of this chapter is understanding why some people are more motivated than others to maintain healthy habits. Only after understanding the theoretical foundations, myths, and truths about motivation can researchers, health educators, personal trainers, dietitians, and anyone else concerned with behavior change use the proper strategies for increasing the motivation and improving the health of others.

When it comes to doing the things we know will help us feel better, provide more energy, and improve our long-term physical and mental health and physical appearance, why is motivation even necessary? Why are people motivated to do the right thing and have the knowledge and incentive to look after their health? In order to develop effective interventions to promote exercise habits, it is important to develop positive attitudes toward exercise and other forms of physical activity starting in childhood. This, however, does not always happen, beginning with some practices in school physical education.

Many students have been upset by their experiences in physical education (O'Rourke, 2011). Better-skilled students are picked to participate while students who are less skilled are left out. Learning sport skills is often replaced by free play, in which students are asked to play various sports on their own. Students who have limited sport skills, have less motor coordination, or are overweight are ignored, criticized, or teased. According to a U.S. government report to general requesters covering physical education and sport programs for students in grades kindergarten through 12 (U.S. Government Accountability Office [GAO], 2012), many physical education programs have no or limited fitness components, including an absence of fitness testing and exercise training that would allow students to improve their fitness scores. Recess, which allows students to engage in physical activity during the school day, is disappearing (Armstrong, 2010). No wonder we need to develop a positive attitude toward physical activity and exercise.

Perhaps teacher education programs need to spend more time teaching future physical education teachers how to improve student fitness in elementary and secondary schools in addition to the traditional role of developing sport skills. Lack of exercise is leading to high rates of obesity and type 2 diabetes, resulting in poor health, astronomical health care costs, and a shortened life span. Addressing the Society of Behavioral Medicine Conference in Baltimore, Lavizzo-Mourey (2004) indicated that for the first time in U.S. history, children today will live a shorter, lower quality of life than their parents. Since 1980, the number of overweight children aged 6 to 11 and adolescents has doubled and tripled, respectively. The combination of obesity and a sedentary lifestyle are leading to the widespread onset of diabetes and hypertension, the likely culprits of a shortened life span. Lavizzo-Mourey asserted that obese children and adolescents become obese adults. The culture of health, including more exercise, needs to change—quickly.

FROM RESEARCH TO REAL WORLD

How do middle-aged men and women who exercise regularly, as opposed to a similar group of nonexercisers who lead a sedentary lifestyle, differ in their attitudes toward and experiences in their high school physical education classes? In other words, do attitudes toward high school physical education among middle-aged men and women influence their exercise habits later in life? Dr. Monica O'Rourke (2011) examined this question, studying attitudes toward high school physical education among 433 women and 265 men (average age 41.4 years) to ascertain if these attitudes influenced their lifestyle.

O'Rourke found that adults who were inactive in middle age did not reflect positive experiences in high school physical education; they felt humiliated from their poor sport performance and fitness. In addition, there were relatively few or, more often, no fitness programs in their high school curriculum, despite being evaluated on various fitness components by their physical education teacher. Along these lines, their high school physical education classes consisted of learning sport skills but did not include a strong fitness component. Perhaps not surprisingly, the adult respondents who were currently overweight, inactive, and lacking sport skills reported their high school physical education experiences as less pleasant than adults who currently maintained an active lifestyle. Finally, both active and inactive adult respondents reported that high school physical education did not prepare them for lifetime physical activity. O'Rourke concluded that high school physical education classes play an important role in lifetime attitudes and choices about maintaining an active lifestyle later in life. Schools and their physical education teachers and coaches have a long way to go in this area.

MOTIVATION DEFINED

The term *motivation* derives from the Latin word *movere*, meaning "to move" or "moves you," and it reflects the energy and direction to initiate and maintain behavior. According to Alderman (1974), motivation is the tendency for the *direction* and *selectivity of behavior* to be controlled by its *consequences*, and for behavior to persist until a *goal is achieved*. Let's determine the implications of this definition in exercise settings.

The *direction* of motivation refers to the target a person is moving toward—where is the person's energy directed? Motivated exercisers are energized to engage in a task that they find meaningful, such as engaging in physical activity or some other healthy habit.

We cannot feel motivated toward everything in our environment; we must determine what ignites or drives us to get what we want and need. This decision about where to focus our energy is *selectivity of behavior*. At times, exercise leaders and other practitioners need to help the exerciser focus on the most important task, to separate what is most important in eventually reaching goals. It is the individual who must determine where and how to direct his effort. Motivation is an active and conscious process, not passive and automatic. Motivated behavior requires conscious thought and planning.

Sometimes motivated behavior is a reaction to aversive (undesirable) *consequences*. Making an athlete exercise as a form of punishment, for example, has the undesirable effect of instilling negative attitudes toward exercise and physical training. Examples include threats such as "If you do *x*, you will have to do 20 push-ups" or "Anyone who makes an error has to jog around the field three times." These threats usually lead to motivated behaviors in the short term because they are controlled by their connections to consequences. However, because these threatening statements are examples of aversive control of behavior and represent a negative approach to motivation, they have a relatively short-term effect as opposed to the preferred long-term, even permanent behavior change (Smith, 1993). Long-term consequences of exercise include improved fitness, more energy, better health, and superior performance.

A far superior value of motivation in sport is to encourage exercisers to maintain positive feelings about exercise and other forms of physical activity, positive emotions (e.g., enthusiasm, confidence, happiness), and long-term adherence to an exercise habit. The type of motivation that reflects positive emotions and a long-term commitment to exercise and a more active lifestyle is called *intrinsic* (discussed later in this chapter). *Goals* provide direction for effort, the incentive to persist at a task until the person feels that the goal—a demonstration of competence and mastery—has been achieved. The anticipation of meeting a goal is called a *motive*.

Motives are a function of how important the exerciser considers the consequences of certain actions and how strongly the exerciser desires (*approach motive*) or resists (*avoidance motive*) these outcomes. An example of an approach motive would be anticipating certain favorable responses from others who detect improved physical appearance. Approach motives have better long-term value than avoidance motives; the latter provide motivation only until the threat of a negative outcome has passed (Duda and Treasure, 2010). Approach motives, on the other hand, are highly valued and are consistent with a person's desire and need to achieve. We obtain recognition and approval from approach motives, which is not usually the case with avoidance motives.

One of the most challenging motivational tasks for health and fitness practitioners is to determine ways to motivate their clients and to help them motivate themselves through the process of self-regulation, that is, helping exercisers to conclude that increased effort will lead to meeting desirable goals (Duda and Treasure, 2010). The exerciser who gives 100% every week but still physically struggles, who is not detecting weight loss or improved appearance, or whose goals far exceed her capabilities will not likely be motivated to persist at the activity. These exercisers will be less motivated to give 100%, leading to feelings of helplessness about changing their fitness level. Sustaining pain or injury makes this situation even less motivating (Anshel, 2012).

According to Howley and Franks (2007), the fitness coach can foster the exerciser's incentive to remain vigilant by pointing out specific ways in which certain exercise

---

APPROACH AND AVOIDANCE

Approach and avoidance motives are related to specific types of health- and fitness-related goals. Examples of approach motives, which have better long-term value and are more likely to lead to maintaining an exercise habit, include improved measures of fitness and lipids profile (i.e., various measures of cholesterol and triglycerides), reduced weight and percent body fat, and improved mental well-being. Examples of avoidance motives include reduced chance of obesity, type 2 diabetes, heart disease, and cognitive impairment (e.g., dementia) and increased physical and mental energy.

Sample Goals That Reflect Approach Motives

I will jog around the track nonstop three times.

I will bench press 10 extra pounds after six weeks.

Sample Goals That Reflect Avoidance Motives

I will not be injured this month.

I will avoid eating a meal or filling my stomach with food within two hours of bedtime.

behaviors and adherence to an exercise program can lead to goals and outcomes that the exerciser finds meaningful (e.g., "If you work hard at least three times a week you'll make faster progress than if you exercise on an irregular schedule and do not give 100%"). Exercisers can also improve their incentive to get fit by engaging in types of exercise that they find pleasant and that they plan to continue doing week after week. Losing an extreme amount of weight and resembling a model or actor is not a realistic goal for most people. Improved fitness and weight loss, however, are far more realistic and achievable (Berger and McInman, 1993). The most important form of motivation is based on the desire to perform an activity based on personal satisfaction, pleasure, or even fun, a concept called *intrinsic motivation*.

SOURCES OF MOTIVATION

Where does motivation come from? What are its origins? Motivation is based on the combination of personal and situational factors that create a sense of direction, energy, drive, and incentive to meet certain desirable goals. There are person-centered, situation-centered, and interactive sources of motivation.

Person-Centered Motivation

One approach to understanding sources of motivation in physical activity is to examine the personal dispositions of exercisers. It is thought that motivation sources and intensity reflect the individual's personality traits, orientations, and needs. Traits are personality aspects that are stable, consistent across situations, and often genetically determined. Orientations and styles are learned, influenced by experience, and situation specific. And certain needs are normal and are shared by most people.

Traits

- Need achievement
- Self-esteem
- Stimulus or sensation seeking
- Trait anxiety

- Pain threshold or tolerance
- Neuroticism versus stability

Orientations and Styles

- Goal or win orientation
- Competitiveness
- Coping style
- Attentional style
- Physique social anxiety
- Fear of success or failure
- Mental toughness
- Learned resourcefulness
- Learned helplessness

Needs

- Recognition
- Approval
- Competence
- Social comparison
- Self-control

Taken together, these psychological characteristics motivate the person to act in predictable ways. Thus, the person-centered view is that if people do not have an inner drive, or incentive, to reach goals, achieve at a high level, and perform at their best, other people have a limited capability to influence behavior change in them. Motivation cannot be forced. Individual desire is the first and foremost characteristic of motivation.

Situation-Centered Motivation

Going beyond personal characteristics, situation-centered motivation posits that a supportive environment enhances feelings of motivation to perform a certain task or to meet a goal. This is not surprising; conditions influence motivation level and intensity all the time. For example, exercisers are more likely to exert optimal effort if the exercise environment induces high arousal. An exercise class and its leader may provide verbal incentives to give 100%. Exercising in the privacy of one's home and in a fitness club both have their own rewards and are preferred by some people more than others. In another example, some people are more motivated to exercise in warmer weather than in the winter. Thus, the location of exercise, the type of exercise, and the exercise environment all influence exercise motivation. Table 2.1 lists the situational factors that improve exercise motivation.

The two primary limitations of the situation-centered view of motivation are that situations do not always influence motivation, and personal factors (e.g., the exerciser's personality or personal needs) may be more influential than situational factors in prompting exercise motivation. For instance, some situations are quite unpleasant and demotivating, yet exercisers may remain motivated despite these negative experiences. The results of one study, for instance, (Martin Ginis, Burke, and Gauvin, 2007), indicated that beginning exercisers are demotivated when required to exercise in front of mirrors. Mirrors can be intimidating and distract an exercise novice, whereas fitter exercisers would find a reflection from mirrors more motivating.

Interactive Personal and Situational Motivation

The interaction model, or, a combination of personal and situational motivation sources, forms a third explanation for motivation (Endler and Hunt, 1966). In other words, it is the combination of personal characteristics and situational factors that influences motivational feelings and actions. For example, the motivational factors that influence a person's decision to exercise combine personal factors, such as high levels of self-esteem, confidence, and goal orientation, and situational factors, such as social support (i.e., exercising in the company of others or being encouraged), close proximity of an exercise facility to one's work or home, and a desirable exercise facility and equipment. Determining the sources of motivation to exercise is important in making exercise a lifestyle habit.

Support for person-centered sources, also called the *trait theory of personality* (Allport, 1937), could mean that exercisers are motivated by their own thoughts, emotions, predictions about outcomes, and even limitations (e.g., self-consciousness about physical appearance, undesirable body image or weight, low confidence, pessimism about future outcomes, presence of physical discomfort or injury, attitudes toward exercise, psychopathology). Support for situational sources of motivation could mean that people are driven to exercise based on the messages they receive from others (e.g., "Your exercise technique looks much better"); the location, attractiveness, and quality of facilities and equipment; and the presence of a fitness coach. Thus, motivation is more likely if exercisers possess certain characteristics that move them to meet their goals if they are supported by the proper conditions.

What about feelings of motivation that accompany threat? Exercisers tend to increase their incentive to begin and maintain exercise programs and generally improve physical activity levels if a doctor expresses concern about their health, they wish to lose weight to improve physical appearance, or they want to avoid some other unpleasant consequence, such as social rejection or increased stress.

Table 2.1 Situation-Centered Motivational Sources

Exercise environment	Sources of social support	Sources of incentive
Exercise facility near home or work	Group or class environment	Building relationships with others in the exercise environment
Home, allowing for more privacy	Exercising with a partner	Improved physical appearance
Presence of music and high-quality exercise equipment	Social setting resulting in interactions and friendships among group members	Improved fitness and health test scores
Fun and exciting	Respected, friendly exercise leader	Less strenuous and easier exercise; more enjoyment

Short-term threats to health status have motivational effects. It is also true that sometimes this type of treatment from an authority figure (e.g., physician, personal trainer) is desirable to increase the exerciser's incentive to change from a sedentary to a more active lifestyle.

Negative motivational techniques, however, have two shortcomings. First, these techniques usually have only short-term effects because the exerciser's behavior changes only until the source of threat is removed (e.g., losing weight, feeling better, competing in sport). As indicated earlier, after the threat is removed, the incentive to persist in the activity is minimal. This is one reason so many athletes tend to avoid exercising after their days as a sport competitor have ended.

The second shortcoming, as indicated earlier, is that threatening another person creates extrinsic, not intrinsic, incentive to change behavior. Some intrinsic value will be derived if the person views exercise and fitness as beneficial to her health and quality of life and if the exercise experience is pleasant and reaffirms her sense of competence. Exercise can be an extrinsic motivator, however, if the sole aim is to improve fitness or physical appearance or if an athlete is training for competition or to achieve some other outcome.

In summary, a person's motivation to change health behavior, especially increasing physical activity, depends on meeting personal needs and objectives. At the same time, the individual wants to pursue a certain predetermined course of action and possess the necessary feelings and attitudes associated with performance success. One important goal in fitness coaching is to give all clients a sense of value and purpose so that they see a reason to give 100% effort in attempting to attain personal goals and achieve success.

ACHIEVEMENT MOTIVATION THEORY

According to most personality studies, one characteristic of people who want to get fit and follow healthy habits is a high need to achieve. This need is commonly referred to as *achievement motivation*. The central focus of this theory is that some people derive tremendous satisfaction from success in achievement activities, such as improving fitness. People determine their own achievement behavior, which defines success. Success is based on the individual's perception that optimal effort will lead to achieving a desirable outcome and meeting goals. Duda and Hall (2001) assert that people with a high need to achieve "tend to maintain a fervent and optimistic belief that success is possible" (p. 418). This is one reason high-need achievers prefer challenging rather than easy activities. Duda and Hall conclude that "immense satisfaction may be experienced when it can be seen that trying hard to overcome difficult challenges results in success" (p. 418). Thus, if people view the performance outcome (e.g., improved fitness, lost weight, increased musculature) as due to their effort or skill, then the outcome is interpreted as successful.

The outcome may be interpreted as a failure, however, if it is perceived as a result of low effort or lack of skill. Thus, what is success for one person (e.g., jogging 10 minutes nonstop) may be failure for another person (e.g., "I should have been able to jog longer" or "Jogging is not that important to me"). Of course, in reality, life is a bit more complicated. For example, some people who begin exercise programs make only a minimal effort; they give up due to feeling out of breath, feeling physical fatigue, or being unable to keep up with the pace of others. According to achievement motivation theory, these individuals will not necessarily interpret their exercise performance as failure because their effort was low, they did not feel the predicted outcome was worth the effort, or they felt physically uncomfortable. Still, high-need achievers give extra effort in achievement-oriented conditions. It is this optimal level of effort, and not always the outcome of their efforts, that many high-need achievers interpret as success. Effort and performing one's best are associated with task-mastery goal orientation, whereas performance outcome (completing a task or meeting a goal) is linked to ego (win) goal orientation. Ego and task orientations are covered later in this chapter in more depth.

A psychological profile of high- and low-need achievers has been generated by Nicholls (1984) and Duda (1993) in the area of exercise and sport psychology. The researchers reveal clear differences between high- and low-need achievers. Duda and Whitehead (1998) and Roberts (1992) separate the concept of need achievement from motives for achievement. People can have a high need to achieve but, due to a past history of failure, they have a low motive to achieve. Children with a past history of failure, for instance, should not be expected to possess a high motive for achievement in most exercise or sport situations. In fact, the researchers claim that the expectancy for success would be quite low. This does not mean, however, that their need to achieve is also low. Unless high-need achievers with a low approach motive find success and enjoyment in exercise, they will tend to reduce their activity or even eliminate an active lifestyle altogether. This is the heart of the fear-of-failure (avoidance motive) phenomenon so common among people who do not find pleasure in physical activity.

As depicted in table 2.2, people who are relatively high-need achievers (as determined by psychological inventories) have the following five characteristics (Roberts 2012):

1. Success is highly pleasurable.
2. They experience weaker physiological symptoms of arousal (e.g., increased heart rate, respiration rate, or sweating).
3. They feel responsible for outcomes based on their own actions.
4. They prefer to receive success or failure feedback very soon after performance.
5. They prefer situations that contain some risk about the result.

Typically, high-need achievers are usually fully conscious of the fact that they alone are responsible for how well they perform, they know immediately (through their own perceptions and feedback from teammates and spectators) whether they have failed or succeeded in their endeavor, and an element of risk is always present as to the outcome of their performance (i.e., they might not meet performance goals).

Some exercisers do not consider fitness classes or exercise facilities to be pure achievement settings because the exerciser may be motivated by reasons other than achievement (Roberts, 2012). For example, people may engage in exercise to have fun, enjoy the company of others, or reduce stress, and increased

Table 2.2 Matrix of High and Low Achievers and High and Low Motives to Achieve

	High achievers	Low achievers
High motives to achieve	Prefer challenging goals, prefer to receive success or failure feedback soon after performance, prefer situations that contain some risk about the result, feel responsible for outcomes based on their own actions, feel they alone are responsible for how well they perform, know immediately (through their own perceptions and feedback from teammates and spectators) whether they have failed or succeeded, are highly competitive, and have strong win orientation.	May not consider fitness classes or exercise facilities to be achievement settings, may be motivated by reasons other than achievement, fear failure or success, do not prefer competitive conditions (low competition orientation), do not feel responsible for own actions and outcomes, and performance level is lower than what most test scores would predict; referred to as *underachiever.*
Low motives to achieve	Performance outcome has a degree of risk (e.g., may or may not meet performance goals), success is only moderately pleasurable, physiological symptoms of somatic arousal are weaker, and often lack the arousal level or motivation for prolonged concentration and attentional focusing on correct cues.	Prefer no goals or easy goals, do not desire feedback on performance outcomes or are unaffected by feedback content (not motivated by positive feedback and less affected by negative feedback), have low perceived self-control, have extensive past history of failure (reflecting either actual or perceived outcomes), and tend to underperform (not meeting performance expectations).

fitness may be less of a priority. Certainly exercisers want to get fitter, increase musculature, and perhaps lose weight; however, some are motivated by meeting other needs, such as being seen at exercise facilities, meeting other people, or improving their physical appearance and relishing the attention they receive from an improved physique. These are not abnormal motives to exercise, but an all-out workout is not necessarily desirable for everyone who attends an exercise facility. This aspect of achievement motivation concerns a related area of study called *self-presentation* (Martin Ginis and Mack, 2012).

Self-presentation involves two components, impression motivation (i.e., the general desire to create impressions) and impression construction (i.e., tactics that convey the desirable impressions). Thus, people who exercise to appear more physically attractive, to lose or maintain weight, to improve muscularity, and to develop a fit and athletic image are engaging in self-presentational exercise motives. Exercising for fun (e.g., recreational events), to reduce stress, and to improve health and fitness are examples of non-self-presentational motives. Martin Ginis and Mack (2012) concluded from their review of literature that "people who are motivated to exercise for self-presentation reasons do less exercise than those who are motivated for other reasons" (p. 348). Self-presentation as a form of motivation that helps explain exercise behavior is conceptually related to a more inclusive concept called *achievement motivation*. The thought process that drives a person's goal orientation—that fuels the need to feel competent—is reflected in achievement goal theory.

ACHIEVEMENT GOAL THEORY

Achievement goal theory posits that the desire to achieve a particular outcome, let's say losing weight or improving fitness, provides the basis for engaging in certain behaviors, what Duda and Hall (2001) call *achievement behavior*. Achievement behavior is dependent on "the personal meaning an individual assigns to

perceived success and failure" (p. 417). If, for instance, a person decides to exercise in order to reach a particular goal (e.g., lose weight, feel better, decrease stress) and she reaches the intended goal, she will perceive her exercise behavior as successful and feel a sense of personal achievement. Ostensibly, the sense of achievement improves the performer's sense of competence, which increases satisfaction and, as a result, increases intrinsic motivation. The long-term result will be to maintain participation in the successful activity and to develop an exercise habit. This habit will, in turn, improve the person's adherence to an exercise program and hopefully establish a lifestyle change of increased physical activity. This process is facilitated if the person has a high need to achieve; achieving desirable goals is more motivational and longer lasting for high-need achievers than it is for people with a relatively low need to achieve.

How, then, does a person acquire a high need for achievement? Duda and Hall (2001) list four factors that contribute to the motivation to achieve a desirable outcome:

1. The person's choice of future activity that he wants to continue

2. The amount of effort the person expends on the task

3. The level of persistence the person maintains on task

4. The person's thoughts and emotional responses associated with the resulting behaviors

To Duda and Hall, achievement goals (e.g., weight loss, improved fitness) are critical factors in a person's intent to initiate and maintain behavior in achievement settings such as exercise. For example, if a person follows a rehabilitation program after experiencing an injury, it is important for her to maintain the achievement goal of a full recovery and expect to engage in exercise as a result of completing the rehabilitation program. The person has to link her effort in the rehabilitation program with full recovery, followed by a return to exercising. Weaker or nonexistent achievement goals are more likely if exercisers do not anticipate a full recovery or are unsure if their rehabilitation efforts will lead to desirable outcomes, such as returning to a full exercise program and achieving preinjury fitness levels.

Injury is one of the most common reasons novice exercisers drop out of fitness programs, and they often stop exercising permanently. Injured exercisers have to perceive the rehabilitation process as meaningful and leading to a desired outcome, and they must recognize that not completing (adhering to) the rehabilitation program is undesirable and will inhibit the likelihood of a full recovery and maintaining fitness. This is where personal trainers, athletic trainers, and even family members and friends play a vital role in creating an environment that aids in establishing and maintaining achievement goals; this support system increases the person's incentive to complete the rehabilitation program successfully. The bottom line is that health care workers will promote motivation in clients or patients by providing them with information—often numerical or in some other quantifiable form—that reflects competence, improvement, and achievement (Roberts and Kristiansen, 2012).

GOAL ORIENTATION THEORY

Goal orientation, embedded in achievement motivation, refers to the extent to which exercisers are motivated by setting and then meeting goals as well as the types of goals they prefer to set (Duda, 2010). Goal orientation in an exercise context reflects two thought processes: the person's achievement goals (e.g., "What do I need to do to feel I have accomplished something meaningful and challenging?") and the person's perceived ability to achieve these goals (e.g., "Do I have the skills needed to meet this goal?"). Exercisers with high goal orientation will

- set a challenging yet achievable goal,
- feel a moderate to high degree of certainty about meeting this goal based on their high perceived ability,

- select a task they feel capable of achieving, and
- persist at that task with optimal effort until the goal is met.

Because goal orientation is not a personality trait, it can be more apparent in some situations than in others, it can be learned, and it is affected by previous experiences, particularly past experiences of perceived success and failure. This means that goal orientation can become stronger or weaker for a given time period, for a specific task or goal, or within a given context (e.g., exercise, academic, work, or social settings).

There are two primary orientations of achievement goals, ego (also called *win* or *competitive*) and mastery (also called *task*), which help determine how exercisers perceive their level of competence. Exercisers with an ego orientation are motivated by outcomes, such as weight loss or task accomplishment (e.g., running a certain distance or speed), and they are consumed by superior competence in comparison to others (e.g., winning an exercise or running competition). Athletic competitors with a task or mastery orientation derive a sense of achievement from successful task completion (e.g., completing an exercise class or meeting a short-term exercise goal).

Ego Orientation

Ego orientation represents the degree to which a person is motivated to engage in exercise for the purpose of improved fitness or health. This person is motivated by comparing his fitness level, strength, physique, or some other characteristic with others and demonstrating his superiority of this measure.

Ego-involved exercisers view exercise outcomes rather than the exercise activity itself as most important. This is not always a bad thing; injured exercisers may engage in weeks of rehabilitation and even additional surgery for the primary, sometimes singular purpose of returning to a physically active lifestyle and continuing to exercise or to compete as an athlete. That's desirable and understandable, but the injured person must also concentrate on full compliance with the rehabilitation program by attending all planned rehabilitation sessions and meeting short-term performance goals in the recovery process. This may mean completing one set of strength-building exercises at a time, requiring the person to maintain a task-involved attitude.

Exercisers with an ego orientation are far more likely than their mastery-oriented counterparts to believe that the ability to exercise, in the absence of extreme discomfort, injury, or excessive body weight, is the single most important determinant of successful exercise outcomes. People with perceptions of low exercise ability, perhaps due to low fitness level, excessive body weight, high level of physical or mental discomfort, or injury, thus will have reduced motivation and commitment to succeed over the long term (Duda and Treasure, 2010). These individuals are far more likely to drop out of exercise programs, especially if they are unable to keep up with other exercisers or to reach self-set short-term goals.

Mastery Orientation

Mastery orientation consists of motivation based on effort, improvement, and performance at one's best. Improved fitness or health would be natural outcomes of engaging in regular physical activity.

According to Papaioannou and Kouli (1999), intrinsic motivation is more likely to occur in task-involved (mastery) exercisers than in ego-involved (win) exercisers. This is because task-involved exercisers engage in activity for its own sake—that is, for pleasure or satisfaction. They are focused on the task at hand in attempting to accomplish short-term (e.g., feeling better, reducing stress, enjoying physical exertion) and long-term (e.g., weight loss, improved physique, reduced chance of obesity and disease) goals.

Duda and Treasure (2010) concluded that people whose exercise participation is based on ego orientation are at greater risk of quitting exercise programs if their aspirations (e.g., improved fitness, superior performance compared with others, weight loss) are not successfully achieved in a timely manner. The following lists help in understanding exercise motivation through the achievement goal framework of ego and task orientation. Helping clients regulate their self-talk also has motivational properties (Oliver, Markland, Hardy, and Petherick, 2008), and table 2.3 lists cognitive strategies for motivational self-talk that enhances a person's sense of achievement.

Task-Orientation Characteristics of Exercisers

- Main task is to improve fitness.
- Gain knowledge about proper exercise technique to gain optimal benefits.
- Exhibit optimal effort.
- Demonstrate improvement.
- Reach predetermined behavioral goals.
- Motivation is not based on perceived level of ability, competence, or fitness.

Table 2.3 Self-Talk Statements Associated With Six Achievement Needs

Achievement needs	Self-talk statements
1. Creating challenging goals	"I will complete the 3-mile course in 20 minutes or less."
2. Learning fitness skills that lead to improved performance	"I feel increasingly comfortable and not in danger of injury when lifting weights."
3. Receiving positive and constructive performance feedback while avoiding negative remarks	"I was able to jog one lap around the track nonstop." "I attended three fitness classes this week."
4. Taking risks and learning from the outcomes	"I'm not trying to beat anyone; I just want to give 100% effort and do the best I can."
5. Creating conditions for success	"I love taking that fitness class. We work hard and the time goes by quickly." "I like brisk walking with my workout buddy."
6. Feeling competent and pleased with achievements	"I did it! I completed the program and feel much better."

- Motivation is self-controlled based on a sense of gratification from the activity and is less dependent on external, often uncontrollable factors such as competition or comparing one's performance against others.

Ego-Orientation Characteristics of Exercisers

- Preoccupied with the adequacy of their exercise.

- Desire to demonstrate superior competence compared with others.

- Likely to enter competitive events to determine competence.

- Social comparisons with others are prevalent.

- High performance and persistence are strong motivation sources.

- Outcome goals rather than process goals are of primary concern.

- Motivation decreases when they feel incapable of achieving a goal (e.g., winning a race) or are unable to attain a certain performance level (e.g., running at a particular speed, lifting a predetermined weight).

- Motivation level is susceptible to environmental and conditional factors that are sometimes beyond their control.

COMPETENCE MOTIVATION THEORY

The theory of competence motivation (White, 1959) posits that behavior is selected, directed, and maintained due to "an intrinsic need to deal [effectively] with the environment" (p. 318). White argues that the need for competence is an inherent (i.e., predispositional) part of life starting in childhood. We habitually attempt to master our surroundings, and pleasure derives from successful outcomes of task mastery.

In an update of competence motivation theory, Harter (1981) proposed that children are motivated by mastery, curiosity, challenge, and play in order to satisfy their urge toward competence. Children's rewards for achieving competence are feelings of pleasure based on fun, enjoyment, and personal satisfaction. Harter claims that skill mastery is a primary motivator, particularly in achievement situations, such as exercise and attempts to improve fitness. If children are successful, their experiences related to task mastery result in pleasant emotions and improved self-confidence. In turn, these feelings lead to a continued incentive to exercise, improve fitness, and reach other fitness-related goals (e.g., weight loss, improved physique).

Central to Harter's (1981) theory is that people who perceive themselves as highly competent and in control of their (exercise) environment will exert more effort, persist longer at tasks, and experience more positive feelings than people who have lower perceived competence and self-control. These predictions have been confirmed in both sport

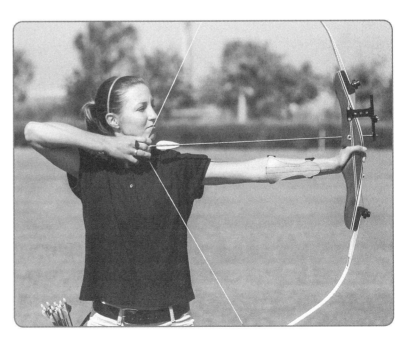

Mastering a task is a positive experience that motivates people to set and reach related goals.

settings (Vallerand and Reid, 1984; Weiss, Ebbeck, and Horn, 1997) and exercise settings (Hackfort and Birkner, 2005).

Improved competence motivation occurs when exercisers feel good enough about their participation to remain physically active regardless of the outcomes (e.g., increased fitness, weight loss). Effort and improvement should be emphasized for building competence motivation using a task orientation, focusing on the outcomes of effort rather than comparing one's characteristics (e.g., weight, musculature) with others (Roberts and Kristiansen, 2012). Fitness instructors should do everything possible to persuade exercisers of all fitness levels to think positive thoughts about linking their current activity to future benefits and desirable outcomes. This is why attempts to increase fitness by learning new exercises and having the opportunity to exercise, perhaps with others, are so important in maintaining motivation. Exercise competition (e.g., participating in races, trying to keep up with a fitness instructor, setting overly ambitious goals) may require more time for instruction and practice before the person is ready to meet new challenges, particularly related to competition.

DECI'S COGNITIVE EVALUATION THEORY

Exercise, as well as other forms of physical activity, is usually performed out of interest, enjoyment, and feelings of accomplishment in attempting to meet a personal goal (e.g., improved health or physical appearance). Rarely do we exercise because we anticipate receiving an external reward such as a trophy, certificate, attention from others, or financial gain. Other than athletes, who must exercise as part of their preparation for competition, and rehabilitation patients, most of us are not required to exercise. This means that repressive, unpleasant environments filled with evaluative pressures (e.g., points off for poor performance or losing a contest), judgments (e.g., exercising for punishment), and selective rewards (e.g., only first-place finishers receive

a prize) undermine the pleasure and benefits we should obtain from exercise.

Most people who exercise regularly are typically motivated to participate in physical activity because it is satisfying, pleasurable, and fun; that is, exercising due to the inherent enjoyment reflects the person's intrinsic motivation. Intrinsic motivation is central to promoting exercise participation and forms the foundation of starting and maintaining exercise participation (Kimiecik, 2002). This is the foundation of Deci's (1975) cognitive evaluation theory and, as discussed later in the chapter, Deci and Ryan's (2000) self-determination theory.

Extrinsic Motivation

Extrinsic motivation is the use of externally imposed incentives to change a person's thoughts, emotions, or actions (Deci, 1975). While most people who exercise regularly do so for external reasons, such as weight loss, better appearance, or socializing with others (Anshel, 2006), engaging in physical activity for intrinsic reasons is preferred for building and maintaining long-term healthy habits. This chapter provides the scientific basis and recommendations for building intrinsic motivation.

Because many exercise beginners are motivated to exercise by external reasons (e.g., weight control, improved appearance, socializing with others), the relatively high dropout rate for this group—approximately 50% within three to six months of starting a new program—is not surprising. A person will not usually engage in any optional activity, such as exercise, without feeling a sense of pleasure or fulfillment. In addition, the satisfying aspects of exercise often take weeks, sometimes months, to achieve. This is due to relatively poor fitness, excessive weight, and the time needed to develop exercise routines. Exercise, however, can be pleasurable for novice exercisers if their short-term and long-term goals are realistic and they do not overexert themselves, which can cause injury. Excessive physical exertion can be uncomfortable and unpleasant.

Intrinsic Motivation

Deci's cognitive evaluation theory defines *intrinsic motivation* as "doing an activity for its own sake, for the satisfaction inherent in the activity" (Ryan and Deci, 2007, p. 2). Ryan and Deci contend that intrinsic motivation has a dual meaning: On one hand, it concerns a person's innate tendency to act rather than being externally initiated and directed. On the other hand, it refers to the fact that the rewards accrued from an activity are inherent in the activity rather than being important to reducing biological drives (e.g., sleep, eating, drinking). The act of engaging in a given activity, not just the outcomes from that activity, creates its own rewards. For example, a person who finds pleasure from exercising without relying on specific outcomes from the activity (e.g., weight control, improved fitness) would be described as intrinsically motivated. Thus, intrinsic motivation consists of the exerciser's decision to engage in an activity due to feelings of satisfaction, personal fulfillment, and pleasure. Engaging in an activity for reasons unrelated to pleasure or satisfaction reflects extrinsic motivation. See figure 2.1 for an illustration of processes that increase and decrease intrinsic motivation according to Deci's theory.

Controlling and Informational Aspects

Deci claims that two components can influence intrinsic motivation—the controlling aspect and the informational aspect. The *controlling aspect* is more apparent, for example, when the person's motivation level is controlled by the reward's location, or locus (internal or external). In receiving an external reward, such as pleasing others or avoiding ridicule about physical appearance, the controlling aspect is external. The controlling aspect would be internal, however, if the person decided to sign up for a fitness club membership on his own volition in order to receive personal training, use quality equipment, and improve energy and general health. The second source of intrinsic motivation occurs when the *informational aspect* is more apparent than the controlling aspect in response to feelings of competence (e.g., "I am capable of meeting exercise goals") and self-

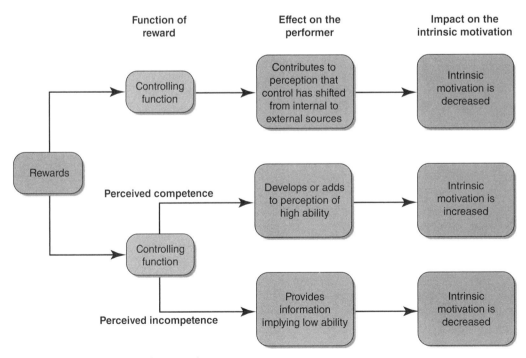

Figure 2.1 Deci's cognitive evaluation theory.

determination (e.g., "I have decided to exercise to improve my health").

People tend to attribute their fitness level to high effort, particularly if they are highly fit; they simply try hard and overcome initial fatigue. They are past the point of experiencing unpleasant feelings associated with exercise, and they view their experience as enjoyable—even fun. Perhaps not surprisingly, exercise becomes a habit, and the motive to continue exercising is intrinsic. Taken together, intrinsically motivated behaviors are more persistent, more enjoyable, and more likely to enhance the person's self-esteem than extrinsically motivated actions.

But what happens to intrinsic motivation when a person is offered extrinsic rewards (e.g., money, trophy, points)? Why, for instance, do people participate in playground games and other forms of physical activity for the fun of it and then, when placed in a competitive situation, it becomes important to win or receive recognition rather than enjoy the activity? Deci's cognitive evaluation theory proposes two processes by which extrinsic rewards can affect intrinsic motivation: the controlling function and the information function.

Controlling Function

People are intrinsically motivated to engage in an activity under conditions of high enjoyment and self-control, such as starting an exercise program. However, if the motive of engaging in an activity shifts from internal to external reasons, extrinsic motivation may override intrinsic motivation—that is, the performer engages in an activity for external reasons; the purpose of the activity is to gain approval, recognition, money, or some other externally derived source rather than for the inherent enjoyment of the activity. This occurs for most adults who enjoyed physical activity as children or adolescents but eventually stopped finding enjoyment from and time for physical activity. Most adult exercisers need reasons to exercise, such as reducing body weight, improving physical appearance, and reducing stress, among other external reasons.

Rewards and other sources of extrinsic motivation may be used constructively to convey information about a person's competence or achievement. For example, exercisers can be rewarded for their effort, attendance at fitness classes, improved fitness, improved

---

TURNING PLAY INTO WORK

A man was about to go take a nap. His bedroom window was next to a small field where children often played. While trying to fall asleep, a group of children were playing outside the window, making a lot of noise and keeping him awake. At first, he did what most people would have done; he asked the children to play quietly so he could take his nap without the noise. The children remained quiet for only minutes before they made more noise, preventing him from napping. The next time, in a raised voice, he asked the children to play someplace else and to leave the area. They did, but the next day they returned and, again, the man could not get to sleep.

The third day the children returned and played loudly outside his window, he decided to turn play into work. He offered to pay each of them 50 cents if they would make as much noise as possible for as long as they wanted, and they agreed. The next day they returned, and again, the man offered to pay them to make as much noise as they could, but this time he could only afford 25 cents instead of 50. He said he would try to pay them 50 cents each tomorrow. Although the children were a bit disappointed with the reduced payment, they accepted the money and made a lot of noise outside the man's window.

The next day the children returned to receive yet more payment to make a lot of noise. One child said, "Hey, Mister, can we have our 50 cents so we can make as much noise as we can?" The man said, "Kids, I'm sorry but I have no more money. I cannot pay you anything today or for the rest of the week." With that, the children expressed their deep disappointment and shouted, "Hey, if you can't pay us to make noise, we're leaving this place. Goodbye!" And with that, the children never returned to make noise and the man was able to take his daily nap in peace and quiet.

exercise performance, and so on. In each of these examples, the person should feel rewarded for accomplishing a task, meeting a goal, or demonstrating competence. Intrinsic motivation increases when the person is recognized for improved competence, perhaps through an award.

Information Function

Feelings of competence and self-determination are other factors that reflect the influence of extrinsic rewards on increasing intrinsic motivation. Deci (1975), in support of White's competence motivation theory (1959), contends that perceptions of high competence are central to increasing intrinsic motivation. People are attracted to and are far more likely to engage in activities in which they feel competent, perceive that the successful outcome was due to high ability (e.g., fitness level) or effort, and achieve desirable outcomes. Rewards can also improve intrinsic motivation if the person's feelings of competence and self-worth are increased. Rewards, therefore, can actually foster intrinsic motivation if they provide participants with recognition for demonstrating success, such as improved performance; showing high effort; or demonstrating competent skill execution. Finally, the second component of the information aspect is called *self-determination*, consisting of the individual's perception that she voluntarily decided to engage in the activity.

SELF-DETERMINATION THEORY

Self-determination theory (SDT) addresses the extent to which behaviors are autonomous, or self-determined (Ryan and Deci, 2000, 2007). The premise of SDT is that people have fundamental psychological needs for *autonomy* (i.e., a sense of independence and making self-serving decisions), *competence* (i.e., meeting self-set standards and desirable performance outcomes), and *relatedness* (i.e., environments in which they feel a sense of connectedness and belonging), and they actively pursue these needs. Thus, experiencing competence and

autonomy are both necessary conditions to promote a sense of satisfaction and pleasure from exercise, which leads to intrinsic motivation. Increased exercise involvement is associated with greater levels of self-determined motivation.

The relative absence of motivation or intention to engage in exercise (e.g., lack of perceived exercise skills, history of quitting, feeling exercise is unnecessary or unimportant) is called *amotivation*. Previous research has supported the validity of SDT to explain and predict exercise behavior (see Hagger and Chatzisarantis, 2008, for a review). For instance, exercisers who do not feel that their effort is sufficient to improve their fitness and reduce body weight will feel less self-determination and, therefore, will be less intrinsically motivated than exercisers who feel that their effort is a primary reason for improved fitness and weight loss.

Exercise leaders and personal trainers can foster exercisers' feelings of self-determination and personal responsibility for exercise outcomes by consulting with them about forming an effective fitness program and using proper exercise techniques. Central to promoting self-determination (and intrinsic motivation) is encouraging all-out effort and preventing feelings of hopelessness (e.g., "I'll never get fit or lose this weight"). The exerciser's perceptions of low self-control and feelings of helplessness foster alienation and markedly reduce or eliminate intrinsic motivation. SDT predicts that people who exercise to improve physical appearance, which is a common exercise motive (i.e., low self-determination), are less likely to adhere to their exercise regimen than people who exercise for their own pleasure (i.e., high self-determination).

In their revision of Deci's (1975) cognitive evaluation theory, Deci and Ryan (1985) proposed a third primary component, *functional significance of the event*. High functional significance reflects an aspect of the situation that the person perceives as most important. Most events include both controlling functions (e.g., "I made the decision to exercise regularly) and informational functions (e.g., "I feel myself getting fitter; exercise is becoming easier").

Functional significance of the event influences perceived control of the situation (internal or external), perceived ability to perform in that situation (high or low), and feelings of intrinsic motivation (versus extrinsic motivation). According to Deci and Ryan (1985), the combination of self-control (choice), perceived competence, autonomy (self-determination), and positive feedback result in increased functional significance. The source of positive feedback is an important factor in improving motivation for adhering to the exercise program.

Intrinsic motivation, that is, high self-determination, has been shown to be related to several beneficial outcomes. There are, however, several factors, referred to by researchers as *mediators* (Thomas, Nelson, and Silverman, 2010), that accompany support for SDT. For example, Hein and Koka (2007) concluded that sport coaches and physical education teachers are important sources of competence-related feedback and influence the learner's self-determined motivation. In another study, Lutz, Lochbaum, and Turnbow (2003) found that an SDT program resulted in a significant elevation in positive mood state.

In the context of exercise and health psychology, the strength of exercisers' needs at least partly determines their direction toward and persistence in engaging in specific healthy habits. Exercisers engage in certain goal-directed behaviors that will result in meeting predetermined outcomes such as weight loss, improved fitness, increased energy, reduced stress or anxiety, and improved self-esteem. Thus, when exercisers associate high effort with positive outcomes from an ongoing exercise program, such as desirable physical appearance, high energy, and improved fitness, they are likely to maintain their exercise habit (Vansteenkiste, Soenens, and Lens, 2007).

Researchers (e.g., see Pelletier and Sarrazin, 2007, for a review) have pointed out limitations of SDT. Lack of valid and reliable measures to ascertain each component of the theory, lack of identification of the mechanisms responsible for determining how the components of the theory influence cognitive and performance

FUNCTIONAL SIGNIFICANCE IN ACTION

A 15-year-old elite baseball player performed admirably in games and received considerable positive feedback and attention from family, peers, and the local media on his performance. His coach, however, was confused about his poor effort, negative mood, and lack of enthusiasm in practice, conditioning, and game preparation. The athlete was chronically late for practice, indicated that he hated exercising to improve his conditioning, and seemed to lack concentration at pregame team meetings when the coach signals and team strategy were reviewed. Only in the presence of his father did the player give 100% and appear to be fully engaged.

Repeated conversations with the athlete indicated that his motive to compete came not from himself but rather from his father's pressure. This explained the athlete's lack of passion about exercising; it was not part of his mission to become an elite athlete. "My dad wants me to get a college scholarship," he said, and "My dad expects me to hit over .300 every season." When asked, "But what do *you* want from baseball?", he responded, "I don't really like baseball all that much. I have no life outside of baseball and a lot of times I prefer to just hang out with my friends."

It was obvious that the controlling aspect was most important to this athlete. The result was his perceived low self-control (i.e., an external perceived locus of causality), undermined intrinsic motivation (i.e., a lack of personal satisfaction and fulfillment), increased extrinsic motivation (i.e., dependence on his father's approval and love), and defiance (i.e., resisting the challenging practice schedule that took time away from socializing with friends). When the athlete's father, a source of extrinsic motivation, was absent from practice, he experienced minimal satisfaction from the activity and, hence, no incentive to maintain optimal effort. This athlete, who had the performance potential to receive a college scholarship, dropped all sport participation by the time he was 16 years old.

outcomes, and lack of understanding the content (e.g., frequency, duration, intensity) of SDT interventions that improve exercise participation and long-term exercise adherence require further clarification and study. Additional research in testing the self-determination model is also needed to explain the motivational factors and optimal intervention strategies that promote exercise participation and long-term adherence. As Levy and Cardinal (2004) concluded in their study on the use of mail delivery to improve exercise motivation, "There is an ongoing need to develop and test individually adapted exercise behavior change programs that can be widely disseminated" (p. 347).

SDT is best represented in figure 2.2, which incorporates factors that explain the relationship between intrinsic and extrinsic motivation.

Exercisers who enter a facility feeling excited, enthusiastic, optimistic about meeting personal goals, and focused on the series of tasks at hand (e.g., determining the proper exercises, developing and carrying out routines related to the fitness program) will feel a sense of belonging, self-motivation, and security. They are on a mission to change their life, they are enjoying the journey, and they are likely to adhere to their exercise program. Conversely, people who enter a fitness facility feeling intimidated, disconnected from the program, uncomfortable and insecure in the environment, and awkward in physical appearance (e.g., overweight, unfit) and who have not developed an exercise routine will not return. This latter set of feelings explains the high dropout rate for many people who start exercise programs (Wang and Biddle, 2007).

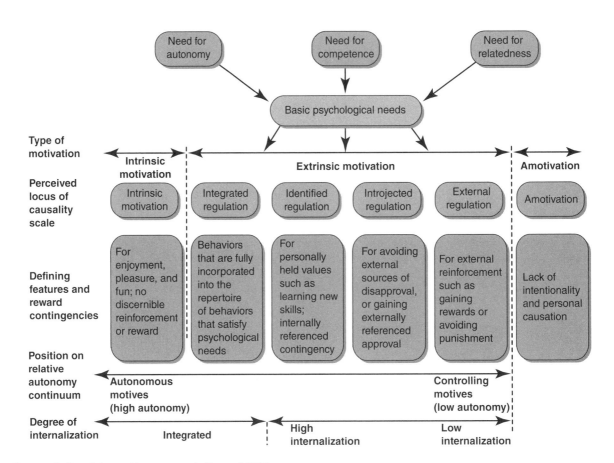

Figure 2.2 Schematic representation of SDT.

Reprinted, by permission, from M.C. Hagger and N. Chatzisaranis, 2007, *Intrinsic motivation and self-determination in exercise* (Champaign, IL: Human Kinetics), 8.

At the heart of SDT is the issue of transferring an individual's source of motivation from less to more self-determination, that is, from feelings of low self-control and autonomy to optimal self-control and autonomy. Self-determination and intrinsic motivation are accompanied by positive feelings such as confidence and a general positive mind-set (Amorose, 2007). Self-determination fuels intrinsic motivation and is therefore highly desirable for exercise programs, particularly among novice participants. High intrinsic motivation is a strong predictor of long-term exercise adherence.

ATTRIBUTION THEORY

How do we determine if we are successful at something, such as improving our fitness or reaching a fitness goal? What strategies keep us on track to improve our fitness and health? How can a health coach motivate clients by helping them conclude that they are responsible for their own success? The area that concerns how we explain the causes of our performance outcomes—successes and failures—in achievement settings is called *making causal attributions* and is central to Weiner's (1985) attribution theory.

Exercisers, for example, may attempt to complete a certain number of repetitions, lift a particular weight, or move at a certain speed that reflects improved fitness. At the same time, exercisers will designate these outcomes as successful or unsuccessful based on their own interpretation of the outcome. How the exercisers explain the primary causes of their perceived success or failure is referred to as *making causal attributions*.

Attribution theory, therefore, provides a framework that describes the ways in which a person explains (appraises) the causes of performance outcomes in achievement settings. It is important that people make accurate causal attributions because certain explanations have strong motivational value while the wrong explanation can lead to reduced motivation and even quitting the activity. It is essential that people who exercise attribute the benefits of an exercise habit to their effort and to their

perceived ability to exercise correctly and effectively. After several days or weeks of exercise, or even after a single exercise bout, the exerciser should attribute the positive outcomes to the effort it took to accomplish these outcomes, such as more energy, better concentration, or improved appearance. Exercisers drop out of their programs due to perceptions of high task difficulty (e.g., "I'm just not built to be fit, so why bother?").

Questions many exercisers ask include, "Did I perform according to my expectations and goals?", "Was I responsible for my success in starting this exercise program?", "Am I capable of performing the proper exercise techniques and meeting the demands of improved fitness?", "What do others think about my exercise participation? Am I out of place among these thinner, fitter exercisers?", and "To what extent is the outcome of my continued exercise program due to my skills and desire to meet my needs?" The answers to these questions have great motivational value in determining the individual's willingness to persevere and maintain an exercise program or any other attempt to improve health and well-being.

What about motivation level in response to making attributions following performance failure? Motivation is greatly affected if you believe you did not meet your exercise goals because it was a difficult task or you had bad luck. Attributing the cause of undesirable outcomes to low effort or, worse, low ability (i.e., "I just don't have the desire or the capability to exercise regularly and lose weight") can markedly decrease motivation. Low-ability causal attributions maintained over time can induce a phenomenon called *learned helplessness*, in which people feel little control over their destiny in achievement settings, and quitting becomes inevitable. Most of us will quit an activity if we feel incapable of performing it successfully. For example, child athletes often quit their sport if they conclude they do not have the proper skill level, especially after repeated performance failures.

In short, the ways in which people explain or interpret their performance directly influence motivation (e.g., intrinsic, extrinsic, achievement, or competence). Fitness coaches can help their exercise clients determine the causes of exercise outcomes (e.g., "Your commitment to getting fit is the reason you've lost 10 pounds over the past six weeks since you started this program. Well done!").

WEINER'S ATTRIBUTION MODEL

Bernard Weiner and his colleagues (1971) first suggested that we perceive and explain success and failure in terms of four categories: ability, task difficulty, effort, and luck. The content of these causal attributions often influences a person's future motivation and performance effectiveness. Researchers have shown that people who conclude that their poor performance is due to low ability (e.g., "I do not have the endurance to jog 20 minutes nonstop," "Moving in rhythm to music during exercise is hard for me") are more likely to reduce their effort or even quit their exercise program than if they interpret the performance limitation as due to task difficulty ("Moving in rhythm to music during intense exercise is difficult to do"), low effort ("I have to try harder to keep up with the fitness instructor"), or even luck ("I'm just having a bad day").

Some dimensions of Weiner's model have more long-term implications than others. For example, exercisers can attribute success (e.g., meeting a particular goal or expectation) to high effort (e.g., "I worked hard to lose this weight") or good luck (e.g., "I have the right genes"), but an attribute of high ability or perceiving the task as difficult after achieving success is longer term and less changeable. It is understandably important, therefore, to make the right causal attribution due to its relatively long-lasting effects on motivation. Making low-ability attributes (e.g., "I'm just not good enough to lose weight," "What's the use of trying, I know I'll never meet my fitness coach's expectations") is devastating to an exerciser's long-term commitment to improving fitness. Chapter 8 discusses the application of Weiner's attribution model for promoting exercise.

Attributional Bias

The concept of attributional bias, also called *self-serving attributional bias* or *hedonistic bias*, reflects the tendency of highly fit or skilled people to reflect internal controllability after successful outcomes and external controllability after unsuccessful outcomes. The *bias* in this concept is that outcomes are explained according to what is in the person's best interests or is most motivational. Perceived failure in achievement settings, such as sport or exercise, is explained by task difficulty (e.g., how well opponents performed rather than how poorly the athlete performed). Winning, however, is usually attributed to high effort and ability, talent, or skill. Thus, attributional bias refers to making internal attributions following perceived success and external attributions following perceived failure. Sometimes that's a good thing; attributing high ability or good effort following success builds self-esteem. However, not taking the blame for failure comes at a cost.

Inappropriate self-blame (e.g., "It's my fault," "I'm really awful at that and I won't improve") can reduce motivation and self-esteem. Feelings of hopelessness and eventually quitting exercise or other forms of physical activity can result. Distorting causal attributions (e.g., externalizing the reasons for failures) can also be damaging to future motivation if the exerciser's failure to meet goals and to experience high physical exertion and discomfort do not provide incentives to practice hard, overcome early struggle in improving fitness, and try to perform better next time. Exercisers need to learn how to make more accurate, constructive, and motivational causal attributions that have motivational properties.

Emotions and Expectations

Weiner (1985) added two other dimensions to his reformulated model—the roles of *emotions* and *expectations* that occur between the times of a person's acknowledged causal attribution and her future behavior. For example, after completing a workout, the person will have an emotional reaction that Weiner calls *outcome dependent*. If the performance is successful or meets the person's expectations, she will have relatively positive emotions, whereas negative emotions will follow the perception of unsuccessful performance. After this point, the person searches for reasons that help explain the outcome, such as, "Why did this happen? Was it due to my hard work, commitment, and perseverance, or did I make the task (or goal) too easy by not giving 100% and just getting by?" After the causal attribution has been made, the person processes it further.

For example, after explaining the cause of a performance outcome, such as completing a predetermined number of exercise repetitions, the person then determines if she should take responsibility for this outcome (i.e., the controllability dimension); if the outcome was due to something that will be consistent over time, such as motivation or fitness level (i.e., the stability dimension); or if the outcome was due to rapidly changing factors, such as the combination of effort (i.e., "Did I give 100%?") and controllability (i.e., "Did I control the cause of this outcome?"). The combination of these dimensions with the performer's emotional reactions and future expectations jointly determine future behavior, according to Weiner (1985).

SUMMARY

The human organism is driven by motivation. Processes of growth, maturation, and improvement are derived from people's conscious decisions about their behaviors. Motivation is the ignition for producing energy, which in turn drives behavior. Motivation is required for replacing unhealthy habits with more desirable behavior patterns.

Theories that at least partially explain ways in which we generate and maintain motivation include achievement goal theory (i.e., the desire to achieve a particular outcome provides the basis for engaging in certain behaviors), goal orientation theory (i.e., people are motivated in varying degrees by setting and then meeting goals), attribution theory (i.e., motivation is driven by the manner in which we explain the causes of performance outcomes, primarily ability, effort, task difficulty, or luck), competence motivation theory (i.e., behavior is selected, directed, and maintained due to an intrinsic need to deal effectively with the environment), cognitive evaluation theory (i.e., some people perform an activity for its own sake and have an innate tendency to act rather than being externally initiated and directed), and SDT (i.e., people have psychological needs for autonomy, or making self-serving decisions; competence, or meeting self-set standards and desirable performance outcomes; and relatedness, or environments in which they feel a sense of connectedness and belonging). Though all motivational theories at least partially reflect the individual's personality and other characteristics, they also incorporate situational and environmental factors that help explain and predict lifestyle choices and health behavior change.

STUDENT ACTIVITY

Developing a Client Action Plan

Without motivation, particularly intrinsic motivation, the exerciser is unlikely to reach goals, improve fitness, and maintain an exercise habit. The primary goal of every person who provides any type of health care service (e.g., fitness coach, registered dietitian, mental health professional, medical practitioner) is to establish a relationship with each client based on trust, mutual respect, credibility, sincerity, sensitivity, and honesty. This type of relationship takes time, effort, and planning. This activity does not address recruiting clients; that's the responsibility of marketing and management. The primary goal of fitness and health professionals is to strongly encourage clients to psychologically buy into the program and to invest time and energy in their long-term health.

Your Task

Your client action plan is intended to increase the client's intrinsic motivation and long-term adherence to an exercise habit.

1. *Pretesting:* Would you pretest your client on specific measures? Which measures, and why did you select these?

2. *Perceived competence:* Perceived competence is a vital element of long-term commitment to an exercise program. What exercise guidelines would you provide your client that would likely lead to increased perceived competence and success?

3. *Goal setting:* What short-term and long-term goals would you help your client generate? How would you measure achievement of these goals?

4. *Motivational strategies:* How would you encourage the development of various types of motivation? Specifically, how would you increase task (not ego) orientation and intrinsic (not extrinsic) motivation? How might sources of extrinsic motivation be used to improve intrinsic motivation?

5. *Action plan:* Describe a full action plan for your client that includes cognitive strategies (i.e., client thoughts and emotions) and behavioral strategies (e.g., testing, goals, ways to improve fitness, instructional techniques, inclusion of coaches with various types of expertise).

6. *Measurement of adherence and success:* Indicate how you will measure your client's success at improved fitness, adherence, and other outcomes.

REFERENCES

Alderman, R.B. (1974). *Psychological behavior in sport.* Philadelphia: W.B. Saunders.

Allport, G.W. (1937). *Personality: A psychological interpretation.* New York: Holt.

Amorose, A.J. (2007). Coaching effectiveness: Exploring the relationship between coaching behavior and self-determined motivation. In M.S. Hagger and N.L.D. Chatzisarantis (Eds.), *Intrinsic motivation and self-determination in exercise and sport* (pp. 209-227). Champaign, IL: Human Kinetics.

Anshel, M.H. (2006). *Applied exercise psychology: A practitioner's guide to client health and fitness.* New York: Springer.

Anshel, M.H. (2012). *Sport psychology: From theory to practice* (5th ed.). San Francisco: Benjamin-Cummings.

Armstrong, A. (2010). Weighing wellness initiatives: Having a policy isn't enough. *The Illinois School Board Journal, 78*, 10-14.

Berger, B.G., and McInman, A. (1993). Exercise and the quality of life. In R.N. Singer, M. Murphey, and L. Keith Tennant (Eds.), *Handbook of research on sport psychology* (pp. 729-760). New York: Macmillan.

Deci, E.L. (1975). *Intrinsic motivation.* New York: Plenum Press.

Deci, E.L., and Ryan, R.M. (1985). *Intrinsic motivation and self-determination in human behavior.* New York: Plenum Press.

Deci, E.L., and Ryan, R.M. (2000). The "what" and "why" of goal pursuits: Human needs and the self-determination of behavior. *Psychological Inquiry, 11*, 227-268.

Duda, J.L. (1993). Goals: A social-cognitive approach to the study of achievement motivation in sport. In R.N. Singer, M. Murphey, and L.K. Tennant (Eds.), *Handbook of research in sport psychology* (pp. 421-436). New York: Macmillan.

Duda, J.L. (2010). Motivational processes and the facilitation of quality engagement in sport. In J.M. Williams (Ed.), *Applied sport psychology: Personal growth to peak performance* (pp. 59-80). New York: McGraw-Hill.

Duda, J.L., and Hall, H. (2001). Achievement goal theory in sport. In R.N. Singer, H.A. Hausenblas, and C.M. Janelle (Eds.), *Handbook of sport psychology* (2nd ed., pp. 417-443). New York: Wiley.

Duda, J.L., and Treasure, D.C. (2010). Motivational processes and the facilitation of quality engagement in sport. In J.M. Williams (Ed.), *Applied sport psychology: Personal growth to peak performance* (6th ed., pp. 59-80). New York: McGraw-Hill.

Duda, J.L., and Whitehead, J. (1998). Measurement of goal perspectives in the physical domain. In J.L. Duda (Ed.), *Advances in sport and exercise psychology measurement* (pp. 21-48). Morgantown, WV: Fitness Information Technology.

Endler, N.S., and Hunt, J.M. (1966). Source of behavioral variance as measured by the S-R Inventory of Anxiousness. *Psychological Bulletin, 65*, 336-346.

Hackfort, D., and Birkner, H. A. (2005). An action-oriented perspective on exercise psychology. In D. Hackfort, J. L. Duda, and R. Lidor (Eds.), *Handbook of research in applied sport and exercise psychology: International perspectives* (pp. 351-373). Morgantown, WV: Fitness Information Technology.

Hagger, M.S., and Chatzisarantis, N. (2008). Self-determination theory and the psychology of exercise. *International Journal of Sport and Exercise Psychology, 1*, 79-103.

Harter, S. (1981). The development of competence motivation in the mastery of cognitive and physical skills. Is there still a place for joy? In G.C. Roberts and D.M. Landers (Eds.), *Psychology of motor behavior and sport – 1980* (pp. 3-29). Champaign, IL: Human Kinetics.

Hein, V., and Koka, A. (2007). Perceived feedback and motivation in physical education and physical activity. In M.S. Hagger and N.L.D. Chatzisarantis (Eds.), *Intrinsic motivation and self-determination in exercise and sport* (pp. 127-140). Champaign, IL: Human Kinetics.

Howley, E.T., and Franks, B.D. (2007). *Fitness professional's handbook* (5th ed.). Champaign, IL: Human Kinetics.

Kimiecik, J. (2002). *The intrinsic exerciser: Discovering the joy of exercise.* Boston: Houghton Mifflin.

Lavizzo-Mourey, R. (2004, March). Childhood obesity. Keynote address presented at the Society of Behavioral Medicine Conference, Baltimore.

Levy, S.S., and Cardinal, B.J. (2004). Effects of a self-determination theory–based mail mediated intervention on adults' exercise behavior. *American Journal of Health Promotion, 18*, 345-349.

Lutz, R., Lochbaum, M., and Turnbow, K. (2003). The role of relative autonomy in post-exercise affect responding. *Journal of Sport Behavior, 26*, 137-154.

Martin Ginis, K.A., Burke, S.M., and Gauvin, L. (2007). Exercising with others exacerbates the negative effects of mirrored environments on sedentary women's feeling states. *Psychology and Health, 22*, 945-962.

Martin Ginis, K.A., and Mack, D. (2012). Understanding exercise behavior: A self-presentational perspective. In G.C. Roberts and D.C. Treasure (Eds.), *Advances in motivation in sport and exercise* (3rd ed., pp. 327-355). Champaign, IL: Human Kinetics.

Nicholls, J. (1984). Achievement motivation: Conceptions of ability, subjective experience, task choice, and performance. *Psychological Review, 91*, 328-346.

Oliver, E.J., Markland, D., Hardy, J., and Petherick, C.M. (2008). The effects of autonomy—supportive versus controlling environments on self-talk. *Motivation and Emotion, 32*, 200-212.

O'Rourke, M. (2011). *Predictors of attitudes toward physical activity as a function of secondary school physical education experiences among adults.* (Unpublished doctoral dissertation). Middle Tennessee State University, Murfreesboro, Tennessee.

Papaioannou, A., and Kouli, O. (1999). The effect of task structure, perceived motivation climate, and goal orientations on students' task involvement and anxiety. *Journal of Applied Sport Psychology, 11*, 51-71.

Pelletier, L.G., and Sarrazin, P. (2007). Measurement issues in self-determination theory and sport. In M.S. Hagger and N.L.D. Chatzisarantis (Eds.), *Intrinsic motivation and self-determination in exercise and sport* (pp. 143-152). Champaign, IL: Human Kinetics.

Roberts, G.C. (1992). Motivation in sport and exercise: Conceptual constraints and convergence. In G.C. Roberts (Ed.), *Motivation in sport and exercise* (pp. 3-29). Champaign, IL: Human Kinetics.

Roberts, G.C. (2012). Motivation in sport and exercise from an achievement goal theory perspective: After 30 years, where are we? In G.C. Roberts and D.C. Treasure (Eds.), *Advances in motivation in sport and exercise* (3rd ed., pp. 5-58). Champaign, IL: Human Kinetics.

Roberts, G.C., and Kristiansen, E. (2012). Goal setting to enhance motivation in sport. In G.C. Roberts (Ed.), *Motivation in sport and exercise* (pp. 207-228). Champaign, IL: Human Kinetics.

Ryan, R.M., and Deci, E.L. (2000). Self-determination theory and the facilitation of intrinsic motivation, social development, and well-being. *American Psychologist, 55*, 68-78.

Ryan, R.M., and Deci, E.L. (2007). Active human nature: Self-determination theory and the promotion and maintenance of sport, exercise, and health. In M.S. Hagger and N.L.D. Chatzisarantis (Eds.), *Intrinsic motivation and self-determination in exercise and sport* (pp. 1-20). Champaign, IL: Human Kinetics.

Smith, R. E. (1993). *Psychology.* Minneapolis, MN: West.

Thomas, J.R., Nelson, J.K., and Silverman, S.J. (2010). *Research methods in physical activity* (6th ed.). Champaign, IL: Human Kinetics.

U.S. Government Accountability Office (GAO). (2012). K-12 education school-based physical education and sports programs. Washington, DC: Author.

Vallerand, R.J., and Reid, G. (1984). On the causal effects of perceived competence on intrinsic motivation: A test of cognitive evaluation theory. *Journal of Sport Psychology, 6*, 94-102.

Vansteenkiste, M., Soenens, B., and Lens, W. (2007). Intrinsic versus extrinsic goal promotion in exercise and sport: Understanding the differential impacts on performance and persistence. In M.S. Hagger and N.L.D. Chatzisarantis (Eds.), *Intrinsic motivation and self-determination in exercise and sport* (pp. 167-180). Champaign, IL: Human Kinetics.

Wang, C.K.J., and Biddle, S.J.H. (2007). Understanding young people's motivation toward exercise: An integration of sport ability beliefs, achievement goal theory, and self-determination theory. In M.S. Hagger and N.L.D. Chatzisarantis (Eds.), *Intrinsic motivation and self-determination in exercise and sport* (pp. 193-208). Champaign, IL: Human Kinetics.

Weiner, B. (1985). An attributional theory of achievement motivation and emotion. *Psychological Review, 92*, 548-573.

Weiner, B., Frieze, I., Kukla, A., Reed, I., Rest, S., and Rosenbaum, R.M. (1971). *Perceiving the causes of success and failure.* Morristown, NJ: General Learning Press.

Weiss, M.R., Ebbeck, V., and Horn, T.S. (1997). Children's self-perceptions and sources of competence information: A cluster analysis. *Journal of Sport and Exercise Psychology, 19*, 52-70.

White, R.W. (1959). Motivation reconsidered: The concept of competence. *Psychological Review, 66*, 297-331.

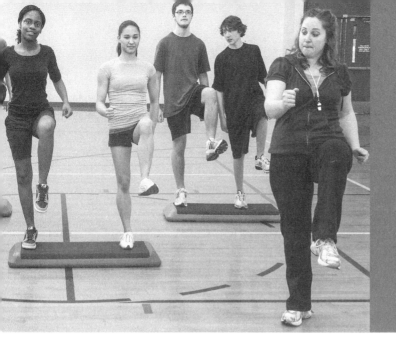

CHAPTER 3

Theories and Models of Exercise Behavior

> ❝ *I am not judged by the number of times I fail, but by the number of times I succeed; and the number of times I succeed is in direct proportion to the number of times I can fail and keep on trying.* ❞
>
> Tom Hopkins, author and speaker

CHAPTER OBJECTIVES

After reading this chapter, you should be able to:

- identify the psychological and emotional benefits of exercise and other forms of physical activity, particularly aerobic exercise;
- apply the theories and models that describe, explain, and predict exercise behavior;
- differentiate between stress and anxiety; and
- understand theoretical explanations of the stress- and anxiety-reducing properties of aerobic exercise.

The four primary reasons people voluntarily engage in health behavior change are to

1. prevent illness,

2. improve general health,

3. manage disease to receive a better diagnosis, and

4. receive treatment or rehabilitation in restoring health or reducing disease progression (e.g., Clark and Becker, 1998; Ockene, 2001).

Researchers and practitioners are interested in determining which interventions are most effective at improving health behavior and replacing unhealthy habits with more desirable ones. Most of the intervention research has been guided by various theories and models that explain and predict improved health outcomes. Personal, environmental, and situational factors influence these outcomes, further challenging researchers to determine the best explanations of why people persist in their self-destructive behavior patterns, refusing to change or dropping out of interventions.

No doubt some people question the applied usefulness of theories and models to their learning about exercise and their development as professionals. The primary purpose of theories and models is to explain, describe, or predict behavior in the attempt to advance knowledge.

A *theory* is usually defined as a set of general principles that attempts to explain and predict a person's thoughts, emotions, and behavior, often by combining environmental (e.g., exercising in a fitness club as opposed to alone at home), situational (e.g., performance under competitive versus noncompetitive conditions), and personal (e.g., a person's level of self-confidence or level of skill or fitness) factors. Predicting behavior is a powerful tool in trying to promote or increase some actions while inhibiting or eliminating others. How, for instance, can we increase the number of people who engage in regular physical activity while reducing the factors that contribute to dropping out of exercise programs? The value of theories is to help answer those types of questions. The key element of a theory is the intention to *predict* future behavior.

For example, Dr. Albert Bandura (1977) published his popular self-efficacy theory that explains behavior change and maintenance as the result of one's expectations about the outcomes that will result from engaging in behavior and expectations about one's ability to engage in or execute the behavior. His concept of *outcome expectations* consists of beliefs about whether certain behaviors will lead to particular outcomes. *Efficacy expectations*, on the other hand, consist of beliefs about how capable one is of performing the behavior that leads to those outcomes. Bandura's theory reflects a person's beliefs about capabilities and the connections between behavior and outcome. He contends that a person's expectations vary as a function of the particular task and its context.

Bandura's theory has direct implications for exercise behavior. A person's motivation is less enduring, less intrinsic (i.e., satisfying), and therefore will lead to less persistence if his exercise behavior is based solely on outcome expectations (e.g., losing weight, running at a certain speed or distance). On the other hand, the person's efficacy expectations are based on his belief that he is capable of investing the time to exercise by scheduling it in advance, creating a routine and performing the exercise routine, and working hard through exertion to overcome fatigue. These feelings of confidence lead to success in meeting goals and to feelings of satisfaction (i.e., greater intrinsic motivation, longer exercise adherence).

Whereas a theory pulls together an array of factors that predict certain outcomes, usually based on many studies that have tested and confirmed the theory, a *model*, on the other hand, is a visual representation of the thoughts, attitudes, emotions, and behaviors in a series of structures (i.e., the boxes in the figure of the model), each connected by one or more processes (i.e., the arrows that connect two or more structures), that eventually lead to a predetermined outcome. The structures are stable and permanent, while the processes are changeable and may be influenced by interventions such as using mental skills or changing thought content. For example, a model might illustrate that a person's positive or negative self-talk content influences attitudes toward exercise, emotional content during exercise, and exercise performance. The research question is, does self-talk content influence the person's attitude toward exercise and her exercise intensity and endurance?

Theories and models are needed to

- improve our understanding of the interrelationships among a person's thoughts (also called *cognitions*), emotions (also called *affect*), and behaviors;
- help explain behavioral phenomena, that is, why certain actions occur under particular circumstances;
- predict future behavior;
- simplify complex and abundant information into a coherent and organized structure that improves our understanding of these processes; and
- test the effectiveness of interventions that can improve certain outcomes.

Students and practitioners who aspire to careers in applied exercise psychology need to understand the foundations of health and exercise behavior, interpret client behaviors, apply selected aspects of theories in practice, and interpret and explain the results of studies.

Each theory or model has been met with limited success in promoting behavior change, particularly with respect to initiating and maintaining exercise behavior. However, each theory or model has also been criticized for having certain limitations that prevent its widespread effectiveness. For example, one limitation of most theories and models of health behavior change has been the assumption that each participant in a study desires a change in behavior. This, sadly, is not true. Following is a review of the most common and well-studied theories and models that are intended to change and improve health behavior. Despite the age of their original publication, many of these models are still being tested and, to some degree, supported.

HEALTH BELIEF MODEL

Do most people behave in a manner that they view as good for their health? According to the health belief model (HBM; Becker and Maiman, 1975), yes, they do. Conversely, most people will avoid actions if they perceive them to lead to unhealthy outcomes. Thus, the perception that engaging in regular exercise will maintain good health, prevent poor health, reduce body weight or maintain proper body weight, and contribute to other desirable outcomes will be likely to induce exercise behavior.

Ostensibly, the HBM predicts healthy behaviors if people are concerned about poor health, feel susceptible to health problems, and feel empowered to prevent or control health problems. The HBM posits that people make decisions that affect their health—either to initiate or to avoid actions that are in their best interest. Decisions about changing health behavior are predicted based on a balance between perceptions of the seriousness of one's condition versus the level of effectiveness the behavior change will bring in reducing the threat to one's health. The challenge in promoting an exercise habit by applying the HBM is that the undesirable effects of not exercising and leading a sedentary lifestyle do not appear for many years; there is no immediate threat to one's health and well-being. Experiencing a heart attack or receiving a life-threatening diagnosis from a medical practitioner, on the other hand, is far more likely to cause people to adopt and maintain an exercise habit or other health-promoting behavior. This process is evident when observing and interviewing members of a program that focuses on rehabilitation, such as cardiac rehabilitation exercise.

Thus, in support of the HBM, initiating an exercise program is far more likely when there is a sense of urgency about one's current health status—ostensibly due to a specific, clearly identified health problem—and the perception that the problem will be remedied with exercise. Other factors such as motivation, familiarity with and attitudes toward exercise, and social support (e.g., exercising with others, being encouraged to exercise by friends and family, having transportation to an exercise venue), also validate the HBM.

The HBM has received moderate support by researchers. In their review of literature, Berger, Pargman, and Weinberg (2007) concluded that the HBM was most predictive of health-related behaviors among younger populations and reflected research conducted in the 1970s and early 1980s. Oldridge and Streiner (1990) tested the extent to which the HBM predicted adherers and dropouts of cardiac rehabilitation programs. They found that the HBM correctly classified 80% of the patients. The researchers also found that predicting a person's readiness to exercise was most predictive if exercise was perceived as effective in improving general health.

Clearly, the HBM can predict exercise participation only to the extent that a person links exercise habits with improved health. For people who do not perceive their health as at risk, however, the HBM is less effective at predicting future health and exercise behavior. Adolescents and young adult males, for example, are particularly known to engage more frequently in high-risk behaviors, such as using tobacco products, mind-altering drugs, and alcohol; they drive faster than the rest of the population as well. The HBM, therefore, does not seem as powerful in predicting health behaviors of relatively younger people.

Another limitation of the HBM, according to Buckworth and Dishman (2002) in their literature review, is that it is based on avoiding illness rather than explaining exercise behavior. The authors contend that "the model is more useful for preventive health behaviors and compliance with medical regimens and less successful when applied to exercise" (p. 224). The results of several studies, in fact, have shown that perceived susceptibility is inversely (negatively) associated with exercise adherence. In other words, people who perceive themselves as less susceptible to health problems are more likely to adhere to exercise programs than people whose perceived susceptibility to health problems is high. Buckworth and Dishman surmise that one explanation for this result is that exercise is not universally

perceived as a health behavior. In addition, the motives to exercise go beyond improving one's health; other reasons include social interaction, enjoyment, stress reduction, competition, and improved physical appearance.

A final limitation of the HBM is that it does not suggest intervention strategies that increase rates of exercise participation and adherence. In this way, the HBM does not explain low exercise adherence very effectively.

THEORIES OF REASONED ACTION AND PLANNED BEHAVIOR

The theory of planned behavior (TPB; Ajzen, 1985) is an extension and modification of the theory of reasoned action (TRA; Janzen and Fishbein, 1974). Both theories attempt to determine and predict the factors that influence a person's actions in social settings. To Janzen and Fishbein, behavioral decisions reflect people's beliefs about the appropriateness of their actions, the outcomes they expect from their actions, and the importance they place on these outcomes. At the center of the TRA for predicting health behavior, including exercise, are three components:

1. The person's *attitudes* about the behavior (e.g., "I enjoy exercising because . . .")
2. The person's *social norms* of that behavior (i.e., its acceptability and commonality among friends and culture)
3. The person's *intentions* to perform the health behaviors (e.g., "I intend to take a brisk walk nightly after coming home from work," "I will not fill my stomach within two hours of bedtime")

Attitudes toward exercise, for instance, reflect the person's beliefs about its benefits versus any negative consequences.

The second component of the TRA consists of subjective, social norms about the behavior. This reflects the individual's perceptions about the importance that others place on the behavior and his incentive to meet others' expectations. Thus, a person who is surrounded by family or friends who habitually exercise or support the person's exercise habit is more likely to exercise regularly than someone whose friends and family have negative attitudes toward exercise. This is why it is important for exercisers, especially novices, to surround themselves with others who support their exercise habit. As Janzen and Fishbein (1974) conclude, sometimes attitude is the primary predictor of intentions, while other times it is the social norm component.

In his modified follow-up of the TRA, Ajzen (1985) contended that a third component predicts exercise behavior: *perceived behavioral control*. According to Ajzen, it is important for people to conclude that they have the personal resources (e.g., skills, general ability) and the opportunity to perform the health behavior or to attain the goal. Thus, people with realistic expectations about their exercise performance or exercise outcomes will possess high perceived control of their destiny and will be more likely to feel motivated and committed to achieving health-related goals. Unmet expectations, on the other hand, will lead to disappointment and feelings of low self-control about the apparent inability to meet fitness-related goals. The likely outcome will be to quit further exercise participation.

In summary, then, the TRA and TPB posit that people who believe that exercise participation will produce the expected benefits are more likely to be physically active. Believing that exercise will not result in meeting desired goals or have intended benefits or having past exercise experiences that were unpleasant (e.g., athletes who feel burned out from overtraining, students who are forced to exercise by their physical education teacher as a form of punishment) will be more likely to result in negative attitudes toward physical activity.

In a meta-analysis to determine the extent to which the TRA and TPB successfully predict

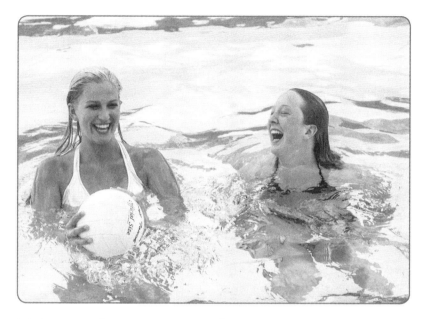

It is important for exercisers, especially novices, to surround themselves with others who support their exercise habit. How may this support differ between friends who enjoy physical activity for fun during their free time and those who engage primarily in sedentary activities?

exercise behavior, Hausenblas, Carron, and Mack (1997) concluded that attitude strongly influences intention to exercise and that intention to exercise predicts exercise behavior. However, one factor that influences this link (i.e., what researchers call a *moderator variable*) is people's perceived control over their behavior. To Hausenblas et al., "Individuals have the greatest commitment to exercise when they hold favorable beliefs about exercise and believe that they can successfully perform the behavior" (p. 45). Ironically, these favorable beliefs and attitudes toward exercise also form one limitation of the model.

Buckworth and Dishman (2002) question the validity of the TRA and TPB. They claim that a person may believe exercise is needed for all its benefits yet offer several excuses for not exercising (e.g., lacking time, not living near an exercise facility, needing to first lose weight, living in an unsafe neighborhood for walking). In addition, the results of several studies have shown that *intention to exercise* does not account for all exercise behavior (Mackinnon, Ritchie, Hooper, and Abernethy, 2003). The final argument against the TRA and TPB is that the literature lists other common barriers to exercise (e.g., physical discomfort, lack of a convenient exercise facility, intimidation of observers), each of which is accompanied by the person's positive attitudes and intentions toward regular exercise (Lox, Martin Ginis, and Petruzzello, 2010).

It is apparent that the components of the TRA and TPB—attitude, norms, intention to exercise, and perceived behavioral control—do not necessarily predict exercise behavior. A favorable attitude toward exercise must first be developed before a person engages in regular exercise. This is no easy task given the sedentary nature of many cultures today. However, understanding the benefits of exercising and the costs of not exercising will help promote the desirable attitude to initiate and maintain an exercise program. Although the TRA and TPB may partially explain the factors that increase regular exercise, these theories offer no behavioral interventions that promote starting and sustaining an exercise program.

SELF-EFFICACY THEORY

Self-efficacy is a set of beliefs and expectations about how capable a person feels in performing certain behaviors that will lead to desirable outcomes (Bandura, 1997). Self-efficacy is specific to performing a particular set of behaviors in specific situations. A person can feel high self-efficacy about the ability to gain strength through weight training yet feel low self-efficacy when it comes to performing aerobic exercise. High self-efficacy about exercise results in a higher likelihood that the person will exercise, but this feeling will not necessary be generalized to other types of tasks (e.g., competitive sport, work, injury rehabilitation) or situations (e.g., running competition, exercising with a partner).

Not surprisingly, people who believe they are capable of performing the required actions to meet situational demands are more likely to engage in those actions. These expectations affect the person's selection of activities (e.g., sport or walking rather than remaining inactive), the degree of effort expended on the activities, and the extent to which he will persist at the activities, especially after experienc-

ing failure and the unpleasant consequences (e.g., weight gain) of not meeting expectations. Thus, exercisers who do not experience rapid success and quickly meet goals will presume that the task is too difficult or that their actions are ineffective, and quitting exercise is more likely, perhaps due to low self-efficacy.

Based on their review of over 100 studies on the effects of self-efficacy theory on exercise behavior, McAuley and Mihalko (1998) concluded that self-efficacy best predicts exercise participation and maintenance under four conditions, when the person

1. selects the type of exercise behavior undertaken, called *perceived choice*;

2. possesses certain *thought patterns*, such as optimism, positive self-talk, intrinsic motivation, and feelings of competence and enjoyment;

3. *expends optimal effort* and feels capable of redoubling efforts in the face of barriers and challenges; and

4. has *reasonably high expectations* of successful performance and desirable outcomes.

To McAuley and Mihalko, the strongest influence of self-efficacy on exercise behavior is *performance accomplishments*, that is, mastering tasks that the individual perceives as difficult.

Not surprisingly, McAuley and Mihalko (1998) acknowledge that one weakness of self-efficacy theory is that even when self-efficacy beliefs about exercise are high, "the decision to embark on an exercise program . . . is fraught with challenges especially when individuals are sedentary, older, or recovering from a life-threatening disease" (p. 372). Engaging in physical activity at the correct level of exertion, duration, and frequency to obtain sufficient health and medical benefits is too unpleasant for many people, particularly given the sedentary lifestyle that is common in many societies. Thus, the benefits of remaining sedentary and not exercising (e.g., having more time to do other things, not experiencing the discomfort associated with vigorous exercise) are often greater than the consequences of a sedentary lifestyle.

IMPLICATIONS OF THEORIES AND MODELS FOR CONSULTANTS

Taken collectively, the theories and models described here may be applied by consultants in promoting client health and fitness. All of these theories and models have one thing in common: the attempt to promote exercise and other forms of physical activity.

Self-efficacy theory indicates that exercise behavior is more likely if clients maintain reasonably high expectations about the positive outcomes that will result from engaging in exercise. In addition, clients should feel they have the skills and perseverance to engage in exercise. Therefore, they should receive instruction about correct exercise technique and be reminded that getting in shape requires considerable time, effort, and patience. The client's motivation to exercise should improve based on the following types of statements coming from fitness coaches: positive outcome expectations (e.g., "You should be able to do five jog–walk intervals for the next 15 minutes"), confidence in meeting those expectations (e.g., "Your fitness test scores and current body weight indicate you should feel confident in completing this task"), and the belief that following a certain exercise regimen will lead to particular outcomes, called *efficacy expectations* (e.g., "If you persist with this exercise program, you should be able to lose at least a few pounds by the end of this month"). Consultants need to convincingly and sincerely inform their clients that they are capable of performing the behaviors that lead to desirable outcomes and that these outcomes will likely be achieved.

For example, it is essential that people engage in exercise that they enjoy and that is not too strenuous and is convenient in terms of location and times of the day and week. Forcing or requiring novice exercisers to engage in a certain type of exercise at a specific location or time of day will only demotivate them from developing a favorable attitude toward regular exercise and eventually will lead them to quit. These types of demands have formed one important limitation of numerous exercise studies in which a program dropout was defined as someone who did not attend a specific group exercise session held at a fitness facility. It was possible, however, that the person decided against exercising at the researcher's required program (e.g., group fitness classes or aerobics rather than a program performed alone or nonaerobic exercise) or location (e.g., at a specific health club rather than having a choice of locations).

TRANSTHEORETICAL MODEL

The transtheoretical model (TTM; Prochaska and DiClemente, 1983), also called the *stages of change model*, was originally constructed and published in reference to addictive behaviors and was later modified (Prochaska and Marcus, 1994) to describe a series of stages that begin with thinking about exercise and end with engaging in a regular exercise habit.

The TTM posits that making the decision to start and then sustaining an exercise habit is a long-term process. The model is cyclical (i.e., stages can be repeated), not linear, because the decision to change behavior is not always permanent; changes in dieting and smoking habits are two examples. There are five stages to the model, each defined by a set of repeated behavior patterns. A complete description of the TTM goes beyond the scope of this chapter; however, each stage of change will be described for application purposes. A more complete explanation of the TTM may be obtained from a book coauthored by Marcus and Forsyth (2003).

• *Precontemplation.* For at least six months, the sedentary person has no intention of exercising. Common reasons include no perceived need to exercise; unpleasant experiences with previous attempts at exercising; lack of social support, whether verbal or nonverbal, direct or indirect, from significant others to engage in regular exercise (e.g., no verbal approval from family and friends, no partner, no transportation to an exercise venue); self-consciousness about exercising in a public facility in the presence of fitter, younger people; inability to afford exercise equipment or fitness club memberships; or living too far away from available programs and facilities.

- *Contemplation.* At this stage, the person intends to start a regular exercise habit, usually within the next six months. Often she has learned about the advantages of exercise through written materials, advice from a physician, or friends or family members. A health care provider may have prescribed exercise, or the individual may feel the need to improve her relationship with a partner. She becomes enlightened that the costs of not exercising are becoming excessive and damaging, while the benefits are increasingly more attractive. Prochaska and Marcus (1994) report that "on the average, individuals stay in this relatively stable stage for at least 2 years, telling themselves that someday they will change but putting off change" (p. 162). These individuals are called *chronic contemplators.*

- *Preparation.* The person is now more serious about an exercise program and intends to start exercising in the near future, usually within a month. Typically, an action plan is formulated, either by the exerciser or by a fitness coach, although the plan may not be carried out to obtain the optimal benefits (e.g., exercising only once a week rather than at least three times a week, not exercising at sufficient intensity). The person is not yet fully committed to the plan because the disadvantages of exercising (e.g., not enough time, physical discomfort due to exertion, cost of a fitness club membership or equipment) still outweigh the advantages.

- *Action.* The person has finally initiated an exercise routine for less than six months. Although extensive energy now goes into the exercise regimen, quitting and reverting to an inactive lifestyle (called *relapsing*) is still very possible. This stage endures for about six months. One uncertainty about this stage concerns the criteria that constitute action—how is *action* defined? Is it exercising at least three times per week at a given intensity and duration, or is it any consistent and enduring change in exercise behavior? As Prochaska

and Marcus (1994) conclude, "Problems exist in areas for which there are no agreed upon criteria" (p. 163).

- *Maintenance.* After six months, there is now less likelihood that the person will quit exercising. There is uncertainty in the literature, however, about the operational definition of *maintenance.* Writers in the medical literature (e.g., Rand and Weeks, 1998) have used terms such as *partial adherence, ideal adherence, appropriate adherence, erratic adherence,* and *involuntary adherence* for the criterion of maintenance (i.e., adherence) to accurately reflect a person's intended and planned exercise behavior. Thus, exercising once per week instead of the planned three times per week reflects partial adherence, and not exercising due to injury is an example of involuntary nonadherence. Prochaska and Marcus (1994) claim that an exercise period of at least five years is the likely criterion for establishing a permanent exercise habit and not returning to a nonexercise lifestyle.

- *Termination.* At this stage, there is no temptation to engage in the former behavior pattern of inactivity. A review of the addiction literature, however, where the TTM was derived, reveals that reverting to previous habits is always possible. The likelihood of reverting to the previous no-exercise habit is often a function of the same perceived barriers that prevented exercising in the first place (Marcus, Bock, Pinto, and Clark, 1996). Perceived barriers include high demands on time, injury, one or more unpleasant exercise-related experiences, poor weather, broken equipment, other activities that are more tempting that replace exercise, absence of encouragement from others (i.e., lack of social support), failure to meet goals, increased exercise difficulty due to weight gain or aging, and lack of financial resources to afford a fitness club membership or purchase the proper footwear.

The model, although replete in the health psychology literature, is not without limitations. For example, Bandura (1997) expresses concerns that the TTM fails to reflect fundamental tenets of traditional stage theory, that is, the stages are not distinct, clearly separated, and practical. In addition, Rosen's (2000) meta-analysis indicated that readiness for exercise may not be a discrete variable (i.e., yes or no) but a continuous variable (i.e., not at all, very little, somewhat, very much, or extremely likely). In addition, testing the efficacy of the TTM requires providing people with intervention strategies that are compatible with their particular exercise stage and then measuring their exercise behavior over a prolonged length of time, perhaps several years. Finally, in their review and critique of the model, Buckworth and Dishman (2002) concluded:

> The usefulness of the transtheoretical model for exercise interventions has been mixed. Targeting specific processes of change to facilitate progression of exercise behavior across stages is based on the assumption that differences between adjacent stages found in cross-sectional studies point to processes that need to be changed to progress to the next stage. However, the efficacy of targeting specific processes to promote stage progression has yet to be adequately tested; there have been few longitudinal prospective designs and the instruments to measure stage and processes of changes have been poorly validated for exercise. (p. 223)

RELAPSE PREVENTION MODEL

The relapse prevention model was created by Marlatt and Gordon (1985) to promote abstinence from addictive behaviors. The model reflects self-controlled (self-regulation) efforts needed to maintain exercise behavior and to resist feelings and situations that promote reversion to former undesirable behavior patterns. With respect to exercise, people are taught to use cognitive (e.g., positive self-talk, visualization) and behavioral (e.g., music, goal setting, social support, record keeping) strategies to deal productively with exercise relapses.

High-risk situations, such as feeling uncomfortable entering a fitness facility or not knowing how to use exercise equipment properly, initiate the relapse process. Situations that challenge people's confidence in their ability to meet exercise goals or a lack of support from others also promote relapse. A particularly damaging event that predicts relapse is called the *abstinence violation effect*, in which the person misses several exercise sessions, perhaps due to illness, injury, or some other reason beyond their control and then quits the exercise habit permanently. The reaction might be to give up all hope (i.e., a state of hopelessness) of reaching exercise goals or maintaining fitness rather than regaining control of the situation and remaining patient with the retraining process.

Another characteristic of the abstinence violation effect reflects all-or-none thinking. The individual views his participation as either full adherence to an exercise regimen or failure to maintain an exercise habit; there is no in-between state. To make matters worse, the person defines himself as a failure and feels guilty over the dilemma of wanting to exercise and not doing so, but he has failed to take responsibility for the perceived failure (called *self-blame*). The relapse prevention model is intuitively appealing in promoting exercise behavior and adherence. Exercise relapse is clearly a significant problem, and any approach to minimize this process is needed.

Buckworth and Dishman (2002) point out that "the model was developed for maintaining cessation of high-frequency undesired behaviors, and exercise is a low-frequency, desired behavior" (p. 225), so it is difficult to detect an exercise lapse or to deal with a lapse in a timely manner to prevent people from quitting permanently. In addition, the model does not account for overcoming an adherence violation effect, in which missing one or more exercise sessions leads the person to permanently abandon future exercise habits. Factors such as lifestyle imbalances and prioritizing self-gratification (e.g., leading a sedentary lifestyle) over devotion to more health-enhancing activities also are not adequately addressed by the model. Thus, while the model provides valuable insights into strategies for promoting exercise adherence, it lacks the incentives and emotions needed to overcome the "benefits" of not committing to regular exercise.

DETERRENCE THEORY

Unintended for exercise behavior, not unlike most theories and models applied in exercise settings, deterrence theory (Paternoster, 1987) was originally intended to explain criminal behavior. The theory posits that a person contemplates committing a crime by weighing its costs and benefits. If the punishment for the act is highly certain and severe, and it outweighs the perceived benefits of the act, the person is more likely to conclude it is not in her best interests to commit the act. On the other hand, if the perceived benefits outweigh the costs, the crime becomes more desirable and is more likely to be executed. Thus, the individual's subjective perceptions rather than the objective reality of legal sanctions determine future behavior.

For example, an obese person might conclude that despite his excessive weight, test

---

FROM RESEARCH TO REAL WORLD

An exercise intervention that consultants should consider using to improve behaviors related to exercise is called the *self-monitoring checklist*. This checklist is not a theory or a model because it does not explain, describe, or predict thoughts, emotions, or behaviors. Checklists list specific thoughts and actions that people should follow to guide their behavior, usually in a predetermined sequence for the purpose of improving one or more outcomes. Checklists are always practical and reflect concrete actions; they are not theoretical or abstract. Their purpose is to provide reminders or guidelines about one's preparation, thoughts, emotions, or actions (Anshel, 2006). A checklist is a kind of to-do list; it consists of a list of reminders to maintain a particular set of actions until the person develops routines that eventually become habits.

Checklists should be reviewed as often as required until checklist items become automatic and completed consistently as part of one's regular (e.g., daily, weekly) routine. The term often used in the research literature that refers to following a certain set of mental or physical tasks is *self-monitoring*.

Self-monitoring is a common practice in the diet and nutrition literature in terms of the type, amount, and timing of food intake. Thus, a checklist is a list of things to do, while self-monitoring is the process of following, or monitoring, that to-do list.

Fitness coaches use checklists to prescribe fitness routines for both aerobic exercise (e.g., alternate three minutes of jogging and 30 seconds of walking for five intervals) and strength training (e.g., lift 75 lb for eight repetitions, rest for one minute, lift another eight repetitions, rest for one minute, and lift a final set of eight reps). Fitness coaches may also develop checklists to help clients prepare for their exercise session, for example, avoiding meals within two hours of aerobic work and maintaining water intake during the day, during an exercise session, and immediately after exercise. The self-monitoring checklist was shown to be an effective strategy in one study (Anshel and Seipel, 2009) in which novice exercisers used the checklist, combined with live coaching, to complete a 10-week strength training program. See form 3.1 for a sample exerciser checklist.

Following are eight guidelines for generating and using exercise checklists:

1. *A checklist should be focused in its goals and purpose.* Is it strictly an information tool? Does it provide insights into exercise preparation and execution? Is it about developing healthy lifestyle habits? Does it address a particular type of exercise or the needs of a special group or population?

2. *Keep the checklist relatively brief and clear to the intended audience.* Users should be able to go through the checklist quickly, yet it should provide a complete list of tasks that need to be done in order to experience a successful exercise session.

3. *Begin the checklist with instructions that are brief and easy to comprehend.*

4. *Keep the scoring consistent for all items.* For easy use, circling a *1* should always represent a low, undesirable score, while *5* reflects a score that is high and desirable. That is, clients should be able to add up their scores and conclude that achieving a higher score represents improvement or achievement over time.

5. *The checklist should be easy to read.* Similar to validating an inventory for research purposes, be sure that intended users understand the instructions and each item. Give the checklist a trial run by having several clients read it and indicate if there are any words with which they are unfamiliar, if they are unsure about how to complete the checklist, or if they do not know what they must do to improve their score.

6. *Allow for individual differences.* Some items may not even pertain to the client. For instance, some people prefer to exercise alone, and they should not feel compelled to exercise with others (if that were a checklist item). If certain items are not relevant, the client should delete those items rather than self-reporting low scores.

7. *Provide live support for using the checklist.* Health care professionals, fitness coaches, dietitians, or anyone else associated with generating and using the checklist should work with the client in reviewing each response and how to improve item scores. Then, the client and professional should agree to meet and carry out certain segments of the checklist to help improve item scores.

8. *Provide clients with positive feedback.* Inform clients with messages about improvement and effort in carrying out checklist items. It is essential that clients feel they are achieving goals toward improved health and fitness.

data (e.g., blood pressure, cholesterol) indicate he is in good health. Therefore, he sees no reason to change his behavior and begin an exercise program. If this same person, however, were to follow a behavior pattern intended to prevent poor health, identify the benefits of exercising regularly and losing weight (e.g., more energy, less risk of type 2 diabetes), and view his excessive body weight as unattractive or unhealthy, he would be more likely to start a new exercise habit. Although deterrence theory has not been examined with respect to exercise behavior, the link between deterrence theory and exercise is more closely evident in Strelan and Boeckmann's (2003) drugs in sport deterrence model.

FORM 3.1 EXERCISER CHECKLIST

Please indicate how much you agree or disagree with each of the following statements concerning your exercise routine. The ratings range from **1** (the statement is not at all like me) to **5** (the statement is very much like me). Higher scores are viewed as more desirable than lower scores. You want to improve your score over time.

1	2	3	4	5
Not at all like me		Somewhat like me		Very much like me

I. Exercise Preparation

1. I think about exercising with enthusiasm.   1 2 3 4 5
2. I look forward to the next exercise session.   1 2 3 4 5
3. I do not make excuses for avoiding exercise.   1 2 3 4 5
4. I view exercising as a challenge, not a chore.   1 2 3 4 5
5. I feel healthier and happier for exercising.   1 2 3 4 5
6. I make time for exercise.   1 2 3 4 5
7. I am confident in my exercise technique.   1 2 3 4 5
8. My family and friends support my exercise habit.   1 2 3 4 5
9. I have a weekly exercise schedule.   1 2 3 4 5
10. I know the physical and psychological benefits of exercising regularly.   1 2 3 4 5
11. I would describe my lifestyle during the week as physically active.   1 2 3 4 5
12. I feel comfortable exercising alone or in the presence of others.   1 2 3 4 5

Subtotal: _____

II. Day of Exercise

13. I look forward to exercising with great enthusiasm.   1 2 3 4 5
14. I am committed to my scheduled exercise time.   1 2 3 4 5
15. I have prepared a proper diet and fluid intake today.   1 2 3 4 5
16. I am feeling positive about exercising.   1 2 3 4 5
17. I am aware of the benefits of my exercise program.   1 2 3 4 5
18. Within 2 hours of exercising, I will not consume any food, coffee, or alcohol.   1 2 3 4 5
19. If I feel sick, I will not exercise today.   1 2 3 4 5
20. I have a planned route to the exercise venue.   1 2 3 4 5
21. I have prepared my exercise gear in advance.   1 2 3 4 5
22. I have organized my day to accommodate my exercise session.   1 2 3 4 5

Subtotal: _____

III. Preexercise Activity

23. I arrive at the exercise venue on time and with enthusiasm.	1	2	3	4	5
24. I remember my goals and plan to meet them.	1	2	3	4	5
25. As I prepare to exercise, I feel energetic.	1	2	3	4	5
26. I plan to have adequate water intake when I exercise.	1	2	3	4	5
27. I have an exercise plan.	1	2	3	4	5
28. I remember the reasons why exercise is good for me.	1	2	3	4	5
29. I will do as much of the exercise session as I can.	1	2	3	4	5
30. I use positive self-talk just before I exercise ("I can do it," "I'm ready," "Stay with it!")	1	2	3	4	5

Subtotal: _____

IV. During the Exercise Session

31. I really enjoy my exercise session.	1	2	3	4	5
32. I feel good during my stretches.	1	2	3	4	5
33. I use positive self-talk before and during the exercise routine.	1	2	3	4	5
34. I feel good during my warm-up.	1	2	3	4	5
35. As I warm up, I plan to give 100% effort.	1	2	3	4	5
36. I am determined to complete as much of the exercise session as possible.	1	2	3	4	5
37. I try not to think about the stress or strain of exercising.	1	2	3	4	5
38. I feel that my exercise performance is improving.	1	2	3	4	5
39. I do not care what others think of my appearance when I exercise.	1	2	3	4	5
40. I try to perform up to my potential.	1	2	3	4	5
41. I ignore the appearance, age, gender, and other characteristics of other exercisers.	1	2	3	4	5
42. I try to complete as many repetitions as possible of each exercise.	1	2	3	4	5
43. I view each exercise bout as a challenge, not a threat.	1	2	3	4	5
44. If I feel uncomfortable during exercise, I try to ignore my feelings and focus externally.	1	2	3	4	5
45. I remember to try to reach my performance goals.	1	2	3	4	5
46. I feel confident in my ability to give 100%.	1	2	3	4	5
47. If I get tired, I rest and then keep going.	1	2	3	4	5

Subtotal: _____

V. After the Exercise Session

	48. I am generally pleased with my exercise performance.	1	2	3	4	5
	49. I feel that my performance has improved since last time.	1	2	3	4	5
	50. I take responsibility for my performance rather than blaming other factors (e.g., poor instructor, noise).	1	2	3	4	5
	51. I have recorded (physically or mentally) my progress.	1	2	3	4	5
	52. I am open to advice and feedback on my performance.	1	2	3	4	5
	53. No matter what level of performance, I plan to keep exercising next time.	1	2	3	4	5
	54. I feel good after exercising and have a sense of accomplishment.	1	2	3	4	5
	55. I reached my target heart rate if I exercised aerobically.	1	2	3	4	5
	56. I replace lost fluids with water.	1	2	3	4	5
	57. My exercise form has improved.	1	2	3	4	5
	58. I plan to maintain my exercise program.	1	2	3	4	5

Subtotal: _____

Grand total: _____

From M. Anshel, 2014, *Applied Health Fitness Psychology*. (Champaign, IL: Human Kinetics).

DRUGS IN SPORT DETERRENCE MODEL

Strelan and Boeckmann (2003) have applied deterrence theory within the context of athletes' use of banned substances in their drugs in sport deterrence model (DSDM). One assumption of deterrence theory is that people make conscious decisions about acceptable or desirable behavior based on obtaining extensive information, planning, and justifying their decisions. The decision maker's best interests are of paramount importance. This assumption holds true for an athlete's decision to use performance-enhancing drugs. The athlete's dilemma is to weigh the benefits of drug use (e.g., improved performance, increased strength) against the possible costs and consequences of using banned substances (e.g., a ban from future competition, poor health over the long term, ostracism by peers and the public, loss of respect from significant others).

Situational factors, such as culture and the influence of peers and significant others, also influence behavioral predictions of the cost–benefit trade-off. Legal sanctions, current organization policies and laws, availability and cost of the drug, and expected drug testing are additional considerations that influence drug use.

Although the name of the DSDM would be altered with respect to exercise, the concepts are relevant. People would make conscious decisions about engaging in regular exercise (i.e., acceptable or desirable behavior) after obtaining all relevant information about the benefits and justification of exercise and how an action plan could help them plan out an exercise program, particularly with social support (e.g., friend, fitness coach). They would have to conclude that exercise would result in far more improvement in quality of life compared with remaining inactive and refusing to exercise. Situational factors would promote an exercise habit, including involvement in a culture in which physical activity is celebrated and expected, support from peers and significant others, reduced health insurance and health care costs, and nearby fitness equipment or exercise facilities. The DSDM awaits validation in an exercise setting.

The model adequately describes the importance of a person's perceptions of the benefits and costs of certain behaviors that are undesirable, illegal, or immoral. The cost–benefit trade-offs are salient, all of which are mediated (altered or influenced) by situational factors. The DSDM, however, is not an intervention model. It is a conceptual model that describes the factors that underlie drug-taking behavior. Similar factors can be used to describe exercise behavior in which the person determines the benefits and costs of exercising as opposed to leading a sedentary lifestyle.

SUMMARY

Most people want to maintain a healthy lifestyle for various reasons. These include preventing illness, improving or maintaining general health, preventing or managing disease, feeling better physically and mentally, and restoring health or reducing the progression of disease. Practitioners want to use interventions that improve the health behavior of their clients, and they are guided by various theories and models that explain and predict improved health outcomes. Personal, environmental, and situational factors all influence these outcomes, further challenging researchers to determine the best techniques that explain why people persist in self-destructive behavior patterns. Theories and models that help explain, describe, and predict health behaviors include the health belief model (HBM), theories of reasoned action (TRA) and planned behavior (TPB), self-efficacy theory, transtheoretical model

(TTM), relapse prevention model, deterrence theory, and drugs in sport deterrence model (DSDM).

All theories and models have limitations. One such limitation associated with each of these models is that researchers need to reach a consensus about operationally defining *exercise*. Is exercise a casual walk in the park? Is it defined as reaching a certain intensity, duration, and frequency? Most people will report that they exercise if they go for a daily walk; however, a casual walk will not accrue the same physiological benefits as more vigorous exercise. Other people will categorize themselves as exercisers if they lift weights or engage in yoga or Pilates.

The type of exercise reported forms another limitation of most exercise psychology theories and models. Is the theory that predicts exercise behavior addressing aerobic exercise, strength training, or some other form of activity? Optimal benefits of exercise are experienced when a person engages in aerobic exercise. The validity of theories and models in explaining and predicting exercise behavior is clouded by the failure to recognize what type of exercise we are trying to encourage and the characteristics (i.e., intensity, frequency, duration) of the exercise regimen.

Examining evidence of psychopathology, or mental illness, in determining and predicting exercise habits is another necessary future area of study. For example, clinical depression results in reduced energy and self-motivation to engage in regular exercise. Chronic anxiety, low self-esteem, irrational thinking, and other types of mental illness are strong mediators in predicting and explaining exercise behavior. Clinical psychology interventions are needed to detect and treat psychopathological conditions that directly influence attitudes toward exercise and starting and maintaining a regular exercise habit.

STUDENT ACTIVITY

Testing Exerciser Checklist Effectiveness

Will using an exerciser checklist result in better fitness and exercise adherence? To examine this question, form two groups with three to five people in each group: the EC (exerciser checklist) group and the no-treatment (control) group. All participants should be healthy adults with similar characteristics, such as similar fitness level (e.g., all are exercise novices), gender (e.g., all males, all females, or a combination), age (e.g., all young adults, all middle-aged adults, all college students), and approximate body weight (same number of obese and nonobese in each group). The checklist was not developed for people who are recovering from illness or injury, undergoing rehabilitation, or currently under a physician's care.

Both groups should receive fitness pretests by a qualified fitness coach to measure baseline (pretreatment) aerobic and strength fitness. After at least four weeks (longer than four weeks is better), both groups take a posttest to determine changes in fitness. Immediately after the pretest, each participant is given an exercise prescription for the type and frequency of exercise that should improve aerobic and strength fitness.

At the end of each week during the program, the EC group should complete the checklist and submit it to you (the study leader) to determine where the participants are falling short (circling a 3 or less on a checklist item). Review the items with each EC group member to increase their score for each item. The control group does not use the checklist and instead is asked to carry out the prescribed program.

At the end of each week, participants in both groups should inform you how often they exercised that week, a measure of adherence. Full adherence would consist of three aerobic exercise sessions and two strength training sessions. The exerciser checklist is intended to provide novice exercisers with direction and coaching on ways to experience the physical and mental health benefits of engaging in regular exercise. Did it help the EC group?

Results

To determine if the checklist was effective at improving fitness, members of both groups should perform the identical tests they experienced under pretest conditions. Conduct the following calculations:

1. Obtain the average score for each group for each fitness test you conducted on all pretests.

2. Obtain the same information for posttest scores for each group.

3. Obtain what is called a *difference score* for each group by subtracting the pretest average from the posttest average. You now have two scores, one for each group. Which difference score is bigger, the treatment or control group?

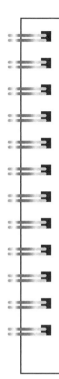

4. If you can, conduct an independent *t*-test comparing the two difference scores on each fitness test to determine if the group differences are statistically significant. This will indicate whether the checklist significantly improved aerobic fitness or strength fitness.

5. To determine if the EC treatment resulted in better exercise adherence compared with the control group, compare the two adherence rates. How often did the EC group exercise (a measure of adherence) as opposed to the control group? Did using the checklist improve the frequency of exercise participation?

6. Did the checklist make a difference? Did the EC group members improve their checklist scores to a significant degree? Compare the grand total on week 1 with the last week of the program, just before the posttest. Use a dependent *t*-test to compare preintervention and postintervention checklist scores. If the scores are much higher on the posttest, then it is likely the checklist contributed to improved fitness and perhaps adherence.

REFERENCES

Ajzen, I. (1985). From intention to actions: A theory of planned behavior. In J. Kuhl and J. Beckman (Eds.), *Action control: From cognition to behavior* (pp. 11-39). Heidelberg: Springer.

Anshel, M.H. (2006). *Applied exercise psychology: A practitioner's guide to improving client health and fitness.* New York: Springer.

Anshel, M.H., and Seipel, S.J. (2009). Self-monitoring and selected measures of aerobic and strength fitness and short-term exercise adherence. *Journal of Sport Behavior, 32,* 125-151.

Bandura, A. (1977). Self-efficacy: Toward a unifying theory of behavior change. *Psychological Review, 84,* 191-215.

Bandura, A. (1997). *Self-efficacy: The exercise of control.* New York: Freeman.

Becker, M.H., and Maiman, L.A. (1975). Sociobehavioral determinants of compliance with health and medical care recommendations. *Medical Care, 13,* 10-24.

Berger, B.G., Pargman, D., and Weinberg, R.S. (2007). *Foundations of exercise psychology* (2nd ed.). Morgantown, WV: Fitness Information Technology.

Buckworth, J., and Dishman, R.K. (2002). *Exercise psychology.* Champaign, IL: Human Kinetics.

Clark, N.M., and Becker, M.H. (1998). Theoretical models and strategies for improving adherence and disease management. In S.A. Shumaker, E.B. Schron, J.K. Ockene, and W.L. McBee (Eds.), *The handbook of health behavior change* (2nd ed., pp. 5-32). New York: Springer.

Hausenblas, H.A., Carron, A.V., and Mack, D.E. (1997). Application of the theories of reasoned action and planned behavior to exercise behavior: A meta-analysis. *Journal of Sport and Exercise Psychology, 19,* 36-51.

Janzen, I., and Fishbein, M. (1974). Factors influencing intentions and the intention-behavior relation. *Human Relations, 27,* 1-15.

Lox, C.L., Martin Ginis, K.A., and Petruzzello, S.J. (2010). *The psychology of exercise: Integrating theory and practice* (3rd ed.). Scottsdale, AZ: Holcomb Hathaway.

Mackinnon, L.T., Ritchie, C.B., Hooper, S.L., and Abernethy, P.J. (2003). *Exercise management: Concepts and professional practice.* Champaign, IL: Human Kinetics.

Marcus, B.H., Bock, B.C., Pinto, B.M., and Clark, M.M. (1996). Exercise initiation, adoption, and maintenance. In J.L. Van Raalte and B.W. Brewer

(Eds.), *Exploring sport and exercise psychology* (pp. 133-158). Washington, DC: American Psychological Association.

Marcus, B.H., and Forsyth, L.H. (2003). *Motivating people to be physically active.* Champaign, IL: Human Kinetics.

Marlatt, G.A., and Gordon, J.R. (1985). *Relapse prevention: Maintenance strategies in addictive behavior change.* New York: Guilford Press.

McAuley, E., and Mihalko, S.L. (1998). Measuring exercise-related self-efficacy. In J.L. Duda (Ed.), *Advances in sport and exercise psychology measurement* (pp. 371-390). Morgantown, WV: Fitness Information Technology.

Ockene, I.S. (2001). Provider approaches to improve compliance. In L.E. Burke and I.S. Ockene (Eds.), *Compliance in healthcare and research* (pp. 73-80). Armonk, NY: Futura.

Oldridge, N.B., and Streiner, D.L. (1990). The health belief model: Predicting compliance and dropout in cardiac rehabilitation. *Medicine and Science in Sports and Exercise, 22,* 678-683.

Paternoster, R. (1987). The deterrent effect of the perceived certainty and severity of punishment: A review of the evidence and issues. *Justice Quarterly, 4,* 173-217.

Prochaska, J.O., and DiClemente, C.C. (1983). Transtheoretical therapy: Toward a more integrative model of change. *Psychotherapy: Theory, Research, and Practice, 20,* 161-173.

Prochaska, J.O., and Marcus, B. (1994). The transtheoretical model: Applications to exercise. In R.K. Dishman (Ed.), *Advances in exercise adherence* (pp. 161-180). Champaign, IL: Human Kinetics.

Rand, C.S., and Weeks, K. (1998). Measuring adherence with mediation regimens in clinical care and research. In S.A. Shumaker, E.B. Schron, J.K. Ockene, and W.L. McBee (Eds.), *The handbook of health behavior change* (pp. 114-132). New York: Springer.

Rosen, C.S. (2000). Is the sequencing of change processes by stage consistent across health problems? A meta-analysis. *Health Psychology, 19,* 593-604.

Strelan, P., and Boeckmann, R.J. (2003). A new model for understanding performance-enhancing drug use by elite athletes. *Journal of Applied Sport Psychology, 15,* 176-183.

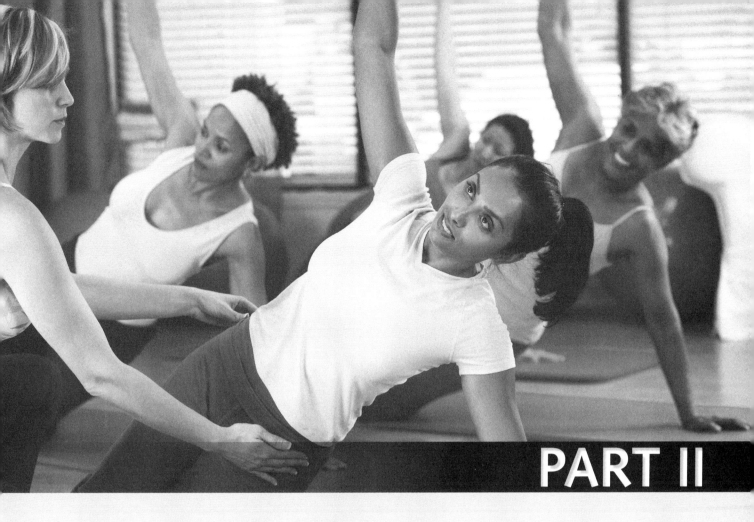

PART II

FACTORS THAT INFLUENCE HEALTH BEHAVIOR

This part of the book addresses a profound question: Why do we do something almost every day that we know is bad for us? In other words, why do we engage in self-destructive behaviors? It begins with chapter 4 reviewing the likely causes of self-destructive behaviors—that's right, researchers, theorists, and practitioners have a good idea why we are our own worst enemy when it comes to unhealthy habits and what health care workers can do to overcome these unwise actions. Chapter 5 explores personal factors in the development and maintenance of healthy habits, and chapter 6 follows with a discus-sion of situational and environmental factors. Finally, chapter 7 discusses cultural, religious, and spiritual considerations for promoting a healthy lifestyle.

These chapters are dedicated to the reasons why so many people refrain from leading a physically active lifestyle and their impli-cations for health care professionals. Our inactive lifestyle is contributing to obesity and disease that is both premature and too common. This part of the book rings alarm bells, setting the stage for part III, which focuses on what health care professionals can do about the problem.

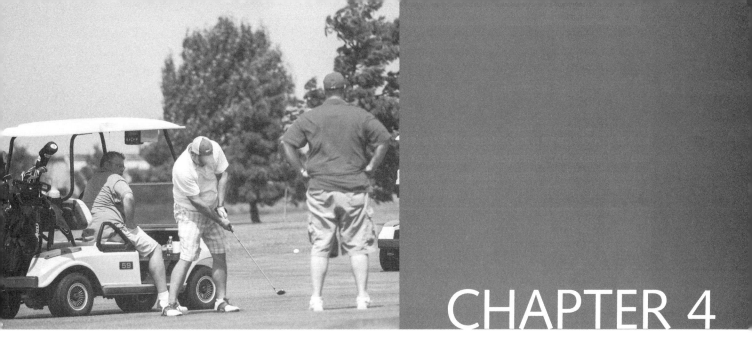

CHAPTER 4

Barriers to Positive Health Behavior

66 *When you have talked yourself into what you want, right there is the place to stop* 99
talking and begin saying it with deeds.

Napoleon Hill (1883-1970), author

CHAPTER OBJECTIVES

After reading this chapter, you should be able to:

- discuss the likely causes that explain why people engage in self-destructive behaviors;

- outline the physical, cognitive, and emotional obstacles to changing unhealthy behavior patterns;

- describe limitations of past intervention research and applications in attempting to change self-destructive behavioral patterns; and

- provide recommendations for future attempts to replace unhealthy habits with more desirable ones.

As discussed in earlier chapters, the consequences of an overweight and inactive society include widespread serious deterioration of health and quality of life. Research conducted in the United States indicates that 63% of U.S. men and women are overweight, and about 33% are classified as obese. Approximately 60% to 70% of adults who begin an exercise program will quit within six to nine months, despite the widespread belief (82%) that exercise is beneficial to good health (U.S. Department of Health and Human Services [HHS], 2004).

The combination of obesity and a sedentary lifestyle, leading to the onset of diabetes and hypertension, is the likely culprit of a reduced life span among obese and inactive people (Nestle and Jacobson, 2000). This undesirable lifestyle begins in childhood. Unlike previous generations in which children were involved in various forms of daily physical activity, particularly after school, children and adolescents in more recent years have remained sedentary during the day. Perhaps not surprisingly, a sedentary lifestyle during childhood leads to obesity. In turn, the combination of a sedentary lifestyle and obesity in childhood significantly predicts similar characteristics in adulthood. Although the causes of obesity are well known, the antecedent undesirable habits that cause obesity have proven to be difficult to change (Hall and Fong, 2003; Nestle and Jacobson, 2000). Effective interventions are needed to promote exercise participation and maintenance, solving a problem commonly referred to as *nonadherence*.

This chapter is about understanding the reasons why so many of us engage in behaviors that we know are unhealthy, even dangerous. Researchers have not been able to determine the causes and remedies in overcoming our unhealthy, self-defeating habits (e.g., overeating, lack of physical activity, poor sleep, lack of hydration, poor stress management) and improving general health. As Glasgow, Klesges, Dzewaltowski, Bull, and Estabrooks (2004) have concluded from their review of literature, "It is well documented that the results of most behavioral and health promo-

tion studies have not been translated into practice" (p. 3). One important reason why theories and the results of studies that test these theories have not contributed to new and effective techniques is the lack of adherence in maintaining these new, more desirable behaviors. New habits are often discontinued within two to four weeks, and it takes six to eight weeks to establish a new habit (Loehr and Schwartz, 2003).

The lack of adherence to new health procedures has been studied for many years. Sackett (1976), for example, found that scheduled appointments for treatment are missed 20% to 50% of the time, and about 50% of patients are remiss in taking their medications as prescribed by their physicians. After six months, other health-related behaviors (e.g., smoking cessation, dietary restrictions, weight-control strategies) have an adherence rate of under 50%. Exercise nonadherence rates are similar (Marcus and Forsythe, 2003). More effective interventions are needed to improve exercise adherence.

One of the most difficult and challenging tasks for professionals in the health care and fitness industries is to help people to change their unhealthy habits and replace them with healthier routines. As Grunberg and Klein (2009) indicate, "Decades of research have made it clear what we should do . . . and what we should not do . . . to enjoy good health. [And yet] it is often difficult to adopt and to maintain a healthy lifestyle" (p. 411).

CAUSES OF SELF-DESTRUCTIVE BEHAVIORS

It seems awkward to contend that humans behave in ways that run counter to maintaining good health, happiness, and a high quality of life. And yet, that is exactly what we do. Behavioral psychologists refer to this phenomenon as *our self-destructive nature*. Hall and Fong (2007), for instance, claim that "human behavior often seems maladaptive, self-defeating, or dysfunctional to the observer" (p. 6). They assert that "behaviors judged to be maladaptive . . . are usually driven by a strongly favorable balance of immediate costs and benefits" (p. 6), an area of health behavior change we will address later in the chapter. The authors assert that unhealthy actions are linked to serious long-term, but not short-term, costs and consequences and few long-term benefits.

Our unhealthy habits are, however, linked to short-term benefits. We crave that bowl of ice cream before bed or even in the middle of the night, which is strongly associated with weight gain and heart disease in the long term. However, the short-term benefit is that we satisfy our hunger; sweets are especially tempting late at night to increase our blood sugar, especially if we have been deprived of calories during the day. We are a culture, therefore, that seeks immediate rather than delayed gratification (Hall and Fong, 2007). The challenge for professionals in health, nutrition, medicine, and fitness is to change unhealthy behavioral patterns—which are costing billions of dollars in health care—to a way of thinking and acting in accordance with what is good for us.

Negative habits are defined as behavioral patterns that a person acknowledges are undesirable or unhealthy (Anshel and Kang, 2007a, b). As depicted by Loehr and Schwartz (2003), *negative physical habits* are persistent actions that lead to low energy, low productivity, unhappiness, or poor health. *Emotional negative habits* are ongoing feelings of unhappiness, dissatisfaction, and generally negative moods that compromise performance and quality of life. *Cognitive negative habits* consist of thoughts that distract the person from the task at hand, multitasking, lack of concentration, and impaired information processing that limit performance. Finally, *spiritual negative habits* reflect thoughts, emotions, and actions that contradict one's deepest values and beliefs about what is important (Super, 1995). For people with spiritual negative habits, life consists of disconnects between their core beliefs and their behavior and thought patterns.

The primary reason people engage in a negative habit is because the perceived benefits of maintaining the habit outweigh the costs and long-term consequences (Loehr and Schwartz, 2003). As Klesges, Estabrooks, Dzewaltowski, Bull, and Glasgow (2005) contend, however, "individual [health-enhancing] behavior change is maximized when benefits of behavior changes are apparent to the individual and have a high probability of occurrence, benefits are realized soon after new behaviors are enacted, and the response cost of behavioral changes is low relative to the benefits realized" (p. 68). People who possess a long-term perspective (e.g., become aware of long-term consequences of unhealthy behaviors) are more likely to engage in actions with health-protective properties (Hall and Fong, 2003).

OBSTACLES TO ADOPTING A HEALTHY LIFESTYLE

For many years, researchers and practitioners (e.g., educators, consultants, fitness coaches, dietitians, mental health professionals) have been challenged by the goal of changing a person's unhealthy habits. It is important, therefore, to examine the multitude of likely obstacles to doing the right thing and not engaging in self-destructive behaviors. Why, for instance, do people remain inactive when they have been informed repeatedly of the advantages of exercise to physical and mental health? Why do so many people eat to the point of obesity and complain of fatigue, painful lower limbs, and difficulty breathing yet not integrate healthier dietary habits? Why do we not get it? Is it arrogance? Denial? Mental illness? A lack of common sense? Acting irresponsibly? Professors Neil Grunberg and Laura Cousino Klein have closely examined the obstacles to adopting and maintaining a healthy lifestyle. When we can identify the obstacles, researchers and practitioners can begin the process of determining the best ways to test and apply techniques to overcome them. These obstacles, or limitations, are divided into biological, physical, cognitive, and motivational categories. The goal is to develop and maintain a healthy lifestyle.

Misinterpretation of Biological Cues

Patients may fail to experience or correctly interpret symptoms of underlying disorders. When they feel fine and conclude there are no problems, they will not feel the need for rest, medications, restricted activities, or dietary changes. Many people who are clinically obese or even morbidly obese (i.e., at least 100 lb or 45 kg overweight) assert there is no need for them to lose weight or change their lifestyle because their vital signs (e.g., blood pressure, absence of pain) are fine. They may also be involved in some type of medical therapy and prematurely discontinue it because they feel good, which can be a dangerous decision. Athletes are also often guilty of this mentality and prematurely return to sport competition before completing their injury rehabilitation. Along these lines, a perception of good health tends to result in people concluding there is no need to improve their health. Feeling fine often is interpreted as meaning there is no need to exercise, especially if a physician has not provided a sense of urgency or medical test data that show the need to change behaviors quickly.

Finally, if the newly adopted healthy habit does not quickly reveal beneficial changes, there is the tendency to discount the need to make the behavioral change. People who adopt a new exercise program expect to see improved fitness, less exertion, and weight loss relatively soon; otherwise they think, "What's the use?" What they do not understand is that changes in physiology, including the effects of physical training, take time—usually a minimum of six weeks and often longer. As Grunberg and Klein (2009) recommend, "These experiences and lack of awareness of bodily states, therapeutic effects, or preventive effects should be addressed and explained to patients" (p. 413).

Physical Limitations

Another obstacle to health behavior change is deficiencies in the ability to move properly. This condition can be due to impairment of a sensory system (e.g., hearing, vision) or limitations in the ability to gather or interpret information from the health care provider. It is well known, for instance, that the ability to store information into working, or short-term, memory deteriorates with age. An array of other physical and mental conditions, as well as the ingestion of various medications, may also alter the ability to process information and respond to external stimuli. Impaired vision slows the ability to read instructions or a prescription. Poor hearing, worsened by the presence of surrounding noise, markedly reduces the ability to process verbal (spoken) information, such as a fitness coach's or dietitian's directions for proper exercise and dietary habits. Physical disabilities that impair movement, breathing, or some bodily function, common in type 2 diabetes, fibromyalgia, and other debilitating diseases, will challenge even the most motivated person to engage in all of the correct health behaviors. This is why the client's medical history and clearance from a health care provider are needed before developing an exercise prescription or diet.

Cognitive Limitations

Cognitive (thought process) impairments can influence a person's ability to begin and maintain a healthy lifestyle. The most serious impairment is dementia, such as Alzheimer's disease. Traumatic brain injuries, including serious concussions, resulting from accidents, falls, and participation in sport, and mental retardation are other serious forms of biological changes in the organism that drastically change thinking processes. One impairment that Grunberg and Klein (2009) do not mention and that is more common among competitive athletes than has been recognized is attention-deficit/hyperactive disorder (ADHD). In this condition, the individual is limited in the ability to process verbally communicated information, resulting in poor retention (Gordon and Asher, 1994). This is important to health care providers because the ADHD client will have poor concentration and does not efficiently remember information that is delivered in verbal form. Taken together, cognitive limitations may lead to a person's unwillingness or inability to follow prescribed exercise and nutritional guidelines or to remember instructions that are delivered in verbal (rather than visual) form.

Motivational Limitations

This area is the most controllable of all obstacles, yet it is often the most common and difficult to overcome. This is also the area researchers have focused on more than any other because lack of motivation is the most common reason for engaging in unhealthy behaviors. As Grunberg and Klein (2009) correctly contend, "Knowledge about nutrition, weight, exercise, long-term health, and the positive effects of taking various medications has little or no value for people who are apathetic or do not care about their current or long-term health status" (p. 415).

It is essential to convince people of the importance of developing a healthy lifestyle to ward off mental illness (e.g., exercise prevents or overcomes certain mental illnesses such as depression and anxiety), increase energy, improve quality of sleep, reduce mental and physical fatigue, maintain a positive mood state, reduce or eliminate chronic pain, and slow the aging process. Strategies to improve motivation are addressed in chapter 3. As Grunberg and Klein conclude, "Motivation is the engine that drives the relevant behaviors and cognitions, and therefore deserves center stage for study" (p. 415). The trick for people in the health care industry is to make the development of healthy habits a priority in the client's journey toward happiness and a high quality of life. Many challenges exist in attempting to overcome these barriers.

EXERCISE BARRIERS AND SOURCES OF NEGATIVE ATTITUDES

As children, we loved physical activity. We called it *play*. Whether it was recess, physical education, after-school playtime, or structured sport, as children most of us were quite happy to be physically active. As adolescents, many of us remained active, but less so, as we drove a car, watched television, sat at the computer, played video games, and stopped or reduced our sport participation. Look at how many people just stand on an escalator going down rather than walk down the stairs as the escalator is moving. Why do people spend much of their time at home sitting as opposed to doing occasional physical activity such as walking, cleaning, and gardening?

Somewhere along the way, we forgot the joy of and need to be physically active. Our desire for physical activity declined and sedentary alternatives turned play into work. As adults, we stopped enjoying physical activity. Positive attitudes toward exercise became negative. Our preferred sedentary lifestyle combined with consuming massive amounts of food has resulted in excessive weight gain and weight-related diseases such as type 2 diabetes (Bauman et al., 2012).

In some parts of the world, however, people of all ages remain physically active and *exercise* is not a four-letter word. Although many cultures breed inactivity and large portions of food, others (e.g., the Scandinavian countries of Sweden, Norway, Finland, and Denmark) encourage physical activity as much as possible and healthy foods in small or moderate portions. During a trip to Sweden, I observed people in their 80s riding bicycles, and exercise, often with musical accompaniment, was a daily ritual in the schools. Paths for jogging or cross-country skiing were carved out in many local parks and rural areas, and they were often used. But in the United States and many other countries, most of the adult world has grown to despise most forms of physical activity, especially exercise. This is why it is so important to encourage clients to simply move, to do anything active such as gardening, walking stairs, or riding a bicycle. When it comes to structured exercise, it is imperative to start slow and build up resistance to fatigue and discomfort.

There are reasons, good and bad, valid and not valid, that explain a person's decision to engage or not engage in regular exercise. Numerous studies have examined the reasons people choose not to engage in an active lifestyle and why they start and then drop out of exercise programs. Here a summary of the literature is presented, covering the main reasons for not starting or for quitting exercise programs. Sadly, being unfit and overweight makes it difficult to enjoy the challenge of becoming fitter, leaner, and healthier. The good news, however, is that health and fitness professionals are in a position to help their clients transition from being unfit and inactive to being physically and mentally healthier. The health or fitness professional can become the client's performance coach by providing information and strategies to overcome perceived barriers to exercise.

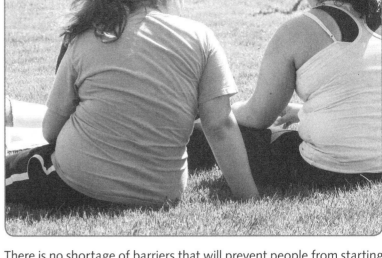

There is no shortage of barriers that will prevent people from starting or maintaining an exercise program. What reasons may someone give for being sedentary while visiting a local park, rather than engaging in physical activity?

Lack of Time

Lack of time is the most common excuse for not exercising or eating a healthy diet (Daskapan, Tuzun, and Eker, 2006). The lack of time is, indeed, a perception (Loehr and Schwartz, 2003). Consider this: Exercise science tells us that we need to exercise at least three hours per week (i.e., three one-hour sessions) on alternate days in order to receive the optimal benefits. There are 168 hours in a week (24 hours per day × 7 days). Three hours is less than 2% of the week, and that's all it takes to receive the health benefits of exercise and to improve fitness. We spend far more time talking on the phone, texting, watching television, and performing other superfluous tasks that contribute to a sedentary lifestyle and actually inhibit good health. Not having enough time to exercise is among the greatest myths of our culture, but it remains an actual excuse for not exercising. As Buckworth and Dishman (2002) have concluded, "Lack of time may be a true determinant, a perceived determinant, the reflection of poor behavioral skills, such as time management, or a rationalization for lack of motivation to be active" (p. 201).

Starting an exercise habit is a challenge. Habits are automatic, and that includes habits that accompany a sedentary lifestyle. Excuses for not exercising regularly abound, and as mentioned, the most common one is not having enough time (Shaw, Bonen, and McCabe, 1991). This is why lack of time is not a valid excuse. Instead, exercise has not been developed into a routine, and it's the lack of an exercise ritual that causes people to never get around to it.

Ill-Matched Fitness Facilities

Clearly, a person who perceives a workout facility as convenient is more likely to exercise at that facility than if the facility were perceived as inconvenient. It is the *perception* of convenience rather than the actual convenience of the facility that is most important in determining exercise behavior (Chenoweth, 2007).

The geographical location, climate, and neighborhood of a facility will influence exercise behavior. Extreme temperatures, precipitation, or an unsafe environment all form valid reasons to avoid exercising. On the other hand, having an exercise facility that is within 3 miles (5 km) of home or work and living in a neighborhood that is perceived as safe increase the likelihood of engaging in physical activity, such as cycling, sport, and jogging (Bauman et al., 2012).

Some people claim they lack the financial resources to purchase a fitness club membership, exercise coaching, and exercise apparel. Others contend they lack transportation to the exercise facility. This issue also relates to not having proper equipment with which to carry out an exercise program. Clearly, lack of income is an exercise barrier to these individuals. However, there are many types of physical activity that are free and contribute to a healthy lifestyle. Examples include doing housework, raking leaves, gardening, taking a walk in your neighborhood, walking your dog (pets need exercise, too), walking stairs, avoiding drive-up windows and instead walking inside restaurants, and lifting weights at home. Try not to miss a chance to move—take steps!

Physical Limitations

It is debilitating and potentially dangerous to exercise when injured or in pain without a doctor's approval. Tissue damage can become more extensive and the level of discomfort can be excessive. Unfit and overweight people are more susceptible to pain and injury compared with their fitter, healthy-weight counterparts (Mackinnon, Ritchie, Hooper, and Abernethy, 2003). Past studies have shown that both aerobic and strength-related fitness improve stability around joints and make us less likely to feel physical discomfort. In addition, lower body weight places less pressure on lower-limb joints, thereby preventing injury in the first place. Clients should work with two people, an exercise coach and a registered dietitian, to reduce body weight and engage in low-intensity exercise several times a week.

For many people, physical exertion is unpleasant. For the overweight or obese person, intense exercise is often unbearable and unsafe, possibly leading to injury and even a cardiac event. In addition, unfit individuals have a lower pain threshold than their fitter counterparts (Skelton and Beyer, 2003). We are who we train to be. If we lead a sedentary lifestyle and become overweight, our body is trained to be comfortable with that lifestyle, and the physiology of our body is not able to immediately adjust to the added stress of increased physical exertion. Poor exercise technique and inadequate footwear (shoes with poor support) make matters worse. Our physiology will adapt to the stress of vigorous physical activity; however, when we are sedentary for much of our lives and do not place physical demands on our tissue, there is no training effect. Exercise becomes difficult and unpleasant, and the result is that some people avoid exercise as much as possible.

Some people have a lean body type with strong musculature, called a *mesomorph* body type, while others have a body type with big bones and a softer, rounder physique, called an *endomorph* body type. These body types are less compatible with aerobic exercise than that of the slightly built person, called an *ectomorph*. Ectomorphs are most compatible with aerobic exercise due to their smaller bone structure, lower body fat, and thin appearance, usually requiring less energy for cardiovascular endurance activities such as jogging and selected sports (e.g., soccer, ice/field hockey, distance running). Body type is collectively called *somatotype*. Thus, body type partially explains the level of a person's attraction toward exercise.

Lack of Fitness Knowledge or Instruction

Exercise is a science consisting of right and wrong techniques. Proper instruction is needed to maintain a safe and effective exercise program to improve fitness. The fields of exercise physiology, sports medicine, and behavioral medicine include scholarly research examining the best approaches and techniques to improve exercise performance and fitness. Too often people walk into a fitness facility without prior instruction on proper technique and go through the motions of exercising. The outcomes of these efforts are usually disappointing because their technique is lacking. Consequently, exercise novices prematurely conclude that their attempts to improve fitness are ineffective. The result is dropping out or injury. Lacking knowledge about exercise technique and how to engage in a properly prescribed exercise program is an exercise barrier.

How can we expect people to feel safe, secure, and motivated to pursue an exercise program and to successfully meet personal goals unless they possess the requisite knowledge and skill? Becoming fitter through a program of regular physical activity requires expert coaching. Going for a casual walk, even daily, will not improve one's fitness. Leading a sedentary lifestyle all week and then jogging or exercising on the weekend also will not lead to reaching desirable fitness goals. Correct exercise technique is a learned set of skills that requires continued practice. Proper instruction on beginning a fitness program, pretests (to use as a baseline against which to compare future test scores), learning correct methods to lift weights and ways to gain strength and cardio fitness safely and without injury are necessary to help prevent people from quitting an exercise program. This rarely happens, however, particularly for novices. New fitness club members, for instance, are often left alone to use the facilities, not knowing proper protocol nor given instruction unless they pay an additional fee beyond club membership. For many people, this added expense is excessive. The fitness club industry can do better when it comes to helping members improve their fitness. High-quality fitness programs and facilities should be accompanied by instruction and feedback on exercise performance quality.

The research literature (e.g., general psychology, sport psychology) clearly indicates that it is human nature to withdraw from activities in which we do not achieve success or perceive ourselves as skilled and capable of success (Anshel, 2012), an area commonly known as *perceived competence*. Unless we provide a comfortable, nonthreatening environment in which to offer instruction to novice exercisers, we can expect high dropout rates from exercise programs.

For many people, physical activity is both unpleasant and unexciting. Imagine an overweight person who leads a sedentary lifestyle walking alone around a track for 20 to 30 minutes or riding a stationary bicycle while perspiring and breathing heavily. Neither of these images creates a sense of excitement and enjoyment for the exerciser whose exercise history may be limited and whose current fitness level and body weight make this undertaking a challenge. The physical challenges of exercise, especially in the early stages of becoming fitter, is one reason it is important to work with a performance coach who offers proper instruction, feedback, and motivation. The absence of a coach's support is a contributing factor to dropping out of exercise programs (Fox et al., 2000).

Unrealistic Goals

It is well known that setting performance goals has a motivational effect on exercise adherence and performance. Sometimes, however, an exerciser, particularly someone at the beginning stages of an exercise program, will set excessively high goals that are unachievable. The result is the perception of failure and lack of progress, soon followed by quitting the exercise routine (Anshel, 2006). Exercisers need to work with a personal trainer or other people who are knowledgeable about fitness and realistic goal setting in order to determine realistic outcomes that are measurable.

Far too many exercise novices want to look like a model or film star or want to meet a goal that is unrealistic, perhaps even dangerous. In fact, a goal such as losing an extensive amount of weight in a relatively short time via a new exercise program can be fatal. Sadly, it is not uncommon for a person to make up for missing weeks or even years of exercise by engaging in an intense program that leads to excessive exertion, injury, negative feelings toward exercise, and other undesirable outcomes (Anshel, 2006).

It takes years to become overweight and unfit, and changing this status will take more than just a few weeks. It is fair to say, however, that based on research in the exercise physiology literature, the minimum time needed to markedly improve fitness after beginning an exercise program is four to six weeks. This also marks the time frame when exercise exertion will feel less intense; there will not be the same feeling of struggle and discomfort. Therefore, health and fitness professionals want to encourage their clients to exercise at least three times a week for four weeks so that they can begin to notice fewer undesirable side effects from physical exertion.

Perceived Lack of Improvement

Most of us have a strong need to feel competent and to achieve, which is the foundation of intrinsic motivation, or what Kimiecik (2002) calls the *intrinsic exerciser*. One primary source of exercise motivation is the perception that some feature of exercise, such as fitness level, body weight, or waist circumference, shows improvement. A lack of perceived progress, especially measured quantitatively (e.g., changes in fitness scores), can result in dropping out.

Returning to the theme of perceived competence and intrinsic motivation, it is imperative that a person's willingness to persist in an activity is based on his perception of improved performance quality and outcomes and that his level of physical exertion is lower (i.e., exercising is getting easier). Exercise becomes more pleasant to perform (Edmunds, Ntoumanis, and Duda, 2007). This is why comparing exercise pretest scores (to establish a fitness baseline before starting a program) with posttest scores has long-term motivational value. As Edmunds et al. concluded, the need for competence is met through perceptions of performance.

Adolescent Experiences and Exercise as Punishment

We cannot turn the clock back, but many people maintain unpleasant feelings toward exercise due to their negative experiences in sport and physical activity as children and adolescents (United States Department of Health and Human Services, 2008). In addition to the reduction of physical education

classes in many countries' schools, including the United States, experiences in these classes have often been negative. In some cases, students are not engaged in sport and exercise programs, and in other cases, only highly skilled students are active, while students who are less skilled or overweight are not included in these classes.

Physical education teachers and sport coaches share responsibility for this problem as culprits who may have contributed to their former students' or athletes' negative attitudes toward exercise. Where did we get this terrible habit of requiring students and athletes to run laps or perform other forms of exercise as punishment for their transgressions? Is there not a better way to discipline a child for misbehavior? The frequent use of exercise by physical education teachers and coaches to discipline inappropriate behavior contributes to the negative attitudes toward exercise we have nurtured over the years (NASPE, 2009c, d). The long-term consequences of using exercise as a form of punishment is the development of a sedentary lifestyle in which students and athletes grow up to despise exercise as adults and parents. By associating exercise with undesirable behavior, this form of punishment fosters a negative attitude toward exercise.

The National Association for Sport and Physical Education (NASPE) has published a position statement titled *Physical Activity Used as Punishment and/or Behavior Management* that addresses instruction and practice guidelines for elementary school, middle school, and high school physical education (NASPE, 2009d). Among the most important statements of this document is that "a student's motivation for being physically active by engaging in the important subject matter content of physical education and sport should never fall victim to the inappropriate use of physical activity as a disciplinary consequence" (p. 1). In addition, "Administering or withholding physical activity as a form of punishment and/or behavior management is an inappropriate practice" (p. 1). Examples of inappropriate use of physical activity include making students run for losing or for poor performance and forcing students to run laps or perform push-ups because of behavioral infractions. Children and adolescents are more susceptible than adults to associating exercise with punishment. Their experiences reinforce the perception that exercise is undesirable and must be avoided. This is not the case in many other countries, such as in Scandinavia, where exercise is enjoyable and often performed to music or in pleasant outdoor conditions. Educators and coaches must find ways to discipline students or alter undesirable behavior other than through physical activity.

The tradition of using exercise as a form of punishment (e.g., "You're late; do 20 push-ups," "Anyone who makes an error makes the team run five laps around the field") has helped create a culture of exercise haters. Performing push-ups and sit-ups, running, and other forms of exercise as punishment build barriers to positive attitudes about physical activity. Exercise should not be associated with undesirable behavior (NASPE, 2009a, b, c). In its *National Standards for Sport Coaches: Quality Coaches, Quality Sports*, NASPE (2005) states that "coaches should never use physical activity or peer pressure as a means of disciplining athlete behavior" (p. 17).

Exercise Burnout

Burnout is characterized by emotional exhaustion and a reduced sense of personal accomplishment about one's work (Maslach and Jackson, 1981). These feelings can also be applied to exercise, in which a person feels physically and emotionally drained of energy and motivation due to overexertion and excessive fatigue. One likely cause of exercise burnout is being in a situation where a person is required to exercise to exhaustion, even at the risk of injury or illness. Athletes, for example, often refrain from engaging in regular exercise after their playing career has ended due to overexertion and excessive exercise intensity and duration when they were competing. This behavior pattern is called *overtraining*. Clearly, sport coaches and physical education teachers who demand repeated, highly intense exercise patterns as an integral part of their program

are promoting negative attitudes toward exercise, and a sedentary lifestyle awaits their athletes and students.

Although physical training and getting in shape for sport competition are important for effective sport performance, sometimes athletes overexercise. Perhaps the person's coach required more exercise than necessary to compete successfully. Exercising an athlete too much (overtraining) can lead to long-term negative attitudes toward physical activity (exercise burnout) after the athlete's retirement from sport. Though statistics on the degree of postretirement exercise habits among former college athletes are not available, my discussions with over 300 former college athletes have confirmed unequivocally that their days of exercising ended when they stopped competing in sport. Overtraining during their playing days was the main reason. Sadly, excessive weight gain is one result of their postretirement negative attitude toward exercise.

From 2007 to 2012 I conducted a study (unpublished) on the number of college athletes who continue to exercise after they retire from sport and the reasons why they discontinue their exercise habit. Only 17 out of 124 athletes (13.7%) who were no longer competing in college indicated that they continued to perform either strength or cardiorespiratory exercise on a regular basis. Thus, 107 out of 124 athletes (86%) indicated that they no longer remained physically active. The main reasons given for an inactive lifestyle included "burned out from exercising as part of my sport training" ($n = 97$, or 78%), "injury and/or pain" ($n = 8$, or 6%), and "not enough time" ($n = 19$, or 15%).

The primary message is that athletes develop negative attitudes about exercise due at least in part to their experiences in sport training. Physical training is an inherent part of preparing for sport competition, but perhaps coaches can take a second look at reducing the unpleasant nature of exercise. One idea is to provide fitness test data to athletes who could detect improved fitness from their pre- and posttest scores. Another strategy is to make exercise more pleasant, perhaps through aerobic games such as soccer or swimming. Third, and very important, is to never use exercise as a form of punishment. As discussed earlier in the chapter, this is all too common in physical education classes and on sport teams.

Lack of Social Support

In the context of exercise and other forms of physical activity, social support is the perceived caring, comfort, and assistance an individual receives from others (Turner, Rejeski, and Brawley, 1997). As discussed further in chapter 6, social support in exercise settings is especially important for novices, who might find the exercise environment lonely, physically challenging, frustrating, and unpleasant. Support from others is essential to overcoming these feelings. In addition, exercise is a science and requires a prescribed program, instruction, and feedback. Coaching, then, is another form of social support. Factors such as the lack of an exercise partner or others who lend verbal and sometimes physical support and the absence of exercise instruction and positive feedback on performance act as exercise barriers.

There is an extensive research base that clearly shows the high motivational value of social support in exercise participation and adherence (Eyler et al., 1999; Oka, King, and Young, 1995). Social support includes receiving verbal and nonverbal positive reinforcement from partners, family, and friends; exercising with a friend; obtaining instruction or coaching; and exercising in an environment that is generally positive and comfortable. Learning a new set of skills, visiting a location that is unfamiliar or threatening such as a fitness facility, and engaging in a task that requires considerable exercise are all predictors of disengagement—that is, starting and then quitting the activity. Social support, then, is the antidote for these factors and a virtual mandate for most exercise novices.

Social support has an important role in exercise adherence because it meets many needs of the exerciser, such as receiving positive feedback, establishing friendships, and engaging in conversation that distracts the exerciser from the exertion and, in some cases, the boredom of performing exercise. Sources of social support include exercising with a partner, exercising in a group setting, meeting others at the fitness club who exercise at the same time and establishing friendships, receiving support from family members, working with a personal trainer, and receiving positive feedback from others, which has reinforcement value and promotes feelings of competence and enjoyment.

MENTAL AND PSYCHOLOGICAL BARRIERS

In addition to physical reasons, there are also psychological reasons for discontinuing exercise. Anshel, Brinthaupt, and Kang (2010) examined the effects of the disconnected values model on changes in fitness and mental well-being among university faculty. In addition to significantly improved fitness, they found desirable changes in mental health, including confidence, self-esteem, and anxiety. Mental state is hugely important to people's willingness to maintain participation in organized, regular exercise. Lack of confidence (e.g., "I have doubts about my ability to perform these exercises correctly"), low self-esteem (e.g., "I do not deserve to be fitter or improve my appearance"), and anxiety (i.e., perceived threat or worry) are strong obstacles to meeting personal goals, feeling optimistic, and maintaining the energy to make exercise a lifestyle choice.

Anxiety

Anxiety, which reflects feelings of worry or threat about a future event (Anshel, 2012), is common in exercise settings, particularly among novices who lack confidence and a sense of improvement and accomplishment (Broman-Fulks and Storey, 2008). Issues such as "Will I succeed?", "I hope I can lose weight," "Can I keep up with the instructor?", "I hope I don't embarrass myself in this fitness outfit," and "What if I look ridiculous in front of all those people?" are sources of anxiety in exercise settings. Longer-term sources of anxiety include feeling concerned about meeting fitness or weight-loss goals, worrying about one's current physical appearance, developing a sense of belonging in exercise facilities and programs, and using one's time to exercise instead of doing something else (e.g., "I could be finishing a report instead of going to the gym"). Exercise has been shown repeatedly to reduce both short-term (acute) and long-term (chronic) anxiety (Wipfli, Rethorst, and Landers, 2008).

Unrealistically High Self-Expectations

Too many people quit exercise programs when their unrealistic expectations (e.g., losing 20 lb or 9 kg in a month, being able to keep up with the fitness instructor after two weeks of working out, eliminating excessive fat from the abdomen or thighs) are not met. Expecting to feel better after exercising reflects what is called the *expectancy hypothesis* (Berger, Owen, Motl, and Parks, 1998). Berger et al. concluded in their study that the expectancy of psychological benefits after exercise may either improve or reduce positive feelings. One approach to experiencing psychological benefits of exercise is to evaluate exercise experiences in terms of performance improvement and not judge performance against unrealistic standards and unachievable outcomes.

Low Perceived Competence

We live in a high-pressure culture filled with lofty expectations to succeed. We almost never persist at any task in which we are not succeeding or we are feeling inadequate. Conversely, we are attracted to tasks at which we feel competent. Therefore, to promote exercise adherence, it is essential for participants to learn the correct exercise techniques and obtain positive feedback on their performance or on the results of their exercise program (e.g., "I feel better," "I dropped a clothing size since I started the program"). Hiring a personal trainer who will provide the proper exercise prescription and instruction is a good investment for many people until they learn to carry out the program independently.

Negative Self-Talk

It is impossible for people to remain motivated and on task if they are engaging in negative self-talk, especially just before or during the exercise session. Examples of negative self-talk include "I don't like this," "I don't feel like exercising," and "I'm tired." Positive self-talk, on the other hand, has arousal-producing effects. Examples include "I can do this," "I feel good," "Just three more minutes to go," and "Hang in there."

Perfectionism

For some people, nothing they do is good enough. Everything they do can always be better. It is important to eliminate that inner voice that reminds them that they are still not good enough. This is an example of negative perfectionism (Anshel and Sutarso, 2010). Although perfectionism can also be positive (e.g., perfectionists are high achievers, persist longer on task, and achieve more than nonperfectionists), its downside includes setting goals that are unachievable, and the person almost never feels satisfied. Negative perfectionists' expectations of others are also excessive. Positive perfectionists set reasonable goals and recognize when they are achieved, especially in exercise settings.

Lack of Confidence

Lacking confidence is a primary cause of not engaging in regular exercise and of dropping out of programs. For example, Anshel (2004) examined the effect of self-monitoring strategies on exercise adherence among the faculty and staff employed at a university. Before the study, consisting of a self-monitoring strategy over an eight-week exercise program during the summer, all 103 participants were interviewed about the factors that might lead them to quit the exercise program and their perceived barriers to adhering to the exercise program. Almost 60% of the respondents indicated lack of confidence and the need for coaching and instruction as factors. Building exercisers' confidence in their ability to main-

---

HEALTH COSTS AND BENEFITS VERSUS COMMON SENSE

Habits, whether healthy or unhealthy, are rarely maintained unless they are perceived as having at least one benefit (Loehr and Schwartz, 2003) that is experienced in the short term rather than farther down the road (Hall and Fong, 2003). These perceived benefits typically outweigh the costs and long-term consequences of the habit. For example, the negative habit of exhibiting anger or impatience in response to others' actions has the perceived benefit of prompting action, maintaining situational control, and releasing unpleasant feelings. The person may acknowledge the costs (e.g., alienating others, poor social relationships, heightened stress) and long-term consequences (e.g., developing heart disease and hypertension, lacking respect and trust from others) of an angry outburst; however, the benefits are viewed as more important and immediate (e.g., mobilizing a person or group to act quickly, getting someone's attention, increasing the listener's level of excitation) in meeting the person's goals. Under these conditions, the negative habit persists.

Although existing theories and models have provided a coherent framework with which to provide explanations, descriptions, and predictions of exercise behavior, their application to increasing exercise behavior has been met with uneven success (Buckworth and Dishman, 2002). This is likely due to limitations in research on the use of interventions to promote exercise or other health-related behavior. There is one additional factor that may explain a person's decision not to engage in regular physical activity that has not been addressed by researchers and writers: lack of common sense, also called *foolishness*.

Explaining a person's behavioral tendencies, particularly when those tendencies are unhealthy and the person knows it, sometimes requires a search for possible motives. Why, for example, would people behave in a manner that they know is potentially dangerous and might lead to harm, poor health, or even premature death? Should we consider taking abnormally high risks (e.g., driving drunk, driving while texting, consistently overeating, ingesting mind-altering drugs) as examples of foolish behavior? Is it possible that people who engage in high-risk behavior do not consider their actions to be high risk? Perhaps most important, what can health care professionals do about people whose high-risk, unhealthy actions demonstrate a lack of common sense regarding their well-being?

Mental and physical health professionals may label actions as foolish or self-destructive, but it is inappropriate to refer to people, their character, or their personality in this manner. People may act foolish or demonstrate ignorance or a lack of common sense, but they are not foolish or ignorant people. Perhaps the bottom line about foolish behavior is that health professionals cannot overcome a person's choice to behave in a certain manner, even if that behavior pattern is contradictory to better health, improved energy, higher quality of life, and greater happiness. Changing health behavior requires cooperation by two parties: the health professional and the client. Health behavior change cannot be forced. The education and expertise of health professionals can be effective only for clients who are motivated to feel better and to maintain a healthier lifestyle.

---

tain an exercise program should be a primary objective of fitness professionals.

HEALTH BEHAVIOR INTERVENTION RESEARCH

Considerable research has been conducted to determine the effectiveness of various treatments and programs on helping people start and maintain healthy habits, including exercise. Though the causes of unhealthy behaviors are known to researchers and practitioners, attempts to change unhealthy behavior patterns through intervention (experimental) research, particularly improving physical activity rates, have been less than successful (Haskell, Lee, Pate, Power, et al., 2007). Even if a particular intervention has been shown to promote starting an exercise program, there is little evidence that the intervention also promotes exercise adherence. In other words, people tend to begin exercise programs but do not continue them. Researchers and practitioners have been frustrated with their failure to find the magic bullet that compels a person to make long-term, permanent changes in healthy lifestyle habits. Perhaps these studies are flawed, and the interventions being tested are ineffective. No one is certain about the causes of the undesirable outcomes of these studies, and therefore more research is needed.

Examining the limitations in existing research has implications for providing more effective interventions in the future. What are the limitations of existing research, and how are these limitations related to creating more effective programs?

• *Absence of a theoretical framework.* In their critique of existing research on promoting exercise behavior, Buckworth and Dishman (2002) criticized the absence of a theoretical framework or model to examine intervention effectiveness intended to promote exercise participation and adherence. In order to explain and predict research outcomes, it is important for researchers to justify what is being tested so that the study (and intervention) can be repeated successfully. You cannot build a home without a blueprint. Buckworth and Dishman correctly conclude, "Without a theoretical framework, the choice of variables cannot be well justified and the ability to interpret [and explain] results is limited" (p. 252).

• *Self-determination versus externally imposed choices.* Another limitation of existing studies is that strategies and programs have often been imposed on the exerciser rather than giving the exerciser choices about the location and type of exercise that is being recorded. Researchers have not controlled for the exerciser's motives and rationale for exercising, preferred type and location of exercise, or commitment to begin and maintain an exercise program. A person who expects to lose considerable weight in a relatively short time, who prefers weight training and is not attracted to aerobic training, or who is forced to exercise in a public facility or to attend a particular program (e.g., group fitness classes) is more likely to drop out than a person who is given an array of choices for an exercise program.

• *Assuming the exerciser desires health behavior change.* Perhaps it is presumptuous of researchers to assume that everyone wants to change certain health behaviors or reach certain performance goals. Researchers have traditionally imposed goals for behavior change on the exerciser rather than having the exerciser set self-determined goals (Marcus and Stanton, 1993). Sometimes the exerciser's goals have differed from those of the exercise leader or coach. This discord can actually demotivate exercisers from adhering to an exercise program.

• *Perceived choice.* If the goal of an exercise adherence study is to foster long-term commitment to exercise, why not give exercisers the opportunity to choose the type of exercise they prefer and the exercise schedule that is most convenient for them? This strategy is referred to as *perceived choice* (Markland, 1999), or what Ajzen (1985) calls *perceived behavioral control.* In typical studies on exercise adherence, exercisers are required to attend group sessions, often at specific times, performing predetermined exercise routines so that the type, length, and intensity of exercise are controlled by the researcher. This has led to high dropout rates and low motivation. Allowing people to select their own exercise type, intensity, and location is preferred and being examined in future studies.

• *Examining mechanisms rather than (or in addition to) outcomes.* Many studies have focused on changes in fitness level, number of sessions attended or amount of exercise time per week, and other outcomes (e.g., changes in attitude toward exercise and level of exercise adherence) rather than the mechanisms (i.e., the underlying reasons) that help explain exercise behavior (Ockene, 2001). For instance, changes in fitness may reflect a high degree of exercise adherence; however, researchers have not examined the factors that may have contributed to adherence rates. What are the reasons for the participants' decision to adhere or drop out? Did participants have a particularly positive or negative attitude toward the exercise program or toward their fitness coach? What are the factors that influence short-term and long-term adherence to an exercise program? Do they include the provision of educational materials? High-quality personal coaching from a person with current knowledge of proper exercise routines and nutrition? The presence or absence of social support? These factors, rather than only the end results, might explain the reasons for performance outcomes.

• *Regimen factors.* One likely factor that promotes health behavior change and exercise adherence is what Oldridge (2001) refers to as a *regimen factor*. In particular, he suggests "keeping the [exercise] regimen straightforward, providing clear instructions and periodic checks, promoting good communication with the patient (client), and reinforcing their accomplishments" (p. 322). Oldridge contends that adherence strategies are seldom effective on their own, and adherence is far more likely if the strategies are implemented as an integral part of one's daily routine. Loehr and Schwartz (2003) refer to regimens as *rituals*, and they claim that establishing rituals leads to healthy habits.

• *Values.* Another area that needs to be considered in building an effective exercise intervention is participants' values and the extent to which their values are inconsistent with their actions, or unhealthy habits (Anshel, 2008). As discussed later in this chapter and in chapter 7 on the influence of religious and spiritual beliefs on health outcomes, the contrast between the lack of an exercise habit and the person's values and beliefs about what is important in life, particularly when those values include health, family, faith, character, and others that reflect a high quality of life (Dunn, Andersen, and Jakicic, 1998), forms an essential source of incentive to establish an exercise habit. Values, then, are a relevant component of any model related to health behavior change.

The process of behavior change is challenging to health care professionals because habits and routines are firmly entrenched in the client's lifestyle (Ockene, 2001). Attempting to increase exercise behavior is particularly difficult because it is accompanied by an array of long-held feelings and attitudes that may reflect negative previous experiences (e.g., a physical education teacher who used exercise as a form of discipline, burnout from too much physical training as a former athlete, injury or perceived failure from previous exercise attempts). Further, vigorous exercise requires effort and physical discomfort in order to obtain benefits.

The degree of discomfort during exercise is directly related to several criteria, including body weight, fitness level, history of past injuries, factors related to aging, and degree to which the person's lifestyle is sedentary. Hunt and Hillsdon (1996) have concluded that "what appears to be lacking at this point is a framework for practitioners to work within which will guide them through the difficult change process and help bring all the successful components [of health behavior change] into one model" (p. 29). A new approach that has been shown to improve the effectiveness of increasing exercise participation, enjoyment, and long-term exercise adherence is the disconnected values model, explained in chapter 9.

FOUR COMPONENTS OF HEALTH BEHAVIOR CHANGE

The main theme of this chapter is to describe reasons why so many of us maintain unhealthy habits and to describe possible ways to replace these comfortable but self-destructive routines with healthier rituals. An overview of the literature on health behavior change reveals four strategies or components that are needed to change health behavior: creating test scores so that exercisers observe numerical data, receiving social support through coaching, establishing routines, and making health behaviors an important value. See chapter 9 for specific strategies to facilitate each of these components.

Data

As Loehr and Schwartz (2003) concluded based on working with clients for over 20 years in a corporate wellness program, and confirmed by Anshel and Kang (2007a, b) in two studies, people are driven by numbers. It is one thing for a person to read an article that promotes healthy habits or for friends, family, or even medical practitioners to offer advice, but the strongest influence on changing health behavior is scores from medical and health tests. Test scores, although not always 100% accurate (e.g., false positives, false negatives), provide information that is objective and meaningful. Numbers typically do not lie! The most common, most effective, and easiest method for obtaining test scores related to exercise include various types of submaximal $\dot{V}O_2$ tests that measure cardiorespiratory fitness, strength tests that measure upper-body and lower-body strength, tests that measure percent body fat (e.g., skin caliper, hydrostatic weighing, Bod Pod), waist circumference (measure of abdominal fat), and a lipids profile that measures good and bad cholesterol, triglycerides, and related measures of blood chemistry that are influenced by food intake.

The key issue concerning the influence of test scores on changing the client's behaviors is the manner in which the health professional interprets test scores. Specialists should interpret undesirable scores with a sense of seriousness, urgency, and even alarm. Let the numbers speak for themselves, inform clients about the long-term implications of the test scores, and prescribe actions and names of specialists who can help them improve future scores. According to Tkachuk, Leslie-Toogood, and Martin (2003), "Behavioral assessment involves the collection and analysis of information and data in order to identify and describe target behaviors, identify possible causes of the behaviors, select appropriate treatment strategies to modify the behaviors, and evaluate treatment outcomes" (p. 104).

Social Support

The inclusion of others in the mission to change health behavior is called *social support* and is reviewed more extensively in chapter 6. The key point of this component is that exercisers, particularly novices, almost always improve their exercise adherence, and consequently their fitness, when they have someone they can depend on for guidance, information, emotional support, and companionship. Coaching in particular allows the person to receive continued information and instruction in addition to encouragement and approval. I have known hundreds of exercise clients over the years who have felt loyalty and accountability toward their fitness and nutrition coaches. These professionals provide instruction and feedback that give their clients a sense of achievement and competence, both of which are highly desirable in long-term motivation and program adherence.

Routines

Routines play the valuable role of structuring one's environment, managing time, and giving a sense of regularity and comfort in carrying out a set of actions that promote good health. All of us develop and maintain routines each day, starting from the time we awaken until we go to sleep. Our day is composed of routines that we regulate in order to maintain a semblance of normality and regularity. If we do not schedule exercise sessions during the week, they are less likely to happen. Routines are at the heart of time management and should be encouraged for maintaining healthy habits.

Values

As described elsewhere in this book, our values reflect our core beliefs about what we consider most important. Most of the time, values guide our behaviors. The value of generosity, for instance, usually results in donations to charity or helping others. The value of faith is often accompanied by attending religious services, maintaining a spiritual belief system, or following a lifestyle consistent with scripture. Health is another value, so if one's value system includes health, then the person is likely to behave in ways that support improved health. As we all know, however, this is not always the case. Although the vast majority of people value their health and happiness, they do not always act in ways that are consistent with these values. Nevertheless, it is imperative for health to become a fixed component of people's character so that they remain open to new ideas and strategies for maintaining a lifestyle consistent with their values.

Ockene (2001) correctly concludes:

Change is a process, not a one-time event, and we can't expect people to make changes at a level for which they're not ready. [Health behavior change] interventions need to be directed to where the individual is. (p. 45)

FROM RESEARCH TO REAL WORLD

Let's take an example of how a practitioner (e.g., fitness coach, dietitian, medical practitioner, physical therapist, cardiac rehabilitation program leader) would apply the four components of health behavior change. Remember, the four components are data, social support, routines, and values.

Test Data

Most people are motivated by numbers, so whether the numbers from test data disclose good news or bad news, people often react to them. Examples of health-related data that would interest most people include fitness tests (e.g., aerobic capacity based on treadmill walking or jogging, strength tests, waist circumference, percent body fat); lipids profiles (e.g., good and bad cholesterol, triglycerides); paper-and-pencil inventories that measure stress, anxiety, various forms of mental illness such as depression, and other psychological dimensions (administered by a properly-credentialed person such as a mental health professional); tracking and rewarding program attendance; and scores on self-monitoring checklists.

Social Support

It is clear that exercisers are more likely to adhere to their program if they exercise with at least one other person or receive instruction from and are monitored by a fitness coach. Practitioners want to provide enough coaching until the client has acquired the skills needed to carry out an exercise program correctly and independently.

Routines

Our whole day, from waking up to going to bed, consists of a series of thoughts and actions that are planned, learned, and carried out efficiently and regularly, sometimes automatically. These regular actions, often carried out one or more times a day, are routines. Sample routines that promote health include presleep rituals of engaging in relaxing tasks, such as reading, going for a slow walk, stretching, and closing one's eyes and engaging in relaxing imagery (visualization), and avoiding behaviors that stimulate the nervous system, such as ingesting caffeine, performing vigorous physical activity, or interacting with others in an unpleasant or hostile manner.

Values

Values reflect what we consider important to live a satisfying life. Values should include good health, family, character, integrity, honesty, faith, generosity, and excellence (see the Values Checklist for a complete list of values). The practitioner's objective is to help clients associate their values with their behavior patterns, particularly with respect to linking health-promoting behaviors with selected values. Reminding clients about their values and beliefs about what is important to them should drive their behavior. Failure to connect values with actions—called a *disconnect*—has costs and long-term consequences.

Along these lines, Glasgow and colleagues (2004) have concluded about the future of research on health behavior change, "If we are serious about evidence-based behavioral medicine and about closing the gap between research findings and application of these findings in applied settings, we cannot continue 'business as usual'" (p. 11). Creative new approaches to changing health behavior, including exercise, are needed. Nicassio, Meyerowitz, and Kerns (2004) suggest that future studies include "specific methodologies for selecting intervention approaches in individual clinical cases" and acknowledging "the mechanisms of action through which interventions achieve their effects" (p. 135). Future research on the effects of cognitive and behavioral strategies to change our food-obsessed mind-set and to overcome our culture's disdain for physical activity, including exercise, is badly needed.

SUMMARY

The consequences of being overweight and inactive include serious deterioration of health, energy, and quality of life. Unhealthy habits, such as poor nutrition, lack of physical activity, inadequate sleep, and prolonged stress, promote poor health and disease, shortening our life span. This chapter attempted to explain the reasons many of us engage in behaviors that we know are unhealthy, even dangerous. One important reason research studies have not resulted in new and more effective techniques is the lack of adherence in maintaining healthier behaviors. New habits are often discontinued within two to four weeks, and it takes six to eight weeks to establish a new habit. Failing to integrate new, desirable behavior patterns into one's lifestyle often reflects physical limitations (e.g., impaired movement), emotional limitations (e.g., impatience with reaching desirable goals, mental illness), and motivational limitations (e.g., apathy toward the long-term effects of unhealthy behaviors, not understanding the consequences of behaviors on long-term health).

Likely barriers to developing and maintaining healthy habits such as exercise include perceived lack of time, lack of social support, exercise burnout (excessive training), exercise used as punishment, perceived lack of improvement, unrealistically high goals, high anxiety, perfectionism, perceived lack of competence in performing exercise correctly, low confidence, and lack of fitness knowledge. Four likely components that would promote health behavior change include test or performance data (people are motivated by numbers), social support (exercising with a friend, fitness coaching), development of routines, and proper values.

STUDENT ACTIVITY

Determining Your Client's Disconnect

The purpose of this exercise is to help your client acknowledge a disconnect between her values and behavior pattern, to state the benefits and consequences of this disconnect (e.g., "I value my good health but I am overweight and do not maintain an active lifestyle"), and then to plan a time management schedule that incorporates time for regular physical activity and proper eating habits. Find a partner and ask him to become your client for the purposes of this activity. Have him mark his three most important values from the Values Checklist and then list one or two of his regular habits that contradict (are misaligned with) any of these values. Ask him why he maintains habits that are not consistent with his values—to list the benefits of these unhealthy habits, to list one or two costs and consequences of maintaining these habits, and to acknowledge that at least one disconnect between values and actions has undesirable consequences. Then, take your client through the 24-hour time management form in which he schedules his typical daily activities, and help him schedule time for exercise at least three times per week, regular meals, bedtime and morning routines, and other daily rituals that promote energy and good health. It should become obvious that if we structure and plan our day, there is time for living our life consistent with our values.

FORM 4.1 VALUES CHECKLIST

Check three of your most important values.

Balance	❏	Happiness	❏
Beauty	❏	Harmony	❏
Concern for others	❏	Health	❏
Character	❏	Humor	❏
Commitment	❏	Humility	❏
Compassion	❏	Integrity	❏
Courage	❏	Kindness	❏
Creativity	❏	Knowledge	❏
Excellence	❏	Loyalty	❏
Faith	❏	Perseverance	❏
Fairness	❏	Respect for others	❏
Family	❏	Responsibility	❏
Freedom	❏	Security	❏
Generosity	❏	Serenity	❏
Genuineness	❏	Service to others	❏

Value	Health	New ritual	Daily brisk walking or resistance training
Value	Family	New ritual	Make phone call at noon to connect with an important other
Value		New ritual	
Value		New ritual	
Value		New ritual	

From M. Anshel, 2014, *Applied Health Fitness Psychology*. (Champaign, IL: Human Kinetics).

FORM 4.2   TIME MANAGEMENT ACTION PLAN

4:00 a.m.		4:00 p.m.	
4:30 a.m.		4:30 p.m.	
5:00 a.m.		5:00 p.m.	
5:30 a.m.		5:30 p.m.	
6:00 a.m.		6:00 p.m.	
6:30 a.m.		6:30 p.m.	
7:00 a.m.		7:00 p.m.	
7:30 a.m.		7:30 p.m.	
8:00 a.m.		8:00 p.m.	
8:30 a.m.		8:30 p.m.	
9:00 a.m.		9:00 p.m.	
9:30 a.m.		9:30 p.m.	
10:00 a.m.		10:00 p.m.	
10:30 a.m.		10:30 p.m.	
11:00 a.m.		11:00 p.m.	
11:30 a.m.		11:30 p.m.	
Noon		Midnight	
12:30 p.m.		12:30 a.m.	
1:00 p.m.		1:00 a.m.	
1:30 p.m.		1:30 a.m.	
2:00 p.m.		2:00 a.m.	
2:30 p.m.		2:30 a.m.	
3:00 p.m.		3:00 a.m.	
3:30 p.m.		3:30 a.m.	

From M. Anshel, 2014, *Applied Health Fitness Psychology*. (Champaign, IL: Human Kinetics).

REFERENCES

Ajzen, I. (1985). From intention to actions: A theory of planned behavior. In J. Kuhl and J. Beckman (Eds.), *Action control: From cognition to behavior* (pp. 11-39). Heidelberg, Germany: Springer.

Anshel, M.H. (2004). Self-monitoring promotes long-term adherence among unfit adults. Presented at the American Heart Association 2nd Scientific Conference on Compliance in Healthcare and Research, Washington, D.C.

Anshel, M.H. (2006). *Applied exercise psychology: A practitioner's guide to improving client health and fitness.* New York: Springer.

Anshel, M.H. (2008). The disconnected values model: Intervention strategies for health behavior change. *Journal of Clinical Sport Psychology, 2,* 357-380.

Anshel, M.H. (2012). *Sport psychology: From theory to practice* (5th ed.). San Francisco: Benjamin Cummings.

Anshel, M.H., Brinthaupt, T.M., and Kang, M. (2010). The disconnected values model improves mental well-being and fitness in an employee wellness program. *Behavioral Medicine, 36,* 113-122.

Anshel, M.H., and Kang, M. (2007a). Effect of an intervention on replacing negative habits with positive routines for improving full engagement at work: A test of the disconnected values model. *Journal of Consulting Psychology: Practice and Research, 59,* 110-125.

Anshel, M.H., and Kang, M. (2007b). An outcome-based action study on changes in fitness, blood lipids, and exercise adherence based on the Disconnected Values Model. *Behavioral Medicine, 33,* 85-98.

Anshel, M.H., and Sutarso, T. (2010). Conceptualizing maladaptive sport perfectionism as a function of gender. *Journal of Clinical Sport Psychology, 4,* 263-281.

Bauman, A.W., Reis, R.S., Sallis, J., Wells, J., Loos, R., and Martin, B.W. (2012). Correlates of physical activity: Why are some people physically active and others not? *The Lancet, 380,* 258-271.

Berger, B.G., Owen, D.R., Motl, R.W., and Parks, L. (1998). Relationship between expectancy of psychological benefits and mood alteration in joggers. *International Journal of Sport Psychology, 29,* 1-16.

Broman Fulks, J.J., and Storey, K.M. (2008). Evaluation of a brief aerobic intervention for anxiety sensitivity. *Anxiety, Stress and Coping: An International Journal, 21,* 117-128.

Buckworth, J., and Dishman, R.K. (2002). *Exercise psychology.* Champaign, IL: Human Kinetics.

Chenoweth, D.H. (2007). *Worksite health promotion* (2nd ed.). Champaign, IL: Human Kinetics.

Daskapan, A., Tuzun, E.H., and Eker, L. (2006). Perceived barriers to physical activity in university students. *Journal of Sports Science and Medicine, 5,* 615-620.

Dunn, A.L., Andersen, R.E., and Jakicic, J.M. (1998). Lifestyle physical activity interventions. History, short- and long-term effects, and recommendations. *American Journal of Preventive Medicine, 15,* 398-412.

Edmunds, J.K., Ntoumanis, N., and Duda, J.L. (2007). Perceived autonomy support and psychological need satisfaction in exercise. In M.S. Hagger and N.L.D. Chatzisarantis (Eds.), *Intrinsic Motivation and Self-Determination in Exercise and Sport* (pp. 35-51). Champaign, IL: Human Kinetics.

Eyler, A.A., Brownson, R.C., Donateller, R.J., King, A.C., Brown, D., and Sallis, F.F. (1999). Physical activity social support and middle-and older-aged minority women: Results from a U.S. survey. *Social Science and Medicine, 49,* 781-789.

Fox, L.D., Rejeski, W.J., and Gauvin, L. (2000). Effects of leadership style and group dynamics on enjoyment of physical activity. *American Journal of Health Promotion, 14,* 277-283.

Glasgow, R.E., Klesges, L.M., Dzewaltowski, D.A., Bull, S.S., and Estabrooks, P. (2004). The future of health behavior change research: What is needed to improve translation of research into health promotion practice. *Annals of Behavioral Medicine, 27,* 3-12.

Gordon, S.B., and Asher, M.J. (1994). *Meeting the ADD challenge: A practical guide for teachers.* Champaign, IL: Research Press.

Grunberg, N.E., and Klein, L.C. (2009). Biopsychological obstacles to adoption and maintenance of a healthy lifestyle. In S.A. Shumaker, J.K. Ockene, and K.A. Riebert (Eds.), *The handbook of health behavior change* (3rd ed., pp. 411-426). New York: Springer.

Hall, P.A., and Fong, G.T. (2003). The effects of a brief time perspective intervention for increasing physical activity among young adults. *Psychology and Health, 18,* 685-706.

Hall, P.A., and Fong, G.T. (2007). Temporal self-regulation theory: A model for individual health behavior. *Health Psychology Review, 1,* 6-52.

Haskell, W.L., Lee, I., Pate, R.R., Power, K.E., Blair, S.N., Franklin, B.A., Macera, C.A., Health, G.W., Thompson, P.D., and Bauman, A. (2007). Physical activity and public health: Updated recommendation for adults from the American College of Sports Medicine and the American Heart Association. *Medicine and Science in Sports and Exercise, 39*, 1423-1434.

Hunt, P., and Hillsdon, M. (1996). *Changing eating and exercise behavior: A handbook for professionals.* Cambridge, MA: Blackwell Science.

Kimiecik, J. (2002). *The intrinsic exerciser: Discovering the joy of exercise.* Boston: Houghton Mifflin.

Klesges, L.M., Estabrooks, P.A., Dzewaltowski, D.A., Bull, S.S., and Glasgow, R.E. (2005). Beginning with the application in mind: Designing and planning health behavior change interventions to enhance dissemination. *Annals of Behavioral Medicine, 29*, 66-75.

Loehr, J., and Schwartz, T. (2003). *The power of full engagement: Managing energy, not time, is the key to high performance and personal renewal.* New York: Free Press.

Mackinnon, L.T., Ritchie, C.B., Hooper, S.L., and Abernethy, P.J. (2003). *Exercise management: Concepts and professional practice.* Champaign, IL: Human Kinetics.

Marcus, B.H., and Forsythe, L.H. (2003). *Motivating people to be physically active.* Champaign, IL: Human Kinetics.

Marcus, B.H., and Stanton, A.L. (1993). Evaluation of relapse prevention and reinforcement interventions to promote exercise adherence in sedentary females. *Research Quarterly for Exercise and Sport, 64*, 447-452.

Markland, D. (1999). Self-determination moderates the effects of perceived competence on intrinsic motivation in an exercise setting. *Journal of Sport and Exercise Psychology, 21*, 351-361.

Maslach, C., and Jackson, S.E. (1981). The measurement of experienced burnout. *Journal of Organizational Behavior, 2*, 99-113.

National Association for Sport and Physical Education (NASPE). (2005). *National standards for sport coaches: Quality coaches, quality sports.* Reston, VA: Author

National Association for Sport and Physical Education (NASPE). (2009a). *Appropriate instructional practice guidelines for elementary school physical education* (3rd ed.). Reston, VA: Author.

National Association for Sport and Physical Education (NASPE). (2009b). *Appropriate instructional practice guidelines for high school physical education* (3rd ed.). Reston, VA: Author.

National Association for Sport and Physical Education (NASPE). (2009c). *Appropriate instructional practice guidelines for middle school physical education* (3rd ed.). Reston, VA: Author.

National Association for Sport and Physical Education (NASPE). (2009d). *Physical activity used as punishment and/or behavior management.* Available: www.aahperd.org/naspe/standards/upload/Physical-Activity-as-Punishment-to-Board-12-10.pdf [June 27, 2013].

Nestle, M., and Jacobson, M.F. (2000). Halting the obesity epidemic: A public health policy approach. *Public Health Reports, 115*, 12-24.

Nicassio, P.M., Meyerowitz, B.E., and Kerns, R.D. (2004). The future of health psychology interventions. *Health Psychology, 23*, 132-137.

Ockene, J.K. (2001). Strategies to increase adherence to treatment. In L.E. Burke and I.S. Ockene (Eds.), *Compliance in healthcare and research* (pp. 43-56). Armonk, NY: Futura.

Oka, R.K., King, A.C., and Young, D.R. (1995). Sources of social support as predictors of exercise adherence in women and men ages 50 to 65 years. *Women's Health, 1*, 161-175.

Oldridge, N.B. (2001). Future directions: What paths do researchers need to take? What needs to be done to improve multi-level compliance? In L.E. Burke and I.S. Ockene (Eds.), *Compliance in healthcare and research* (pp. 331-347). Armonk, NY: Futura.

Sackett, D.L. (1976). The magnitude of compliance and noncompliance. In K.L. Sackett and R.B. Haynes (Eds.), *Compliance with therapeutic regimens* (pp. 9-25). Baltimore: Johns Hopkins University Press.

Shaw, S.M., Bonen, A., and McCabe, J.F. (1991). Do more constraints mean less leisure? Examining the relationship between constraints and participation. *Journal of Leisure Research, 23*, 286-300.

Skelton, D.A., and Beyer, N. (2003). Exercise and injury prevention in older people. *Scandinavian Journal of Medicine and Science in Sports, 13*, 77-85.

Super, D.E. (1995). Values: Their nature, assessment, and practical use. In D.E. Super and B. Sverko (Eds.), *Life roles, values, and careers: International findings of the work importance study* (pp. 54-61). San Francisco: Jossey-Bass.

Tkachuk, G., Leslie-Toogood, A., and Martin, G.L. (2003). Behavioral assessment in sport psychology. *The Sport Psychologist, 17*, 104-117.

Turner, E.E., Rejeski, W.J., and Brawley, L.R. (1997). Psychological benefits of activity are influenced by the social environment. *Journal of Sport and Exercise Psychology, 19*, 119-130.

U.S. Department of Health and Human Services (HHS). (2004). *Healthy people 2010 midcourse review.* Washington, DC: U.S. Government Printing Office.

U.S. Department of Health and Human Services (HHS). (2008). *Physical activity guidelines for Americans.* www.health.gov/paguidelines/guidelines/chapter2.aspx.

Wipfli, B.M., Rethorst, C.D., and Landers, D.M. (2008). The anxiolytic effects of exercise: A meta-analysis of randomized trials and dose-response analysis. *Journal of Sport and Exercise Psychology, 30*, 392-410.

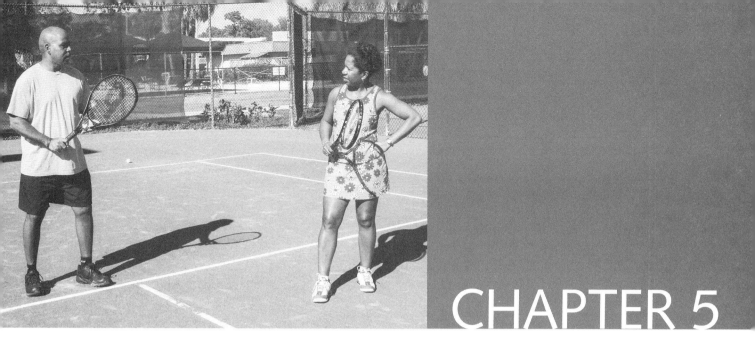

Personal Factors

> 66 *Your biggest break can come from never quitting. Being at the right place at the right time can only happen when you keep moving toward the next opportunity.* 99
>
> Arthur Pine, author

CHAPTER OBJECTIVES

After reading this chapter, you should be able to:

- determine the role of personality in developing and maintaining healthy habits;
- acknowledge the limitations of personality inventories in predicting behavior;
- identify the differences among personality traits, styles or orientations, and behavioral tendencies and know which are susceptible to change and which are not; and
- know which styles or orientations and behavioral tendencies are more closely allied with initiating and adhering to new routines that create a healthy lifestyle.

Researchers and clinicians tell us something we already knew: We are all different. The content area of psychology that concerns the study of personal factors that describe, explain, and predict behavior is called *individual differences*. Journals such as *Personality and Individual Differences* and the *Journal of Health Psychology* devote their entire mission to understanding the ways in which personal factors affect behavior, specifically the development and maintenance of healthy habits. If researchers, educators, and clinicians can show that possessing specific personal characteristics (e.g., personality traits, thinking styles or orientations, behavioral tendencies) accurately predicts changes in health behaviors, then interventions can be used to promote these outcomes.

The high dropout rate of exercise programs—averaging about 50% within six months of starting a program (Stathopoulou and Powers, 2006)—and reversion to unhealthy eating habits are primary reasons health care professionals should be able to identify the factors that best predict success in discarding old habits and developing healthier ones. Although the causes of exercise adherence and dropping out are known to researchers and will be discussed more extensively in chapter 8, at least two factors—exercising with one's partner or spouse (Wallace, Raglin, and Jastremski, 1995) and receiving advice to exercise from one's physician and other medical and health specialists (Heaton and Frede, 2003)—strongly improve exercise adherence and reduce the rate of dropping out of exercise programs from 33% (exercising alone) to 10% (exercising with a partner).

The primary purpose of this chapter, therefore, is to examine the psychological factors that influence exercise behavior and adherence to an exercise habit. What do we mean by *psychological factors*? Much of the literature in this area does not make a distinction between personality and other forms of psychological characteristics, such as orientations, styles, and behavioral tendencies. Clarifying these distinctions, however, is important so that health care professionals can differentiate between long-term, stable characteristics that

are not subject to change (i.e., personality) and psychological characteristics that are changeable, such as the person's *style* (e.g., coping style, attribution style) or *orientation* (e.g., goal orientation, competitive orientation). It is also important to determine how each of these characteristics differs from *behavioral tendencies*, which are the most susceptible to change of these concepts, and how they differ in healthy and unhealthy individuals.

PERSONALITY TRAITS AS PREDICTORS OF HEALTH BEHAVIOR

Personality traits consist of a person's distinctive and enduring psychological characteristics that predispose her to react in a certain way in classes of situations. They can reflect thoughts, emotions, and behavior patterns. Traits are partially determined by the age of six; however, they may be determined genetically (McCrae and John, 1992). Examples of personality traits include depression, trait anxiety, trait confidence, neuroticism, stability, extroversion, introversion, trait anger, and stimulus seeking. Table 5.1 categorizes and defines these personal characteristics.

Although the terms *orientation* and *style* have been used interchangeably in the literature, they may differ according to some theorists. Personality researchers and theorists have distinguished between temperament, which is similar to orientation, and character, which resembles style as described by Cloninger (2003). *Temperament* approximates the concept of orientations and refers to the broad dispositional set points that regulate moods and general tendencies. Competition orientation or goal orientation are examples. *Character*, on the other hand, resembles the concept of styles and refers to more idiosyncratic ways of adapting to specific environmental stimuli and to an individual's identity. Examples include coping style and attributional style, which reflect categories of how we cope with sudden stress and how we explain the causes of performance outcomes, respectively.

Table 5.1 Categories of Personal Characteristics

Psychological factors	Definition	Examples
Personality traits	Underlying stable and enduring thoughts and emotions that predispose a person to act in a certain way	Depression, trait anxiety, trait confidence, neuroticism, stability, extroversion, introversion, trait anger, stimulus seeking
Orientations and styles	A person's preference to have certain thoughts or emotions; may predict future behavior	Goal orientation, task vs. ego orientation, coping style, attribution style, explanatory style
Behavioral tendencies	A person's actions or observable habits, sometimes performed automatically, that reduce information load and are highly predictable	Pregame meal, preperformance routines, warm-up, halftime rituals

Predicting who is more likely to start and maintain an exercise habit based on the results of a personality inventory would be enormously helpful for creating and delivering effective, tailored interventions that target individual needs. Exercisers with certain characteristics—high social physique anxiety and low self-esteem, for instance—might prefer exercising alone rather than in a group setting, and they should especially avoid exercising in front of a mirror. People with high confidence, optimism, and other characteristics are more likely to thrive in group exercise programs. Some people are in greater need than others of individual coaching and being held accountable for adhering to their program. Eaters described as compulsive or emotional (see chapter 12) may react to certain stimuli (e.g., television commercials, social settings) or have particular eating habits (e.g., late-night snacking) that differ from people who do not possess these characteristics. It would be ideal if personality inventories existed that allowed researchers and practitioners to predict certain behavior patterns that influence health. Unfortunately, the general consensus among researchers is that the ability to predict exercise and other health behavior based on personality has not shown much promise (see From Research to Real World for more discussion).

Environmental conditions have a strong influence on behavior (Morgan, 1980). Feeling anxiety (i.e., thoughts of worry or threat) about entering a fitness facility, which is common among exercise novices (Anshel, 2006), does not necessarily result in avoiding that facility. Sometimes anxiety can actually promote exercise behavior by creating the incentive to overcome the barriers of negative thinking and create challenging goals that are more likely to improve exercise performance and adherence (Anshel, 2012).

By definition, personality traits reflect a person's characteristics and behaviors from situation to situation. Traits are relatively stable over time, and each person has the same set of personality traits. Specific environmental factors and situational conditions will elevate, or manifest, certain traits more than others. For example, each of us possesses trait anxiety; however, some of us have higher trait anxiety than others as part of our personality. Certain situations, such as sport competition, for instance, will stimulate anxious feelings more easily and extensively in high trait-anxious people—a reflection of state anxiety—as compared with people who have low trait anxiety. Personality, then, is the relatively stable and unique set of psychological processes and characteristics that influence a person's behavior and reactions to the environment.

Given the stability of personality across situations, can exercise influence it? Can a person actually decrease his trait anxiety or influence any other personality trait through extensive physical training? The explanation that personality traits are always present but that certain environmental factors stimulate, influence, or interact with one or more of these traits partly answers these questions. Perhaps more important, and more realistic and doable, it would be of interest to know if specific personal attributes, or traits, are likely to *cause* or *facilitate* exercise behavior and whether certain attributes or dispositions are likely to *develop as a consequence* of long-term exercise involvement. Not unlike the answers to most complex questions, the answer to the relationship between personality and exercise is that it depends.

The literature concerning the relationship between personality traits and exercise behavior is speculative. There is no specific cause-and-effect relationship. Researchers have not clearly shown an exercise personality profile or that exercisers are likely to have a specific set of personality traits. Also unknown to date is whether engaging in a regular exercise program actually influences a set of personality traits. We cannot become bigger risk-takers or reduce our propensity to feel anxious through prolonged involvement in exercise.

Another example of conjecture in attempting to associate exercise and personality comes from Cattell's (1960) 16 personality factor (16 PF) model, in which his analyses of data showed evidence of 16 personality factors. Cattell speculated that exercisers would score low on certain measures of his inventory, including anxiety and a trait called *neuroticism*. Cattell concluded that exercisers are more emotionally stable and less tense than their inactive counterparts and therefore respond more positively to high exercise intensity.

FROM RESEARCH TO REAL WORLD

There is little support for administering a personality inventory for the purpose of predicting future behavior or talent in the areas of sport and exercise performance. In their review of related literature, Martin Ginis and Mack (2012) concluded that, although personality traits per se do not predict health behavior, "personality and other personal characteristics may lead to physical activity through social-cognitive antecedents of motivation" (p. 344). That is, personal characteristics are background factors that influence a person's motivation to engage in healthy behaviors. Examples of social-cognitive antecedents of motivation include the person's beliefs; intrinsic motivation; level of need to achieve; self-efficacy, which is belief in one's capabilities to organize and carry out activities required to attain one or more specific goals (Bandura, 1997); general beliefs and attitudes; and personal values. A variety of factors influence a person's motivation to act, and personality traits by themselves have relatively little influence.

Another reason personality inventories do not highly predict exercise behavior is that they were not developed for exercise populations. Personality tests were developed to measure personality, of course, but also to diagnose mental illness (American Psychiatric Association [APA], 2000). And even when a study shows an association between exercise behavior and personality, how can these results be applied in clinical or practical settings? Does a high score for the trait called *extraversion* provide information that might influence exercise adherence or give practitioners insight into meeting the client's needs? And finally, some traits are more predictive of healthy habits, such as adherence to exercise or nutritious dietary habits, than others (see Rhodes and Smith, 2006, for a review of this literature).

In summary, researchers suggest providing checklists and other forms of coaching that focus on changing observable behavior patterns, or habits.

Even if this conclusion were valid, the data remain descriptive. This means that exercisers may possess certain personal characteristics that nonexercisers do not share; however, there is no evidence that exercise causes an increase in these personality traits, and these results do not suggest that these qualities are required if a person chooses to engage in an exercise program. The traits (e.g., self-esteem) and mental conditions (e.g., depression and anxiety) discussed in the following sections have been shown to be strong predictors of good health and well-being.

Self-Esteem and Exercise

Whereas *self-concept* is a set of self-perceptions that reflect an accounting of our identity in various settings (e.g., academic self, social self, spiritual self, physical self), *self-esteem* reflects how we feel about who we are, that is, how much we like or value ourselves. Self-esteem consists of an evaluation of our self-concept, or how well the self is doing both in specific areas and in general based on our values and standards. *Self-esteem* is a concept used interchangeably with the related terms *self-regard*, *self-respect*, *self-acceptance*, and *self-worth* (Buckworth and Dishman, 2002). Both self-esteem and self-concept are multidimensional, including physical, religious, social, intellectual, and sport sources of both constructs.

Self-esteem is associated in many studies with psychological well-being and with the use of healthy behavior patterns. Behavior is motivated by a related concept and disposition called *self-enhancement* (Biddle, Gorely, and Stensel, 2004). As Biddle explains, human behavior is driven, or motivated, by actions that result in positive feelings or feelings of competence (i.e., perceived competence) and esteem. We act, in other words, according to how we perceive ourselves, and we engage in behaviors we think will lead to success, happiness, and general well-being. Thus, the combination of positive self-esteem (e.g., "I feel better about myself due to my ability to do this") and self-efficacy (e.g., "I feel confident that I will be successful and reach desirable goals") can predict future health behaviors.

Depression and Exercise

A significant predictor of nonparticipation or dropping out of exercise programs, depression is a mood disorder that ranges from mild to severe and, at more advanced stages, may reflect mental illness. It is an important personal factor influencing health behavior and the decision to maintain unhealthy habits. Most authors in this area depict depression as a depressed mood or a loss of interest or pleasure in all or most activities for at least two consecutive weeks. Symptoms of depression include loss of appetite, weight loss or gain, disturbance of sleep, disruption of psychomotor skills, decreased energy, feelings of worthlessness, guilt, poor concentration, and thoughts of suicide (Leith, 1998). Leith's review of related literature indicates that exercising for 15 to 30 minutes at a time promotes positive mental health, and therefore that is also the time frame for improving symptoms of depression. More than 70 studies across a variety of age groups and both genders have shown that aerobic exercise reduces clinical (severe) depression.

Lox, Martin, and Petruzzello (2010) reviewed the research literature on the extent to which physicians and other health professionals communicate exercise-related information to patients for improving mental and physical health. The authors generated several important findings related to promoting physical and mental health.

- In the United States, 65% of patients would be more likely to exercise to stay healthy at the prompting of their doctor and if they were given resources to help them get started (e.g., educational materials, a fitness coach to follow up on this advice).

- About 25% of Canadians look to health professionals to advise them on how to become physically active.

- Sedentary Australians (*N* = 2,300) said their preferred source of advice on ways to increase physical activity was their physician.

- Activity counseling by physicians occurs among less than 50% of patients.

- However, 85% of 1,750 physicians in a survey indicated that they prescribed exercise for patients suffering from depression.

Thus, while the medical community can be far more involved in prescribing exercise, including follow-up referral to an exercise coach or personal trainer, results of the relatively few studies examining this issue indicate that more and more physicians are informing their patients of the benefits of exercise for improving their physical and mental health. Along these lines, Lox and colleagues (2010) claim that many medical practitioners are forming partnerships with local fitness centers and health clubs and

referring their patients to staff members at these facilities.

Finally, Leith (1998) reported that a lifestyle of regular physical activity may help prevent mental disorders from developing. This is especially important given the costs and physically debilitating effects of pharmaceutical agents in treating depression and the time involved in psychotherapy. Remember that diagnosing depression, a mental illness, and counseling depressed clients is reserved for mental health professionals who are licensed by national organizations and recognized by state governments to help clients overcome mental illness. Consultants are nonlicensed individuals who have expertise in changing unhealthy habits and providing instruction to clients but do not provide formal counseling or deal with mental health issues.

EXERCISE AND MOOD CHANGE

Likely explanations for the benefits of exercise for reducing acute and chronic anxiety, referred to as *mechanisms of change*, include changes in the exerciser's psychophysiology due to the use of stress hormones during exercise (i.e., the serotonin hypothesis), the metabolism of stress hormones during physical exertion (i.e., the norepinephrine hypothesis), attentional focusing toward the exercise activity and away from unpleasant thoughts (i.e., the distraction, or time-out, hypothesis), elevation in body temperature (i.e., the thermogenic hypothesis), and changes in hormones that improve mental well-being (i.e., the endorphin hypothesis, also called *runner's high*).

Changes in the exerciser's psychophysiology, or the *serotonin hypothesis*, reflect the complex relationships between exercise and mood. Though the neural basis for the interaction between exercise and mood remains uncertain, it is predicted that exercise influences antidepressant therapeutic properties in the brain, the same mechanism that is targeted by antidepressant drugs.

The *norepinephrine hypothesis* posits that exercise improves mood and reduces stress because physical activity stimulates norepinephrine neurons in the brain, producing a calming effect. It has also been suggested that stress hormones are used as

fuel (i.e., energy) during physical exertion.

The *distraction*, or *time-out*, *hypothesis* asserts that the anxiety-reducing effects of exercise are due to the distraction from one's normal routine (Bahrke and Morgan, 1978). Because the person is focused on the physical and mental demands of exercise, attention toward other issues, thoughts, or emotions unrelated to the present situation serves as a distractor or time-out from regular routines. Researchers contend that distraction from current life events only partially explains the mechanisms that reduce depression and anxiety due to exercise.

The *thermogenic hypothesis* reflects studies showing that elevated body temperature, a natural result of exercise, produces therapeutic benefits, such as reduced muscle tension and reduced anxiety. Apparently, a muscular relaxation response is triggered when the brain senses increased internal body temperature, which in turn reduces stress, tension, and anxiety (Petruzzello, Landers, and Salazar, 1993).

Finally, the *endorphin hypothesis*, which also explains the runner's high, reflects the well-known state of euphoria during or soon following aerobic activity. The exerciser's blood chemistry changes dramatically, partly due to an increase in hormones called *endorphins* (Hoffmann, 1997).

Anxiety and Exercise

Anxiety consists of feelings of threat or worry. It can either be acute (short term) or chronic (long term). According to the APA (2000), clinical anxiety is a form of mental illness that leads to changes in a person's thoughts and actions, occurs even without some initiating event, and leads to disproportionate and unmanageable responses. Anxiety is actually healthy, even potentially lifesaving, under certain conditions (e.g., crossing the street and looking both ways, walking carefully on snow or ice, competing cautiously against the opposing sport team). However, anxiety can also be a disorder and debilitating to normal thinking, quality of life, happiness, and general well-being.

Behavioral strategies that combat debilitating forms of anxiety have been studied extensively. Several meta-analyses have examined the results of many studies on the effects of exercise on both acute and chronic anxiety. The most extensive review of this literature, conducted by Petruzzello and colleagues (1991), found that exercise, particularly of an aerobic nature, markedly reduced both acute (state) and chronic (trait) types of anxiety. The forms of exercise included walking, jogging, running, swimming, cycling, and group aerobic classes. Measures of reduced anxiety included questionnaires (self-reports), muscular tension (electromyography), cardiovascular measurements (e.g., heart rate), and changes in the central nervous system (electroencephalogram, or brain wave activity). Changes in acute anxiety normally last two to four hours.

ORIENTATIONS, STYLES, AND EXERCISE ADHERENCE

Most authors in the health and exercise psychology literature do not differentiate between personality traits and other personal characteristics called *orientations* and *styles* (terms that are used interchangeably), but there are stark differences between the two. Personality traits are permanent, stable across situations, and partly a reflection of one's genetic predisposition, and therefore they are not subject to change. Orientations and styles, on the other hand, reflect common attitudes or a person's tendency to think or act in a predictable manner. The concepts of attributional style, coping style, and win orientation reflect predictable and persistent ways of thinking and acting under certain conditions. If, for instance, a person who demonstrates success or competence has an internal attributional style, the typical way the person explains success may be internal. That is, she may typically attribute the cause of her success as due to high effort or excellent skills, both internal explanations. Not taking responsibility for success or failure and perceiving the cause as something beyond the person's control reflects an external attributional style, at least for that particular situation (e.g., maintaining high fitness, improving performance on a given task, gaining excessive weight).

Orientations and styles also predict how people perceive the importance of a healthy lifestyle and to what they attribute their good or poor health. An internal disposition could reflect taking responsibility for one's excessive weight or poor fitness as due to poor dietary choices, excessive food intake, and lack of physical activity. Someone with an external disposition will be more likely to attribute weight gain to genetics or similarity to other family members, to not acknowledge there is a weight problem, or to believe that weight gain and consequent diseases (e.g., type 2 diabetes, high blood pressure, heart disease) are normal and part of the aging process. Other types of orientations and styles related to health behavior include self-control, self-awareness, and the interchangeable concepts of self-confidence and self-efficacy.

Self-Control

Self-control refers to the extent to which a person voluntarily and consciously creates, carries out, and maintains thoughts, emotions, and behaviors toward reaching desirable goals, even after encountering obstacles (Rosenbaum, 1990). Self-control behaviors are regulated by deliberate cognitive processes that are under the person's voluntary control. A good example of self-control in exercise settings is time management. Perhaps the primary reason people offer for not exercising is not having enough time (Sternfeld et al., 2009). People with high self-control plan their day and set aside time (i.e., day of the week, hour of the day, length of time) devoted to maintaining an exercise routine.

Self-control also means that the activity itself may be planned. For example, perhaps an exerciser who prefers the company of a friend during a workout plans to meet his friend at the exercise facility. Upon entering the facility, the individual has preplanned an hour devoted to various tasks that compose the exercise workout; specific routines are planned and carried out for the duration of the session, from entering to exiting the facility. The type of aerobic and resistance training may also be predetermined and executed in attempting to reach challenging goals. Presumably, the excuse of not having enough time now becomes having more time to do other things thanks to increased energy and vigor as a function of the workout. People with a high self-control orientation are more capable of carrying out preperformance and performance routines compared with their counterparts with low self-control (Faulkner et al., 2006). People with high self-control are schedule keepers and rarely waste time.

An important situational factor in developing an exercise habit is scheduling one's exercise sessions during the week. This requires good time management skills. Rather than saying, "I'll exercise when I get the time," restate that view with, "I will exercise at x times on the following days." A minimum of three times a week of intense exercise that expands one's fitness capacity and has a training effect (e.g., increased heart rate, increased muscular strength) is needed. However, finding opportunities to become physically active during the day (e.g., taking the stairs instead of the elevator, walking up or down the escalator, taking an evening or lunchtime walk) is also helpful for burning calories and managing weight.

Learned Resourcefulness

The pioneer writer and researcher in the literature on learned resourcefulness is Dr. Michael Rosenbaum (1990). He defined *learned resourcefulness* as "an acquired repertoire of behavioral and cognitive skills with which the person is able to regulate internal events such as emotions and cognitions that might otherwise interfere with the smooth execution of a target behavior" (p. xiv). High scorers on Rosenbaum's Self-Report Scale (Rosenbaum, 1990) are better able to

- tolerate physical discomfort,
- cope effectively with stress,
- succeed in weight-reduction programs,
- prevent or overcome feelings of helplessness,
- comply with medical and other health-related regimens,
- establish and maintain a relatively healthy lifestyle, and
- delay immediate gratification (e.g., binge eating) and understand the value of delayed gratification (e.g., exercising takes time, but the person receives more energy, better health, and improved performance quality).

In general, learned resourcefulness is particularly important in controlling negative thoughts and emotions while engendering desirable cognitive processes such as positive self-talk, optimism, self-motivation, and positive mood states. People high in learned resourcefulness are more confident; more likely to adopt an active lifestyle, including regular exercise; and less likely to engage in self-destructive behaviors (e.g., smoking, taking extreme risks). It is important to note that learned resourcefulness is not viewed as a personality trait. Instead, it is an orientation—a way of thinking that can be influenced through experience, counseling, and situational conditions.

Mental Toughness

Mental toughness is a disposition that represents the ability to reach and sustain high performance under pressure by expanding one's physical, mental, and emotional capacity (Connaughton, Hanton, and Jones, 2010). Mental toughness is learned, not inherited; it's an orientation. One common but false view of many athletes and coaches is that we are born with the right competitive instincts, and people who cannot handle failure lack the genetic predisposition to be mentally tough. The belief in a mental toughness gene is tempting because it absolves the person of taking responsibility for failure. However, the reality is that mental toughness can be taught, improved, and mastered. Exercisers need mental toughness to acknowledge their poor health and the need for physical activity, to withstand the challenges of physical exertion, to overcome physical fatigue, to continue to see the benefits of an exercise program, and to maintain exercise participation as a lifelong habit.

Mentally tough people are self-motivated and self-directed (their energy comes from internal sources; it is not forced from the outside); positive but realistic about handling adversity; in control of their emotions, especially in response to frustration and disappointment; and calm and relaxed under fire (rather than avoiding pressure, they are challenged by it). Mental toughness is also characterized by high energy, physical and mental readiness for action, a strong desire to succeed, relentlessness in the pursuit of challenging goals, superb concentration skills, self-confidence in the ability to perform well, and taking full responsibility for one's actions.

Self-Awareness

Think of self-awareness as the willingness to self-reflect, to engage introspectively, and to look at oneself through the eyes of others. This is not always easy to do, but others give us signals about their expectations and evaluations of us all the time, if we just take a good look. People react to us one way if they want our friendship and we have their respect. They react to us in a completely different way if they reject or disrespect us for whatever justified or unjustified reasons.

Self-awareness is an important component of health behavior because the ability to look inside and to be cognizant of our thoughts, emotions, and behaviors allows us to initiate steps for desirable change. If, for instance, we look in the mirror and see a person who is out of shape, overweight, and even unattractive, we can then begin the process of determining the reasons for our low energy, labored breathing, and general discomfort. Self-aware people also become more aware of the short-term costs and long-term consequences of their bad habits. They do not ignore their poor health and the negative habits that cause their current health status. This is why they are more likely to embrace support and opportunity to make lifelong changes that improve their health and happiness. They refuse to remain stuck in a self-destructive lifestyle. The challenges of self-awareness are addressed by Loehr and Schwartz (2003), who paraphrase John 32:8 from the Bible: "If the truth is to set us free, facing it cannot be a one-time event. Rather, it must become a practice. Like all of our 'muscles,' self-awareness withers from disuse and deepens when we push past our resistance to see more of the truth" (p. 163).

Self-awareness, then, is an orientation. We differ in our willingness to become introspective about who we are and what we need to do to become better. As Loehr and Schwartz (2003) contend, "We must persistently shed light on those aspects of ourselves that we prefer not to see in order to build our mental, emotional and spiritual capacity" (p. 163). The authors also agree, however, that self-awareness can be self-defeating and overwhelming, bringing out negative thoughts, feelings, and emotions if it is absorbed in too big a dose. The right amount and frequency of self-awareness provides sufficient information to keep us on track and to be used as a source of information about what we need to become healthier and happier. As the authors conclude, "Facing the most difficult truths in our lives is challenging but also liberating" (p. 163).

Self-Efficacy

Confidence is a person's general feeling, perception, or belief that she has the capability to be successful in performing a skill and meeting task demands. Self-efficacy combines confidence with self-expectations. *Self-efficacy*, often associated and used interchangeably with *self-confidence*, is defined by Feltz and Lirgg (2001) as "the belief one has in being able to execute a specific task successfully . . . to obtain a certain outcome" (p. 340). They further write, "Self-efficacy beliefs are not judgments about one's skills, objectively speaking, but rather are judgments of what one can accomplish with those skills" (p. 340). Thus, self-efficacy beliefs reflect a person's feelings not about what she can do but rather about what she has already done.

Self-efficacy is enormously important in an exercise setting and for changing and adhering to desirable, healthy behaviors. For example, people who experience self-doubt about their ability to join a fitness class and perform at least most of the exercises will be more likely to stop attending the class and either try some other form of exercise or return to their sedentary lifestyle. It is against human nature to continue participating in an activity in which we perceive our performance as incompetent or we fail to meet self-expectations or experience improved exercise performance and outcomes (e.g., better fitness). Therefore, building self-efficacy in an exercise setting bolsters the exercisers' perception that they are exercising properly, using correct technique, and improving performance. With respect to general health, clients will feel that following a certain set of routines will result or has resulted in superior health-related outcomes (e.g., more energy, positive mood, favorable results from medical tests). The objective of every worker in the health care industry, including fitness and nutrition coaches, is to provide instruction and positive feedback to build the person's self-efficacy about maintaining healthy habits.

Researchers have examined the link between self-efficacy and exercise behavior. Perhaps not surprising is the finding that as a person becomes more committed to an exercise habit, his self-efficacy improves. Self-efficacy is relatively low in the early stages of exercise, when a person is just beginning to develop an exercise routine or starting to make exercise a habit, and it increases dramatically as the person inserts exercise among his daily rituals. What is unknown is whether self-efficacy causes a person to adopt exercise as a lifestyle ritual or whether continued exercise increases self-efficacy. No doubt the two processes interact and self-efficacy is both the cause and the outcome of maintaining a regular exercise habit (Feltz and Lirgg, 2001; O'Leary, 1985).

BEHAVIORAL TENDENCIES

Exercisers have particular behavioral patterns that help them maintain participation and improve health and fitness. Unlike traits, orientations, and styles, behavioral characteristics are more easily learned and changed. An exercise consultant, for example, may suggest that the client initiate specific changes in certain protocol, either physically (e.g., avoid stretching before engaging in light aerobic activity) or mentally (e.g., use positive self-talk before lifting weights). Examples of behavioral characteristics include self-regulation, routines, prayer, and social support.

Self-Regulation

Self-regulation is typically defined as actions that occur when executing a task that allow performers to control or direct their activity through self-imposed rules or regulations. The goal of self-regulation is to adapt performance demands to varying circumstances, situations, or surroundings (Crews, Lochbaum, and Karoly, 2001).

To Zimmerman (1986), self-regulation consists of three subcomponents, each of which has implications in exercise settings. The *metacognitive* component consists of planning, organizing, self-instructing, self-monitoring, and self-evaluating at various stages during performance. The *motivational* component consists of performers perceiving themselves as competent, autonomous, and confident. Finally, the *behavioral* component reflects selecting, structuring, and creating environments that optimize goal-directed behavior—

that is, helping the client to achieve predetermined goals.

To use an exercise example, metacognitive self-regulation could include scheduling exercise sessions for the week; preparing for exercising that day by bringing appropriate clothing and shoes for the anticipated workout; ensuring the proper exercise skills by hiring a personal trainer, reading, or observing others; monitoring exercise intensity, physical fatigue levels, thirst, and performance goals; and finally, assessing performance quality and general well-being. In the motivational component, the person makes self-assessments that reflect competence (e.g., "I am performing the exercise correctly"), the skills needed to complete each task independent of instruction, and confidence or self-efficacy (e.g., "I feel good and have met my fitness goals"). And the behavioral component could consist of exercising at a specific location (e.g., nearby fitness club), in a given environment (e.g., weight room), under specific conditions (e.g., early in the morning before the facility gets crowded), using specific equipment (e.g., weights, jogging track), and obtaining instruction if needed (e.g., getting help from a personal trainer) to achieve personal goals. Keeping records of performance outcomes is also part of self-regulation as a reminder of current fitness capability, detection of performance improvement, and source of personal motivation and competence.

Sadly, it is not uncommon to drop the ball when it comes to self-regulation. Self-regulation is based on the premise that the person is both self-motivated and capable of engaging independently in tasks that will lead to achieving goal-directed performance outcomes. If, for instance, we brush our teeth and floss regu-

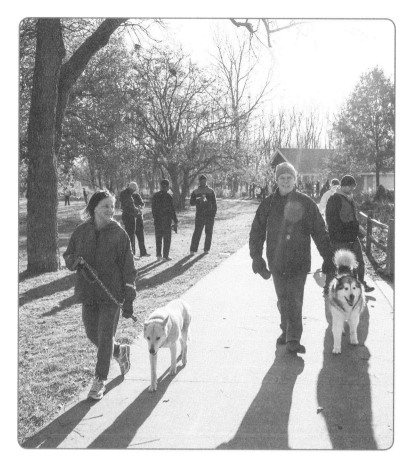

An exercise consultant may suggest making behavior changes, such as planning daily walks, and enlisting social support for longer and more frequent outings.

larly, we will be far less likely to suffer from dental and periodontal disease than if we did not perform these tasks. If an athlete engages in the proper training regimen and practices the requisite sport skills, performance success under competitive conditions is far more likely than if practice and other game preparation are neglected. Self-regulation failure means that a person does not carry out the cognitive and behavioral strategies that are necessary for task success, and goals are not met.

Examples of self-regulation failure related to health behavior abound in our culture. Dentists tell us to floss our teeth, health professionals criticize the bad habits of not eating breakfast and of overeating (especially near bedtime), and we all know the benefits of regular exercise and other forms of physical activity. And yet many of us fail with these preferred habits. Self-regulation means making a conscious decision to develop habits that have desirable outcomes, including improved health, more energy, slower aging, improved mood, and reduced risk of mental illness. Although everyone self-regulates certain behavior patterns, sometimes those behaviors are self-destructive and unhealthy.

In their temporal self-regulation theory, Hall and Fong (2007) attempt to answer the question of why human behavior is often maladaptive, self-defeating, or dysfunctional. Self-regulation failure is associated with a person's conclusion that short-term benefits of negative, unhealthy habits outweigh long-term consequences of these same dysfunctional habits. At the same time, the costs of unhealthy actions are often long-term, with presenting disease and other health problems several years away. This situation, therefore, leads to a lack of urgency about preventing problems that take years to become life-threatening diseases. At the same time, the authors assert that we live in a culture that either rewards or reflects the need for immediate gratification, while delayed gratification is less common. This tendency is seen when a person does not detect rapid results from a fitness program (e.g., lack of significant weight loss, no noticeable change in fitness level, similar difficulty with physical exertion). Self-regulation failure represents one of the biggest challenges facing researchers and practitioners of health behavior change.

Routines

All of us engage in behavioral routines during almost every waking hour. *Routines* are typically defined as thoughts and actions that are carried out almost automatically during the day. At first, before these thoughts and actions become routines, the person repeatedly plans and carries out the thought or action in a conscious manner, particularly within the context of a specific time frame (e.g., "Each evening before bedtime I will make sure my exercise clothing is prepared and placed in my gym bag"), location (e.g., "My gym bag will be located near the door on my way out"), and other situational conditions (e.g., "I will have a backup supply of clean workout clothes, toiletries, and a clean towel available before leaving the house"). Over time and with repetition, these planned, conscious thoughts and actions become second nature (Loehr and Schwartz, 2003). In other words, at first they are highly cognitive (i.e., thought producing), but with time, they become virtually automatic and ritualized.

Routines serve many valuable purposes, including reducing the amount of energy and time spent thinking (e.g., decision making and problem solving) before and during health-related activities such as exercise, maintaining a healthy diet, and receiving adequate sleep (Anshel, 2012). Routines also help exercisers maintain emotional control, especially related to preexercise thoughts (e.g., positive self-talk, psyching up). The development of routines is a critical element in adhering to healthy habits.

SUMMARY

It is apparent that numerous personal factors—traits, orientations and styles, and behavioral tendencies—influence a person's decision to initiate and maintain an exercise program. The primary aim of workers in the health care industry is to promote a healthy lifestyle and to convince their clients or patients to understand the huge short-term and long-term benefits that accrue from engaging in exercise and making healthy choices about food intake and daily physical activity. The factors outlined in this chapter strongly influence people's actions to live a healthy life. One of the most common enemies of health behavior change is denial, or the failure to recognize there is a problem with one's daily routines that eventually will lead to severe consequences. People have to be willing to acknowledge their deepest values (e.g., health, family, character, faith, happiness) and to live their lives consistent with those values.

STUDENT ACTIVITY

State Anxiety Scale—Exercise

Researchers have found that exercise reduces state anxiety and elevates mood. People tend to feel better after exercise, according to an extensive review of the literature and a meta-analysis—a synthesis of results from 124 previous studies—by Petruzzello and his colleagues (1991). In particular, the researchers concluded that aerobic (cardiorespiratory) exercise that was maintained for at least 20 minutes, including interval training consisting of alternating work–rest bouts, improved participants' moods and reduce state (situational) anxiety. Let's test the theory in this mini experiment.

1. Try to conduct this task with a volunteer (who is willing to follow your instructions but is not a personal acquaintance) or with a small group.

2. Meet at a specific location just before you begin engaging in an aerobic form of exercise. Examples of aerobic work include riding stationary bicycles, walking on a treadmill, walking briskly, and jogging.

3. Immediately before exercising, complete the State Anxiety Scale—Exercise (SAS-E) that was generated for this chapter. This inventory was adapted from the Illinois State Self-Evaluation Questionnaire authored by Martens, Vealey, and Burton (1990) that has been used to measure state anxiety in sport settings (see the inventory in form 5.1).

4. Engage in your full aerobic workout. The workout should result in an increased heart rate. For novice exercisers and those who are less fit,

   • engage in interval training in which you work vigorously for several minutes (start slowly, perhaps 2-3 minutes) and then reduce your work intensity for 30 to 60 seconds (to reduce heart rate), and

   • engage in another brief but vigorous bout of exercise again followed by a less intense recovery period.

5. If you feel comfortable increasing the length of your work bout to, let's say, 5 minutes instead of 2 or 3, go ahead. Try to maintain several work–rest intervals (e.g., jog–walk, or high intense–low intense) over at least 20 minutes. Even if you have to slow down later due to physical fatigue, try to stay active for at least this length of time.

6. Retake the SAS-E. Did you notice a decrease in the final score? Decreased scores represent reduced state anxiety. Although this is not a formal study, it is possible that reduced scores from pre- to postexercise indicate that aerobic exercise was at least partly responsible for reduced state anxiety.

FORM 5.1   STATE ANXIETY SCALE—EXERCISE (SAS-E)

Here are items that describe feelings before and after engaging in cardiorespiratory exercise. Next to each statement, circle the number for each item, ranging from not at all to very true, that best describes your feelings right now. Add both sets of numbers (from before and after exercising). Your state anxiety has been reduced if the postexercise number is *higher* than the preexercise number.

1	2	3	4	5
Not at all	Low	Moderate	True	Very true

1. I feel at ease.	1	2	3	4	5
2. I feel confident in my exercise ability.	1	2	3	4	5
3. I have no self-doubts about giving 100% to my exercise effort.	1	2	3	4	5
4. I feel excited.	1	2	3	4	5
5. I feel comfortable I will be able to reach my exercise goals.	1	2	3	4	5
6. I can ignore my surroundings and focus on the exercise task at hand.	1	2	3	4	5
7. I feel enthusiastic.	1	2	3	4	5
8. I feel psyched up.	1	2	3	4	5
9. I do not worry about who is watching me.	1	2	3	4	5
10. I feel content.	1	2	3	4	5

Total: _____

From M. Anshel, 2014, *Applied Health Fitness Psychology*. (Champaign, IL: Human Kinetics).

REFERENCES

American Psychiatric Association (APA). (2000). *Diagnostic and statistical manual of mental disorders* (4th ed.). Washington, DC: Author.

Anshel, M.H. (2006). *Applied exercise psychology: A practitioner's guide to improving client health and exercise.* New York: Springer.

Anshel, M.H. (2012). *Sport psychology: From theory to practice* (5th ed.). San Francisco: Benjamin-Cummings.

Bahrke, M.S., and Morgan, W.P. (1978). Anxiety reduction following exercise and meditation. *Cognitive Therapy and Research, 4,* 323-333.

Bandura, A. (1997). *Self-efficacy: The exercise of control.* New York: Freeman.

Biddle, S.J.H., Gorely, T., and Stensel, D.J. (2004). Health-enhancing physical activity and sedentary behaviour in children and adolescents. *Journal of Sports Sciences, 22,* 679-701.

Buckworth, J., and Dishman, R.K. (2002). *Exercise psychology.* Champaign, IL: Human Kinetics.

Cattell, R.B. (1960). Some psychological correlates of physical fitness and physique. In S.C. Staley (Ed.), *Exercise and fitness* (pp. 138-151). Chicago: Athletic Institute.

Cloninger, C.R. (2003). Completing the psychobiological architecture of human personality development: Temperament, character, and coherence. In U.M. Staudinger and U.E.R. Lindenberger (Eds.), *Understanding human development: Dialogues with lifespan psychology* (pp. 159-182). Boston: Kluwer Academic.

Connaughton, D., Hanton, S., and Jones, G. (2010). The development and maintenance of mental toughness in the world's best performers. *Sport Psychologist, 24,* 168-193.

Crews, D.J., Lochbaum, M.R., and Karoly, P. (2001). Self-regulation: Concepts, methods, and strategies in sport and exercise (pp. 566-581). In R.N. Singer, H.A. Hausenblas, and C.M. Janelle (Eds.), *Handbook of sport psychology* (2nd ed.). New York: Wiley.

Faulkner, G., Taylor, A., Ferrence, R., Urban, S., and Selby, P. (2006). Exercise science and the development of evidence-based practice: A "better practices" framework. *European Journal of Sport Sciences, 6*, 117-126.

Feltz, D.L., and Lirgg, C.D. (2001). Self-efficacy beliefs of athletes, teams, and coaches. In R.N. Singer, H.A. Hausenblas, and C.M. Janelle (Eds.), *Handbook of sport psychology* (2nd ed., pp. 340-361). New York: Wiley.

Hall, P.A., and Fong, G.T. (2007). Temporal self-regulation theory: A model for individual health behavior. *Health Psychology Review, 1*, 6-52.

Heaton, P.C., and Frede, S.M. (2003). Patients' need for more counseling on diet, exercise, and smoking cessation: Results from the National Ambulatory Medical Care Survey. *Journal of the American Pharmacists Association, 46*, 364-369.

Hoffmann, P. (1997). The endorphin hypothesis. In W.P. Morgan (Ed.), *Physical activity and mental health* (pp. 163-177). New York: Taylor and Francis.

Leith, L. (1998). *Exercising your way to better mental health.* Morgantown, WV: Fitness Information Technology.

Loehr, J., and Schwartz, T. (2003). *The power of full engagement: Managing energy, not time, is the key to high performance and personal renewal.* New York: The Free Press.

Lox, C.L., Martin, K.A., and Petruzzello, S.J. (2010). *The psychology of exercise: Integrating theory and practice* (3rd ed.). Scottsdale, AZ: Holcomb Hathaway.

Martens, R., Vealey, R.S., and Burton, D. (1990). *Competitive anxiety in sport.* Champaign, IL: Human Kinetics.

Martin Ginis, K.A., and Mack, D. (2012). Understanding exercise behavior: A self-presentational perspective. In G.C. Roberts and D.C. Treasure (Eds.), *Advances in motivation in sport and exercise* (pp. 327-355). Champaign, IL: Human Kinetics.

McCrae, R.R., and John, O.P. (1992). An introduction to the five-factor model and its applications. *Journal of Personality, 60*, 175-215.

Morgan, W.P. (1980). The trait psychology controversy. *Research Quarterly for Exercise and Sport, 51*, 50-76.

O'Leary, A. (1985). Self-efficacy and health. *Behavior Therapy and Research, 23*, 437-452.

Petruzzello, S.J., Landers, D.M., Hatfield, B., Kubitz, K.A., and Salazar, W. (1991). A meta-analysis on the anxiety-reducing effects of acute and chronic exercise: Outcomes and mechanisms. *Sports Medicine, 11*, 143-182.

Petruzzello, S.J., Landers, D.M., and Salazar, W. (1993). Exercise and anxiety reduction: Examination of temperature as an explanation for affective change. *Journal of Sport and Exercise Psychology, 15*, 63-76.

Rhodes, R.E., and Smith, N.E.I. (2006). Personality correlates of physical activity: A review and meta-analysis. *British Journal of Sports Medicine, 40*, 958-965.

Rosenbaum, M. (1990). *Learned resourcefulness on coping skills, self-control behavior, and adaptive behavior.* New York: Springer.

Stathopoulou, G., and Powers, M.B. (2006). Exercise interventions for mental health: A quantitative and qualitative review. *Clinical Psychology: Science and Practice, 13*, 179-193.

Sternfeld, B., Block, C., Quesenberry, C.P., Block, T., Husson, G., et al. (2009). Improving diet and physical activity with ALIVE: A worksite randomized trial. *American Journal of Preventive Medicine, 36*, 475-483.

Wallace, J.P., Raglin, J.S., and Jastremski, C.A. (1995). Twelve-month adherence of adults who joined a fitness program with a spouse vs. without a spouse. *Journal of Sports Medicine and Physical Fitness, 35*, 206-213.

Zimmerman, B.J. (1986). Becoming a self-regulated learner: Which are the key subprocesses? *Contemporary Educational Psychology, 11*, 307-313.

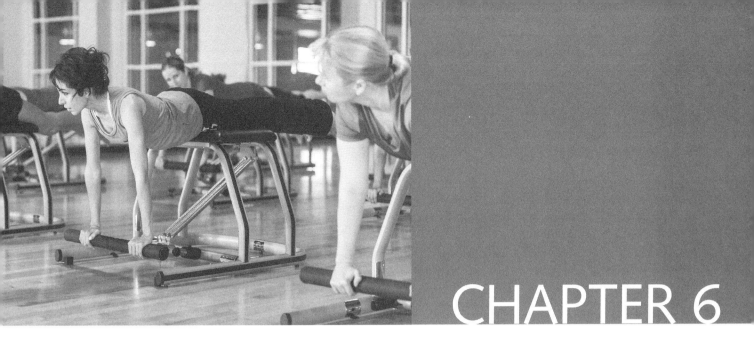

Situational and Environmental Factors

> *We all have dreams. But in order to make dreams come into reality, it takes an awful lot of determination, dedication, self-discipline, and effort.*
>
> Jesse Owens (1913-1980), Olympic gold medalist

CHAPTER OBJECTIVES

After reading this chapter, you should be able to:

- explain the strong influence of situational factors and environmental factors on the promotion of physical activity in general and exercise in particular, and

- understand and apply the role of the person's social environment in developing a healthy lifestyle.

People do not behave in a vacuum; they are exposed to numerous situational factors (e.g., the presence of others, competitive versus noncompetitive situations) and environmental conditions (e.g., exercising in a group setting versus alone or at a fitness club versus at home) that can strongly influence their actions that directly affect health and well-being. This chapter addresses some of the situational and environmental factors that influence a person's desire to begin and maintain an exercise habit and to engage in other healthy habits as well. These external factors include social support, coaching, and a combination of other situational and environmental factors that promote a physically active and generally healthy lifestyle.

SOCIAL SUPPORT OF EXERCISE HABITS

Extensive research has been done on the influence of support from others as part of an exercise habit. *Social support* refers to the degree of perceived physical, mental, or emotional assistance someone receives from other people (Wills and Shinar, 2000). Formal definitions of social support are absent from the literature; however, researchers view social support in two categories, primary (i.e., direct) and secondary (i.e., indirect). An example of primary social support in an exercise setting is a friend who exercises with the person receiving support. Secondary social support might consist of communicating support for another person's exercise habits, recognizing her efforts, and urging her to continue. Researchers in various studies have defined social support in a variety of ways using both primary and secondary criteria.

Another criterion of social support is the amount and type of support provided. The number of people supporting the exerciser is one standard; for example, friends, family, work colleagues, health care providers, fitness class participants, and mental health professionals all are sources of support to the exerciser. Social support has been called "probably the most important type of social influence in exercise and other physical activity settings" (Lox, Martin, and Petruzzello, 2010, p. 102). Providing support to others and being supported by others is a common behavioral tendency among regular exercisers, and it is of particular importance among novices.

Advanced exercisers, who have firmly established an exercise habit as part of their lifestyle, are far less likely to need social support than the novice exerciser who lacks the experience, familiarity, knowledge base, and psychological readiness to engage in and enjoy regularly scheduled exercise or some other form of physical activity. The novice exerciser has much greater need to be supported in this new and sometimes uncomfortable undertaking. Social support has been found to be a crucial component of starting and especially maintaining an exercise program. The results of previous studies indicate positive outcomes from an exercise habit that includes social support. Perhaps Wills and Shinar (2000) have provided the most comprehensive list of forms of social support, several of which are typical of exercisers. Table 6.1 summarizes the various types of social support.

Instrumental support involves providing tangible and hands-on support for another person's exercise regimen. For instance, the fitness coach or other health staff member provides on-site, direct assistance to the exerciser. Examples include fitness testing and prescription, exercise instruction, individual consulting, counseling by mental health professionals, spotting a weightlifter, and other types of direct involvement that improve the exerciser's motivation, confidence, and encouragement while reducing anxiety and other undesirable thoughts and emotions. Exercising with another person and providing the exerciser with transportation to the workout are other examples.

Emotional support consists of encouraging others to exercise or maintain a more active lifestyle through physical activity; praising others for their effort, commitment, and accomplishments; and showing empathy

Table 6.1 Forms of Social Support in Exercise and Health Settings

Type of support	Description	Example 1	Example 2
Instrumental support	Person exercises with someone else.	Fitness coach exercises with or monitors client's efforts or provides and interprets fitness test results.	Person receives a gift fitness club membership; employer gives time off for exercise.
Emotional support	Health expert praises, encourages, or provides feedback to exerciser to increase or maintain an active lifestyle.	Family member praises person (e.g., "Keep up the good work," "You're looking terrific since you started exercising").	Health professional provides test results and suggests ways to improve test scores.
Informational support	Medical or health practitioner provides information.	Person receives health-related advice or instruction from an expert or coach.	Person purchases written or audiovisual material that motivates the person to improve healthy habits.
Companionship support	Person exercises with others (family, friends, coach).	Person exercises with a friend.	Fitness coach monitors the person's exercise technique.
Validation support	Person compares self with others on a particular characteristic.	"I'm doing pretty well compared with that person and my earlier performance."	"I can almost keep up with the exercise leader."

toward others for their attempts to reach goals and overcome discomfort to stay active. Emotional support can also be derived from people who provide strong incentives to maintain an exercise habit.

Two types of people who can provide emotional support but are often ignored by health consultants, mental health professionals, and beginning exercisers themselves are physicians and religious leaders. People in both of these roles have tremendous credibility as sources of information (e.g., medical literature) and inspiration (e.g., scripture and other religious texts). Physicians have access to their patients' medical records and can use test scores (e.g., undesirable cholesterol, high blood pressure) as an incentive for their patients to engage in regular exercise as a means to improve these scores. Religious leaders can reveal the ways that a person of faith lives a life consistent with the tenets of the religion by attaining better health and energy through a proper regimen of physical activity and nutrition. People of faith want to be better managers of their temple (i.e., body) and to overcome spiritual complacency, and the person with the most credibility in this area is the person's religious leader.

Anyone who offers positive, encouraging, motivational, and instructional input to the exerciser is providing emotional forms of social support. Two types of information feedback are almost always possible and highly motivational, no matter how early in the exercise program—giving 100% effort and showing improvement. Anyone at any level of fitness or body weight can give top effort, and that has to be recognized. Improvement is also highly likely if the person is serious about his commitment to exercise. Coaches must find something they can observe to show that the client has improved.

Informational support concerns obtaining coaching, written materials, or health-related information from a medical practitioner that motivates the exerciser to continue the program. Even mental health practitioners provide emotional support during counseling sessions that provides clients with optimism and helps them recognize improvements in their self-esteem and reductions in anxiety or other undesirable states of mind. Friends and family members in particular can remark to the exerciser something as simple as, "You look terrific." Information, whether its purpose is to educate or to provide feedback, is a highly motivational source of support. Exercisers, especially novices, are in great need of information to improve their exercise technique, better prepare themselves for the exercise session, exercise more comfortably, and incorporate new information into their lifestyle and exercise sessions. Positive feedback has high motivational value.

Companionship support comes from exercising with friends, family members, or groups. Understandably, some people prefer to exercise alone and not have to communicate with anyone, and that's fine. Others, however, find that the companionship of other exercisers uplifts them, distracts them from the effort of working out, and helps them adjust to exercising in a public facility in the presence of strangers. Novice exercisers are in far greater need of exercise partners or groups than their fitter counterparts. However, as mentioned, some people prefer to exercise alone, so this is a highly subjective issue. If people want to exercise with a partner, they can ask a friend or family member, join a fitness class, or exercise with others in a fitness facility.

Another form of social support, called *validation*, is similar to a concept in social and sport psychology called *social comparison processes*. This form of social support involves exercisers comparing themselves with others to determine their current fitness status, appearance, or improvement. Comparing oneself with others on a particular characteristic serves to affirm, or validate, their self-appraisal. An example of self-talk might be, "I'm doing pretty well compared with that person" or "If they can do it, so can I." This is also why it can be so difficult for obese family members or people from particular cultures to change their unhealthy habits; it is perceived as normal to be overweight or obese based on norms that nurture physical inactivity and overeating.

Are you fitter or exhibiting other desirable personal changes over time as compared with others? People of all ages, especially children who want to determine their own level of competence, compare their current status with that of others. Validation also includes

exercising with people of a similar health status (e.g., heart patients, obese exercisers, people in rehabilitation), fitness level (e.g., introductory fitness courses), age (e.g., exercise for senior citizens), or gender (e.g., women's fitness classes).

FITNESS COACHING FOR EXERCISE PARTICIPATION

One of the most powerful situational factors that influence exercise participation, particularly in the early stages of developing an exercise habit, is fitness coaching. Based on their extensive review of related literature, Martin Ginis and Mack (2012) assert that "the fitness leader is often cited as the single most important determinant of an exerciser's motivation to continue in an exercise program" (p. 349). A *fitness coach*, also often called a *personal trainer*, is a person with knowledge of proper exercise testing, exercise technique, and fitness training who provides instruction and guidance to others for the purpose of reaching fitness-related goals (Anshel, 2006). A fitness coach, therefore, has demonstrated mastery of the exercise science literature and applies that knowledge in helping others improve various forms of fitness. Fitness coaching is a reflection of that knowledge; good fitness coaches are good teachers.

Improving fitness is a science; there is a right way and a wrong way to exercise and to improve fitness. Due in part to our sedentary lifestyle, we pay a steep price for trying to get back in shape and improve our fitness. In fact, for many people, improving fitness and developing a more active lifestyle is simply too challenging to do on their own. This is why coaching is so important in the process of reversing self-destructive habits and replacing them with healthier, more desirable routines.

Without question, most people who want to begin or maintain an exercise program and improve their fitness will almost always benefit from fitness coaching to help them get

CHARACTERISTICS OF A HIGH-QUALITY FITNESS COACH

Fitness coaching is both an art and a science. It's an art with respect to communicating well, leading and modeling exercises in both group and individual settings, providing motivation and incentive to exercisers of all fitness levels, and showing enthusiasm for improving the health and well-being of others. But effective fitness coaching is also a science. The fitness coach needs to know and communicate proper exercise technique, provide valid fitness testing, and correctly interpret test results. Here is a list of the qualifications of high-quality fitness coaches based on an overview of the literature.

- *Physical appearance.* Fitness coaches should reflect good health by maintaining proper body weight and fitness and also by simply looking healthy. An overweight, unfit personal trainer lacks credibility with clients and may not be taken seriously. The fitness coach must appear tidy, clean, and appealing to clients, who will likely view the coach as someone they aspire to be like. Well-kept hair, nails, teeth, and general cleanliness (no body odor) are also expected in building a relationship of trust and respect.

- *Healthy habits.* Excessive alcohol, tobacco, and drug use, as well as other unhealthy habits, must be avoided. Getting proper sleep and maintaining healthy dietary habits will improve the coach's energy.

- *Knowledge.* The fitness coach must demonstrate mastery of the exercise literature. This includes knowing up-to-date information reported in recent research journals or textbooks about fitness techniques. Fitness coaches should have obtained a university degree in this area or have successfully completed a nationally recognized certification program that indicates mastery of requisite knowledge related to all forms of fitness. Issues related to continuous versus interval training, exercise for special populations, and coaching exercisers at various fitness levels requires mastery of a unique segment of the literature.

- *Skills for working with special populations.* Exercise coaches will be asked to assist people with unique characteristics and needs in improving their health and fitness. Example of special needs populations include pregnant women and people with various diseases and conditions, such as diabetes, cancer, depression, anxiety, asthma, menopause, and heart or pulmonary disease. Specific age groups also have unique needs, including children, adolescents, and the elderly.

- *Communication skills.* Fitness knowledge has little meaning if coaches are unable to effectively communicate their knowledge and instruct clients on proper exercise techniques and programs. This is referred to as having *pedagogical skills*, and it means that the fitness coach is able to effectively teach exercise techniques, and clients can understand and carry out their instructions to improve their fitness.

- *Personal skills.* Do fitness coaches demonstrate passion about their role in helping others? Are they compassionate about making a difference in their clients' lives? This area concerns the coach's ability to consistently appear and act professional and to be passionate about improving the health and fitness of others.

- *Administration and organization skills.* High-quality fitness coaches keep accurate and detailed records of their clients' beginning fitness status, current status, test scores, exercise progress, and special needs or desires (e.g., exercising on a certain day or at a certain time, working with a male or female coach, avoiding the use of particular exercises or equipment, having injured or uncomfortable body parts). In-depth records of each client are highly desirable.

- *Skills for leading exercise sessions.* Many fitness coaches will be asked to lead group exercise sessions, sometimes to music. They will also be asked to coach small groups of exercisers. Each person will have unique exercise needs and require special attention, which good coaches are capable of offering. Leading group classes of any type is a skill that requires far more than the instructor's high level of fitness and the use of motivational techniques. Instructors should participate in as many group exercise classes as possible to become familiar with the ways other instructors carry out this important responsibility.

- *Mental skills (cognitive strategies).* Fitness coaches need to have mastery of the exercise psychology literature that includes the use of mental skills to improve exercise performance (see chapter 9). Strategies such as positive self-talk, psyching up, visualization, association, and dissociation may be used to improve the participant's emotions and thought processes to facilitate exercise performance. As the term indicates, *mental* skills are not directly observable; they consist of specific thought content that influences emotion, cognitive processing, and ultimately, exercise performance.

- *Behavioral strategies.* Unlike cognitive strategies, behavioral strategies are directly observable. They consist of actions that are intended to facilitate exercise performance or improve fitness. Examples include goal setting, use of music, self-monitoring checklists, and social support (see chapter 9 for an in-depth discussion). Setting goals, in particular, is primarily a science; there are right ways and wrong ways to set goals, and the fitness coach needs to know this literature.

- *Familiarity with related literature and practice.* Though fitness coaches should not claim to be experts in multiple fields of study and practice (unless they have acquired the appropriate credentials), good fitness coaches know something about diet and nutrition, ways in which food intake can improve energy, exercises for injured patients or for people involved in physical rehabilitation programs, and even signs of mental health issues, such as depression, anxiety, low self-esteem, and vast mood swings, each of which could result in referral to a mental health professional. Coaches should not claim similar expertise as registered dietitians, medical practitioners, or mental health professionals.

Clearly, fitness coaching is a profession that requires mastery of several bodies of literature, in addition to having excellent communication and personal skills to help meet the challenge of improving clients' health, energy, well-being, and quality of life. Peoples' lives are depending on high-quality fitness coaching.

started. Effective fitness coaching consists of any or all of the following:

- Pretesting strength and aerobic fitness to obtain scores for comparison with posttest scores after a certain length of time, such as three to six months, to detect changes in fitness
- Providing clients with an exercise prescription for the next few months
- Helping clients set and attain short-term (within three months) and long-term (after three months) goals that indicate improved fitness
- Providing instruction on proper exercise techniques
- Helping clients gain the self-motivation to persist in the program and not give up
- Holding clients accountable for attending exercise sessions regularly and adhering to the program

Coaches can also supply the client's physician and insurance company with fitness and attendance data. Coaches in general provide a powerful source of support and should be incorporated into the initial phase of the client's exercise habit.

Coaching to promote fitness is only one of several types of coaching that promote health, performance, and well-being. Other types of coaching include the following:

- Nutrition coaching
- Sport coaching
- Mental skills coaching
- Life skills coaching
- Executive coaching
- Performance coaching

SITUATIONAL FACTORS THAT PROMOTE PHYSICAL ACTIVITY

In addition to the influence of personal characteristics, such as motivation, personality, anxiety, body image, and confidence (see chapter 5), there are situational factors that influence the decision to initiate and maintain an exercise habit. Examples of situational factors include the availability of an exercise facility and equipment; time management for scheduling exercise sessions; participation in fitness classes; availability of fitness coaching; financial resources for purchasing home fitness equipment, proper exercise footwear, and clothing; transportation to exercise facilities; closeness of the exercise facility to home or work; an environment that is compatible with engaging in physical activity (e.g., safety and low traffic volume for walking in the neighborhood, availability of a sidewalk or jogging path); availability of written materials to learn more about exercise techniques, nutrition, and ways to maintain a healthy lifestyle; and job incentives that promote healthy behaviors such as reduced health insurance costs, health-related gifts, complimentary or reduced fitness club membership costs, or free t-shirts.

An important strategy that counters the number one reason for not exercising—not having enough time—is finding an exercise facility and equipment that are readily accessible. A ventilated, temperature-controlled exercise room filled with proper fitness equipment and located inside one's place of employment or near one's home will far more likely lead to a regular exercise routine than the absence of these facilities. One of the strongest sources of social support in the fitness industry is participation in group exercise classes. Although some people are intimidated by exercising in the presence of others and trying to keep up with a highly fit instructor, others consider the group environment enjoyable and a distraction from the boredom of exercising alone. Fitness clubs schedule group classes during the day and night.

Researchers have found that engaging in regular exercise at a fitness facility is far more likely if the facility is located not more than 3 miles (5 km) from the person's home, place of employment, or travel between home and work. This is perhaps one reason why having a fitness coach and exercise equipment in the work environment is a strong source of developing an exercise habit (Howley and Franks, 2007). For various reasons, some people do not have transportation to an exercise facility. This is especially true for people who are older or physically impaired. Clearly, one facilitating factor of engaging in regular exercise is the availability of transportation to the exercise venue, and a primary reason for nonadherence to exercise programs is the lack of transportation (Chenoweth, 2011).

Exercise adherence using home equipment is not promising, with at least 50% of novice exercisers no longer using their home equipment within six months (Chenoweth, 2002). Perhaps this is due to the lack of instruction; absence of others (i.e., observers) to create a more pleasant environment and improved

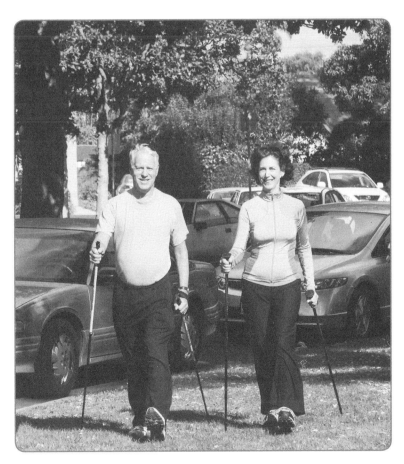

A safe, low-traffic neighborhood with parks or walking paths promotes exercise.

exercise performance, a concept from the sport psychology literature called *social facilitation* (Anshel, 2012); lack of proper instruction; boredom; or the fact that home is usually associated with relaxation and recovery rather than hard physical exertion. It is essential that home exercise equipment be accompanied by knowledge about how to use the equipment correctly and good time management skills for establishing scheduled exercise routines (Mackinnon, Ritchie, Hooper, and Abernethy, 2003).

Proper fitness and nutrition to maintain good health and energy is a science. As with any form of science, there is considerable knowledge about the dos and don'ts of exercise and dietary intake. The availability of fitness and nutritional coaches are strong situational factors that influence adherence to healthy habits. As discussed earlier, fitness coaches, preferably certified by a national organization, serve many important functions. These include helping others learn exercise techniques, providing fitness tests, improving health and fitness, avoiding injury, maintaining exercise motivation, and developing positive attitudes toward an active lifestyle. The end result is that clients develop and adhere to a long-term exercise habit. Nutrition coaches, on the other hand, help others eat strategically so that food intake is pleasant and promotes good health and energy. They also avoid artificial diets that have a relatively brief life span. Fitness and nutrition coaches may provide clients with information on health-related topics in the form of written materials, lectures, books, magazine subscriptions, and classes (Booth et al., 1992).

ENVIRONMENTAL FACTORS THAT PROMOTE PHYSICAL ACTIVITY

There are numerous ways in which the environment, including neighborhoods, roads, jogging and biking paths, and parks, can be constructed to enhance an active lifestyle. Some neighborhoods have more space for parks and physical activities such as bicycling,

jogging, and walking. In addition, neighborhoods with less traffic volume promote more daily physical activity than neighborhoods that are more congested and allow their residents less access to physical activity. These are essential features of the social-ecological models of friendly environments that promote physical activity among residents (McLeroy, Bibeau, Steckler, and Glanz, 1988).

Social-ecological models for health and physical activity, first developed by Bronfenbrenner (1989), acknowledge that several environmental factors that are beyond the person's control may influence the decision to engage in regular exercise (see figure 6.1). Although the individual is primarily responsible for the decision to exercise, several environmental conditions also play an important part in maintaining an active lifestyle. Health care professionals need to incorporate these external conditions when assisting clients to develop a healthy lifestyle action plan. Examples of social-ecological conditions favorable to an active lifestyle include availability of public transportation to activity venues; fitness equipment and facilities; partners or groups; paths for walking, jogging, or biking; parks and other recreational areas; lighting for evening outdoor activities; and sport and recreational programs, all in areas considered safe and accessible. These conditions are more integrated into some cultures (e.g., Scandinavian countries such as Sweden, Norway, Denmark, and Finland) than others. From a personal perspective, in Sweden I witnessed lighted outdoor jogging and cross-country skiing paths in local parks and biking paths along streets in most towns and cities. Elderly men and women were biking as a form of transportation. Physical activity was heavily integrated into daily lifestyle and culture.

Researchers have studied the role of geographical factors that might promote physical activity and have concluded that neighborhood planning can influence the activity level of residents. According to their review of research in this area, Humpel, Owen, and Leslie (2002) concluded that availability of sidewalks, parks, and jogging paths has been

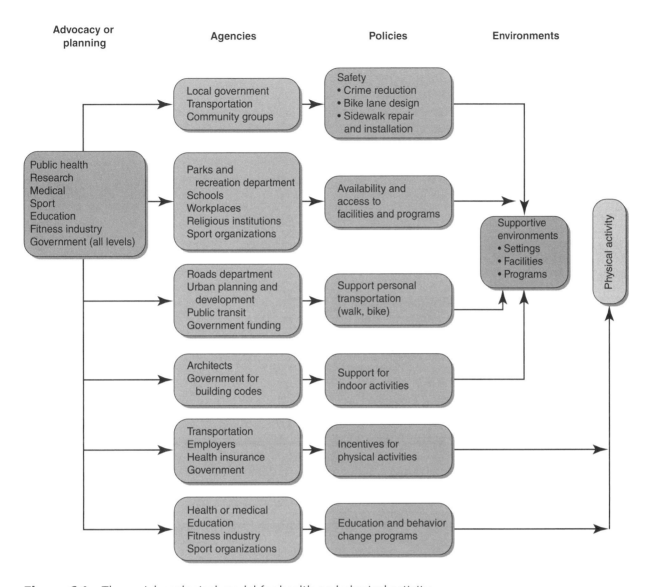

Figure 6.1 The social-ecological model for health and physical activity.

Adapted from *American Journal of Preventive Medicine,* Vol. 15, J.F. Sallis, A. Bauman, and M. Pratt, "Environmental and policy interventions to promote physical activity," pg. 388. Copyright 1998, with permission from Elsevier Science.

shown to result in superior health outcomes. Thus, physical activity rates increase when community residents perceive opportunities and accessibility to environmental features such as walking, jogging, and biking paths and the presence of green and recreational space.

In one study, for instance, Maddison and colleagues (2009) examined the influence of the physical and perceived environment (e.g., walkability, access to physical activity facilities) on physical activity patterns within the home and in the community among adoles-

cents aged 12 to 17 years. Physical activity was assessed using the ActiGraph accelerometer and the Physical Activity Questionnaire for Adolescents (PAQ-A). The results showed that perceptions of an active environment and actual activity level were both higher in response to more environmental opportunities to be physically active within the home and in the community. The researchers concluded that the number of pieces of exercise equipment in the home was associated with higher self-reported physical activity among

According to the social-ecological model, physical activity will increase if local governments, businesses, and agencies develop policies that provide environments that support active forms of transportation. There are numerous strategies that could be initiated by community leaders and health care professionals to make it easier for citizens of all ages to become more physically active in their community.

Create an Active Physical Environment

- Install sidewalks and bicycle paths along roads that include adequate lighting.
- Create walking and bicycle paths in parks and other low-density environments.
- Offer public transportation service to areas of high employment volume.
- Include a health-related column or weekly health feature in the community newspaper.
- Encourage community leaders (e.g., government, religious, medical) to provide verbal support of healthy habits to their constituents and members.

Improve Daytime Exercise Options

- Install fitness facilities in work environments, particularly factories and other locations with a large number of employees.
- Sponsor special (corporate) rates for fitness club use.
- Promote fitness clubs in populated areas.
- Install equipment in school playgrounds that, if possible, may be open for public use after school hours.

Provide Program Opportunities

- Sponsor after-school sport and exercise programs.
- Provide an evening lecture series on health-related topics at a local recreation facility, school, or other convenient location.
- Offer health courses in local schools.

Get the Government Involved

- Develop policies and legislation to establish financial incentives for organizations and communities to provide opportunities to be involved in various forms of physical activity, including lower health care costs on paychecks for fitness club memberships, absence of unhealthy habits (e.g., smoking), and improved scores on medical tests.
- Provide financial incentives (e.g., reduced payroll deductions) to government employees who join a fitness club or exercise program or obtain or improve upon a health-related test score, or reduce health care premiums for employees who do not smoke, are not morbidly obese, or who obtain the counsel of a registered dietitian, personal trainer, mental health professional, or some other expert who contributes to better health.
- Use public messages to encourage the use of stairs or at least walking up and down escalators in government buildings.
- Promote taking public transportation at reduced rates for employees.
- Mandate physical education classes and recess in all public schools.
- Encourage restaurants to include healthy menu choices, such as salads, fresh fruits, and low-calorie options.

Research Results on Community Environmental Influences on Physical Activity

- There is a strong relationship between ecological factors and rates of physical activity by community members. For example, living in an attractive neighborhood, particularly within walking distance of shops, increases rates of physical activity (Humpel et al., 2002).

- Environmental changes, such as organizing sport leagues, establishing walking or jogging groups, developing neighborhood walking and bicycling routes, and increasing access to swimming pools, increase rates of physical activity among local adults (Cochrane and Davey, 2008).

- Rates of community and neighborhood physical activity increase for neighborhoods where crime rates are low, walking paths and sidewalks are clearly designated, parks are accessible, and public transportation is available. In other words, user-friendly neighborhoods will result in higher levels of physical activity by residents than less attractive neighborhoods (Nathan, Wood, and Giles-Corti, 2013).

- Stanley, Boshoff, and Dollman (2013) asked children aged 10 to 13 years to indicate the factors that would promote after-school physical activity. Results indicated that safety in the neighborhood and home settings, distance to and from places, weather, availability of time, enjoyment of physical activity, perception of competence (i.e., motor skills) in the activity, and the influence of peers and parents were primary motivators of after-school physical activity.

adolescent girls and boys. Conversely, high crime rates, personal safety concerns, and a poor transportation infrastructure (e.g., many roads to cross, high traffic density or speed) were associated with decreased rates of physical activity. The From Research to Real World highlight box lists several strategies that communities and health coaches can use to provide opportunities to get people moving (Andersen et al., 2006; Booth et al., 1992; Brownell, Stunkard, and Albaum, 1980; Marcus et al., 1998; Pate et al., 2003).

JOB INCENTIVES THAT PROMOTE HEALTHY LIFESTYLE CHOICES

Workplace wellness has become increasingly popular over the past 10 to 15 years, as more and more employers are convinced that a fitter workforce has more energy, reduced absenteeism, and lower health care costs than a workforce that is primarily overweight and unfit. Examples of job incentives include reduced health insurance costs, availability of employee fitness programs or exercise facilities, low absentee rates resulting in better work productivity, employer incentives (financial and otherwise) to engage in regular exercise or nutrition programs for encouraging weight control and improved health and fitness, and employer support for taking time off during work hours for exercise (Chenoweth, 2011).

Several studies have confirmed that a company that encourages healthy habits among its employees, particularly improved fitness, proper diet and nutrition, time for recovery, and reduced stress, will improve worker productivity and reduce illness, absenteeism, sickness, and disease. In addition, company health care and health insurance costs will be markedly reduced (see Quick, Quick, Nelson, and Hurrell, 1997, for a review of this literature).

The availability of an employee fitness program or exercise facility increases the likelihood of employee exercise due to its convenient location and the social support of exercising with work colleagues. Instead of merely encouraging employees to follow healthy habits, companies that sponsor programs that result directly in improved fitness, such as fitness facilities, programs, and staff, will reap even more benefits. If an exercise facility is not physically or financially feasible, then working with local fitness clubs who offer reduced monthly (corporate) rates is an option (Chenoweth, 2011).

Numerous incentives can be used to promote regular exercise, proper nutrition, and programs that improve health, energy, quality of life, and work performance. Reducing monthly health care deductions from the employee's salary is one such incentive to engage in healthy habits. As described in chapter 2, the motivation to engage in a healthy lifestyle must be intrinsic—it must come from within based on a sense of enjoyment, achievement, and perceived competence. At the heart of intrinsic motivation is the drive to perform certain tasks (e.g., regular exercise, healthy dietary habits) based on feelings of enjoyment, satisfaction, perceived success, and the sense of achievement it generates. Building intrinsic motivation among employees involves achieving challenging but realistic health-related goals (e.g., improved fitness, reduced body fat) and developing feelings of success and satisfaction (e.g., recognizing employee exercise adherence). Incentives related to financial gain and time off from work will help drive desirable behavior, such as developing and adhering to exercise and nutritional action plans.

Employer support for taking time off to exercise during work hours will likely lead to improved employee health, energy, recovery from active work demands and mental fatigue, social interaction, and job satisfaction. Several companies realize the value of fitter, leaner employees in terms of energy, self-esteem, reduced health care costs, decreased absenteeism, and increased company loyalty. As Chenoweth (2011) advises, one job condition that encourages involvement in exercise and dietary programs is to provide these services during work hours rather than expecting employees to add one or two additional hours to their work day. This may not always be possible due to work demands and limited employee resources. However, assuming that a minimum of three exercise sessions per week is desirable, providing work time to exercise only twice per week is needed if employees can fit in that third exercise session on their own time. Employees will be devoted to management in terms of effort, perseverance, and self-motivation if they perceive that management cares about their health and happiness.

SUMMARY

Developing and maintaining healthy habits do not happen automatically and are strongly influenced by an array of external—situational and environmental—conditions. The most common and, perhaps, important external factor in the development of healthy habits, including exercise, is called *social support*, the degree of perceived physical, mental, or emotional assistance a person receives from others. Social support is divided into two categories, primary (e.g., exercising together) and secondary (e.g., providing positive verbal feedback, encouragement, or transportation).

Another form of external support is called *coaching*. Many forms and sources of coaching play an important role in promoting proper skills, time management, and motivation to establish long-term healthy routines.

Finally, numerous environmental and situational factors influence exercise behavior and other healthy habits. These include the availability of a nearby fitness facility, fitness and nutrition coaching, fitness classes, fitness equipment, transportation to exercise facilities, an environment that is compatible with engaging in physical activity (e.g., safety and low traffic volume for walking in the neighborhood, availability of a sidewalk or jogging path), and job incentives that promote health behavior (e.g., time off work for exercise, reduced health care costs, exercising with colleagues, free or reduced-cost health club memberships, employer-sponsored competitive sport teams with colleagues). Each of these external factors contributes to the likelihood of greater self-awareness about the importance of maintaining a healthy lifestyle.

STUDENT ACTIVITY

Using a Time Management Worksheet for Developing Healthy Habits

Select a person to act as your client for the purposes of this activity—perhaps a classmate, friend, or family member who wishes to develop healthy habits, including exercise and improved nutrition. The goal of this task is to help the client develop a time management schedule that designates a certain time of day and days of the week to initiate and maintain specific healthy habits. Using the provided time management template, sit down with your client and begin to insert tasks that will be performed at specific times. Specifically, insert the time of day your client can exercise, go for a walk (as a form of relaxation and recovery), consume meals and snacks, go to bed and wake up (including presleep rituals such as no TV, no full meals, no stress, and reading relaxing material), and take breaks during the day. The key goals are planned exercise and food intake.

Ask the person to commit to this schedule for two weeks. For some people, it would be easier to start one new ritual at a time, let's say scheduling exercise at least three days a week and not eating a full meal within two hours of going to sleep. Keep in touch with your client once per day through texting or e-mail with encouraging and uplifting messages, and give positive feedback in response to their successes. After six weeks, the new ritual should become automatic and part of the client's lifestyle.

FORM 6.1   STUDENT ACTIVITY TIME MANAGEMENT WORKSHEET

Make a copy of this schedule for each day of the week.

Day: _____

4:00 a.m.		4:00 p.m.	
4:30 a.m.		4:30 p.m.	
5:00 a.m.		5:00 p.m.	
5:30 a.m.		5:30 p.m.	
6:00 a.m.		6:00 p.m.	
6:30 a.m.		6:30 p.m.	
7:00 a.m.		7:00 p.m.	
7:30 a.m.		7:30 p.m.	
8:00 a.m.		8:00 p.m.	
8:30 a.m.		8:30 p.m.	
9:00 a.m.		9:00 p.m.	
9:30 a.m.		9:30 p.m.	
10:00 a.m.		10:00 p.m.	
10:30 a.m.		10:30 p.m.	
11:00 a.m.		11:00 p.m.	
11:30 a.m.		11:30 p.m.	
Noon		Midnight	
12:30 p.m.		12:30 a.m.	
1:00 p.m.		1:00 a.m.	
1:30 p.m.		1:30 a.m.	
2:00 p.m.		2:00 a.m.	
2:30 p.m.		2:30 a.m.	
3:00 p.m.		3:00 a.m.	
3:30 p.m.		3:30 a.m.	

From M. Anshel, 2014, *Applied Health Fitness Psychology.* (Champaign, IL: Human Kinetics).

FORM 6.2   SOURCES OF SUPPORT TO CARRY OUT NEW RITUALS

List the client's responses to each area (names of people providing support), whether the support is primary (direct involvement by exercising together) or secondary (indirect by providing verbal or emotional support), and details about how the support will be carried out.

Family Members _____

_____

_____

_____

_____

Personal Friends _____

_____

_____

_____

_____

Acquaintances at the Exercise Venue_____

_____

_____

_____

_____

Colleagues_____

_____

_____

_____

_____

Additional Sources _____

_____

_____

_____

_____

From M. Anshel, 2014, *Applied Health Fitness Psychology.* (Champaign, IL: Human Kinetics).

FORM 6.3   POTENTIAL BARRIERS TO DEVELOPING
AND MAINTAINING NEW RITUALS AND STRATEGIES
FOR PREVENTING AND OVERCOMING THEM

Most Likely Potential Barrier to Exercise Initiation and Adherence _____

_____

_____

Preventing or Overcoming the Barrier_____

_____

_____

_____

_____

_____

Second Most Likely Potential Barrier to Exercise Initiation and Adherence_____

_____

_____

Preventing or Overcoming the Barrier_____

_____

_____

_____

_____

_____

Additional Barriers _____

_____

_____

_____

_____

_____

Strategies for Preventing or Overcoming the Barriers_____

_____

_____

_____

_____

_____

From M. Anshel, 2014, *Applied Health Fitness Psychology*. (Champaign, IL: Human Kinetics).

REFERENCES

Andersen, R.E., Franckowiak, S.C., Zuzak, K.B., Cummings, E.S., Barlett, S., and Crespo, C.J. (2006). Effects of a culturally sensitive sign on the use of stairs in African American commuters. *Soz Praventiv Med, 51,* 373-380.

Anshel, M.H. (2006). *Applied exercise psychology: A practitioner's guide to improving client health and exercise.* New York: Springer.

Anshel, M.H. (2012). *Sport psychology: From theory to practice* (5th ed.). San Francisco: Benjamin-Cummings.

Booth, M., Bauman, A., Oldenburg, B., Owen, N., and Magnus, P. (1992). Effects of a national mass-media campaign on physical activity participation. *Health Promotion International, 7,* 241-247.

Bronfenbrenner, U. (1989). Ecological systems theory. *Annals of Child Development, 22,* 723- 742.

Brownell, K.D., Stunkard, A.J., and Albaum, J.M. (1980). Evaluation and modification of exercise patterns in the natural environment. *American Journal of Psychiatry, 137,* 1540-1545.

Chenoweth, D.H. (2002). *Evaluating worksite health promotion.* Champaign, IL: Human Kinetics.

Chenoweth, D.H. (2011). *Worksite health promotion* (3rd ed.). Champaign, IL: Human Kinetics.

Cochrane, T., and Davey, R.C. (2008). Increasing uptake of physical activity: A social ecological approach. *Journal of the Royal Society for the Promotion of Health, 128,* 31-40.

Howley, E.T., and Franks, B.D. (2007). *Fitness professional's handbook* (5th ed.). Champaign, IL: Human Kinetics.

Humpel, N., Owen, N., and Leslie, E. (2002). Environmental factors associated with adults' participation in physical activity. *American Journal of Preventive Medicine, 22,* 188-199.

Lox, C.L., Martin, K.A., and Petruzzello, S.J. (2010). *The psychology of exercise: Integrating theory and practice* (3rd ed.). Scottsdale, AZ: Holcomb Hathaway.

Mackinnon, L.T., Ritchie, C.B., Hooper, S.L., and Abernethy, P.J. (2003). *Exercise management: Concepts and professional practice.* Champaign, IL: Human Kinetics.

Maddison, R., Vander Hoorn, S., Jiang, Y., Mhurchu, C.N., Exeter, D., Dorey, E., Bullen, C., Utter, J., Schaff, D., and Turley, M. (2009). The environment and physical activity: The influence of psychosocial, perceived and built environmental factors. *International Journal of Behavioral Nutrition and Physical Activity, 6,* 119-136.

Marcus, B.H., Owen, N., Forsyth, L.H., Cavill, N.A., and Fridlinger, F. (1998). Physical activity interventions using mass media, print media, and information technology. *American Journal of Preventive Medicine, 15,* 362-368.

Martin Ginis, K.A., and Mack, D. (2012). Understanding exercise behavior: A self-presentational perspective. In G.C. Roberts and D.C. Treasure (Eds.), *Advances in motivation in sport and exercise* (pp. 327-355). Champaign, IL: Human Kinetics.

McLeroy, K.R., Bibeau, D., Steckler, A., and Glanz, K. (1988). An ecological perspective on health promotion programs. *Health Education Quarterly, 15,* 351-377.

Nathan, A., Wood, L., and Giles-Corti, B. (2013). Selling neighborhoods as good for walking: Issues for measuring self-selection. *Journal of Physical Activity and Health, 10,* 5-9.

Pate, R.R., Saunders, R.P., Ward, D.S., Felton, G., Trost, S.G., and Dowda, M. (2003). Evaluation of a community-based intervention to promote physical activity in youth: Lessons from active winners. *American Journal of Health Promotion, 17,* 171-182.

Quick, J.C., Quick, J.D., Nelson, D.L., and Hurrell, J.J. (1997). *Preventive stress management in organizations.* Washington, DC: American Psychological Association.

Stanley, R.M., Boshoff, K., and Dollman, J. (2013). A qualitative exploration of the "critical window": Factors affecting Australian children's after-school physical activity. *Journal of Physical Activity and Health, 10,* 33-41.

Wills, T.A., and Shinar, O. (2000). Measuring perceived and received social support. In S. Cohen, L.G. Underwood, and B.H. Gottlieb (Eds.), *Social support measurement and intervention* (pp. 86-135). New York: Oxford University Press.

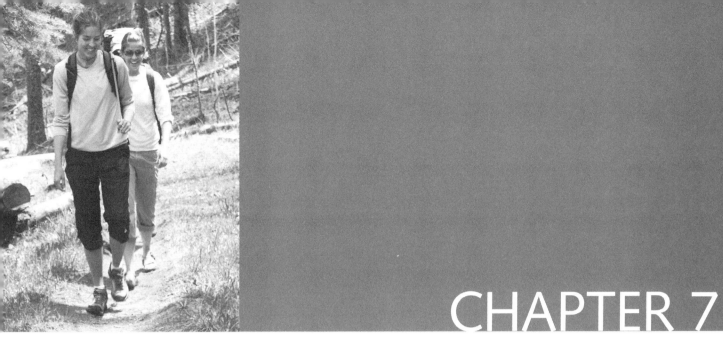

Cultural, Religious, and Spiritual Components

> " *If a man would take care of his body as he takes care of the animal he rides on, he would be spared many serious ailments.* "
>
> Maimonides, medieval philosopher and physician

CHAPTER OBJECTIVES

After reading this chapter, you should be able to:

- know the role that culture, spirituality, and religion play in a client's decision to maintain healthy habits;

- be familiar with the content of various religious texts that recognize the importance of maintaining one's health; and

- understand the role of culture in maintaining health-promoting rituals and the implication of those cultural rituals for health professionals.

The focus of this chapter is not to impose a particular religious view on clients who may or may not hold religious or spiritual beliefs. Instead, this chapter examines the relationships among health status, health behaviors, and religious and spiritual beliefs, followed by a discussion of implications and applications for health practitioners. Results of studies concur that over 90% of Americans believe in a higher power, and other countries have similar rates (Koenig, 2007; Levin, 2001). The contribution of one's spiritual life to health behaviors and the extent to which religion and religious leaders may play a role in removing unhealthy behavior patterns has not been sufficiently explored by health practitioners. Researchers have examined the influence of religion and spirituality on the practice of a healthy lifestyle; however, this area is virtually ignored in the exercise psychology literature. Also ignored is the role of religious leaders in promoting healthy habits in the community.

The terms *religion* and *spirituality* are used interchangeably in this chapter, but they are defined differently. When attempting to understand the role of religion and spirituality and the role of health professionals in maintaining a healthy lifestyle, it is important to understand the difference between these two concepts. *Religion* denotes organized religious institutions and a scholarly field of study. Practicing religion refers to behaviors (e.g., regularly attending religious services), attitudes (e.g., maintaining thoughts and feelings consistent with a specific religion), beliefs (e.g., supporting scripture or other religious texts), and experiences (e.g., worshiping a higher power or interacting with other congregants or within religious institution programs) that are linked to a specific religion or religious institution. *Spirituality*, on the other hand, refers to a state of being that is acquired through religious devotion and observance (Levin, 2001). Attaining spirituality—a connection with a higher power—is the ultimate goal of religion. Spirituality is a subset of religion and is pursued through religious participation. However, as will be discussed, some people

avoid religious services and have no formal ties with a specific religion, yet they describe themselves as spiritual.

Levin (2001) contends that religion consists of organized institutions and buildings that are used for worship, forms a scholarly field of study, and deals with issues related to the person's spirit and matters of personal concern. Along these lines, Koenig (2008) contends that religion is "a system of beliefs and practices observed by a community supported by rituals that acknowledge, worship, communicate with, or approach the Sacred . . . [or] God in Western cultures" (p. 11). Practicing religion, or being religious, then, refers to a person's behaviors, attitudes, beliefs, and experiences that involve this domain of life. Religion consists of a connection between humans and a higher power, such as God.

Religion typically offers a moral code of conduct agreed upon by community members, who attempt to live according to that code. Spirituality, on the other hand, "refers to a state of being that is acquired through religious devotion, piety, and observance" (Levin, 2001, p. 9). Spirituality is the ultimate goal of and a subset of religion; it consists of a union or connection with God or the divine. Spirituality is something to be attained; it is sought through religious participation. In more recent years, however, spirituality has taken on a new meaning as private religious expression such as meditation and feelings of oneness with nature, referred to as "secular transcendent experiences" (Levin, p. 10). In the more current definition, spirituality is the larger phenomenon, and religion is reserved for organized religious activity.

To Koenig (2008), spirituality has cognitive, experiential, and behavioral aspects. It is expressed in the person's search for ultimate meaning through participation in religion and belief in God, family, and other areas of life. Koenig contends that "many people find spirituality through religion or through a personal relationship with the divine" (p. 13). Others, however, may find spirituality through a connection to nature, music and the arts, a set of values, or the attempt to discover scientific truth. Whereas spirituality is a personal relationship with a higher power, religion is the community and institutional aspects, or the expression, of spirituality. Although several scholars and practitioners differentiate between religion and spirituality, for all practical purposes these terms are used interchangeably in this chapter with regard to their relationship to health.

HEALTH CARE IN MULTICULTURAL POPULATIONS

Culture strongly influences the way we think, feel, and act. How could it not influence our attitudes toward food intake, physical activity, and a lifestyle that affects our health? For

---

SAMPLE CULTURAL DIFFERENCES IN TRADITIONAL HEALTH VIEWS

It should be noted that these are generalizations of traditional cultural differences and not all clients from these cultures will hold these views, especially in the younger generations.

Latinos

Illnesses may be attributed to divine intervention, fate, changes in temperature, food ingestion, physical activity, strong emotions, imbalances between the individual and the environment, lack of personal attention to health, punishment from a higher power for committing a sin, or even a curse. Only a high degree of trust between the patient and health care provider, which is fostered if the provider speaks Spanish, will result in full disclosure of clients' beliefs about possible causes of their illness or their decision to initiate treatment.

African Americans

African Americans traditionally endorse two sources of support and healing: family and church. Perhaps this reflects a tendency to embrace a holistic philosophy of health and view the mind and body as inseparable and central to maintaining health. Illnesses are usually attributed to natural factors (e.g., excessive eating or drinking, stress) or unnatural factors (e.g., witchcraft, spiritual causes). Prayer is a common approach to remedying the patient from illness. Folk healers often are the only available or affordable option for rural or low-income people.

Asians

Healthy people must balance themselves within the environment and "balance the forces of yin (inside and in front of the body) and yang (outside and back of the body)" (Huff and Yasharpour, 2007, p. 30). Violating this balance can result in illness. Sample medical practices, some of which are preventive and are familiar to Westerners, include meditation, yoga, acupuncture, herbology, and acupressure. Traditional healers usually employ these methods of diagnosis: feeling the pulse, looking, listening, and inquiring. Perhaps understandably, Asian communities often view Western medical practices as intrusive, unnecessary, and excessive. Asian medicine predates Western medicine by thousands of years.

Native Americans

To many Native Americans, health is closely linked to spirituality. American Indian medicine is holistic. It focuses on behavior patterns and lifestyle and seeks to establish harmony among the person's physical, mental, spiritual, and emotional lives. Techniques to reach these ends include praying, chanting, performing dance rituals, prescribing botanical medicines, and performing physical manipulations.

Middle Eastern and Muslim Culture

Health means wholeness or completeness to this community. Illnesses occur due to natural causes, that is, by forces in nature, such as germs, bacteria, and weather conditions. Some illnesses are explained as punishment from God or the devil. Medical treatment includes both folk-traditional (i.e., home and herbal remedies) and Western biomedical treatments. The sudden onset of illness can be prevented by saying "In the name of God" or "With the power of God" (Huff and Yasharpour, 2007). In addition, Huff and Yasharpour assert that Muslim culture and practice strictly forbid men and women from sharing facilities or interacting while engaging in any form of recreational or physical activity, including exercise.

health care professionals, the implications of working with a variety of cultures are enormous. Here we examine the needs and behavior patterns of selected cultures and the ways in which health care professionals should be sensitive to clients' individual needs. As Huff and Kline (2007) note, "Cultural considerations ultimately may determine whether a particular population or target group will choose to participate in health promotion and disease prevention (HPDP) programs" (p. 4). See Kline and Huff (2007), Purnell and Paulanka (1998), and Aten, McMinn, and Worthington (2011) for more extensive reviews and ideas for practice in this area.

A review of multicultural health promotion includes both Western (what is called *traditional*) forms of health care delivery and alternative forms. Murray and Rubel (1992) designate five categories of practitioners who practice alternative medicine. A detailed review of these categories goes beyond the scope of this chapter, but briefly, these categories of alternative medicine practitioners, some of whom may go against traditional Western medical practices, include

- spiritual and psychological practitioners (e.g., religious faith healers, psychics, mystics who use psychological approaches to try to heal or cure their patients);
- nutritional coaches, including those who use herbal remedies and special diets for healing;
- drug and biological specialists who employ various chemicals, drugs, and vaccines to cure or prevent disease;
- practitioners who provide treatment with physical forces and devices, such as chiropractors, acupuncturists, and massage therapists; and
- therapists who use other techniques that intend to heal patients, such as aromatherapy, iridology, herbology, and colon therapy.

The value in reviewing the health beliefs and medical practices of selected cultures is to note vast differences in the diversity, historical perspective, and medical practices of a multicultural population that need to be considered by health care professionals. Medical and mental health care professionals and coaches must be sensitive to the unique characteristics of their clients' beliefs that are firmly entrenched throughout their lives. Health promoters must suspend their personal beliefs, biases, and judgments about those who are being treated. It is incumbent upon each professional who provides care and treatment to integrate the client's customs when possible and to understand, respect, and work with these individual differences in treating acute and chronic conditions.

RELIGIOUS COMMUNITY AND HEALTH HABITS

Levin (2001) concluded from his review of the religion and health literature that "nearly every religion espouses beliefs that govern behavior regarding health, disease, and death [and] some religions require behaviors related to health while others forbid behaviors related to health or medical care" (p. 22). Religions, for example, promote beliefs that regulate behaviors related to alcohol, tobacco, diet, general hygiene, and medical care. Levin found that commitment to religion "may have a protective effect against subsequent illness . . . prevent or delay (illnesses), and have long-term benefits for physical and mental functioning and health" (p. 23).

The religious community is not immune from the health-related problems derived from an unhealthy lifestyle, however. The obesity epidemic still thrives in the religious and spiritual community (Cline and Ferraro, 2006). For example, the prevalence of obesity increased from 24% to 30% from 1986 to 1994 and likely has become much higher in more recent years among people of faith, that is, people who claim an affiliation with or membership in a denomination or religious institution. One potentially powerful source of health behavior change that has not been recognized in the war against obesity is the importance of religious and spiritual institutions and their leaders.

Next to physicians or other personal care providers, religious and spiritual leaders are some of the most credible people who influence the thoughts, emotions, and actions of a person of faith. People of faith often make a conscious decision to behave in a manner that is consistent with the expectations of their religious or spiritual messages.

In his book, *Medicine, Religion, and Health: Where Science and Spirituality Meet* (2008), Dr. Harold G. Koenig, MD, divides the benefits of religious practice or belief into six health-related areas:

1. Mental health
2. Immune function
3. Cardiovascular function
4. Stress and behavior-related diseases
5. Mortality
6. Physical disability

Based on his review of the research literature in each of these areas, Koenig (2008) concluded that religious practice or spirituality were strongly associated with superior health outcomes. He found, for example, that blood pressure and rates of stroke and cognitive impairment were each highly correlated with religious involvement (e.g., service attendance, frequency of prayer, strength of belief in a higher power). Although not always acknowledged by religious leaders, messages related to maintaining healthy habits are common throughout most religious texts.

To people of faith, arguably no one has more credibility for influencing behavior than their religious or spiritual leader. Should these leaders play a role in promoting healthy habits among congregants and the community at large? How can they address the apparent disconnect between people's religious practices, including a firm belief in religious or spiritual texts, and their lack of self-awareness about practicing healthy habits? And how can health professionals be involved in this process?

Role of Religious Leaders in Promoting and Modeling Healthy Habits

Many religious leaders contend that people who attend traditional ceremonies or services are looking for spiritual fulfillment, and that is the primary role of their institutions. Educating congregants about healthy habits is not. Perhaps this view, and the mission that propels it, needs to be reexamined. All sources of behavioral influence, including school systems, governments, corporations, the food industry, and religious institutions, need to be unified in providing information and incentives to replace self-destructive behavior patterns with healthier alternatives. One source of health behavior interventions that has received only minimal attention is the role of religious and spiritual leaders.

What should religious and spiritual leaders do to promote healthy habits, perhaps with assistance from health professionals? First, they need to look at themselves and determine if the change needs to start with them. Next, they must speak up and encourage their institution members—and other members of the community, when given the opportunity—to have discipline in all areas of their lives. One religious text, the Bible, addresses eating, indulgence, self-control, self-discipline, and gluttony. These topics need to be addressed in religious institutions and services without fear of offending attendees. Leaders of congregants who attend spiritual events and services should encourage their congregants to make lifestyle changes that will ultimately bring glory to God or some other higher power to whom they feel accountable. Religious leaders must stop being intimidated by the risk of losing members by offending them in order to acknowledge the importance of self-care as an inherent component of a religious and spiritual lifestyle (Colbert, 2002).

Perhaps the most serious obstacle to health behavior change in the religious community is persuading people of faith to take responsibility for their health and engage in the free will of healthy lifestyle choices, rather than surrender control to a higher power. Most religious texts, including the Bible, promote taking responsibility for health behavior. Philippians 2:13 states that God works within us to will his Holy Spirit and the free will to desire to create balance in our life—and the will to act on that desire.

For example, as Omartian (1996) contends, "The main reason to exercise is for your health. Without good health you cannot do all that the Lord has for you do to and you cannot be all the Lord wants you to be" (p. 117). Along these lines, Koenig (1999) asserts, "The world's religions encourage healthy living. . . . All established religions discourage . . . any habit or activity harmful to the human body, which has traditionally been viewed as sacred, created in the image of God" (p. 72). And as Levin (2001) concludes, "All religions endorse the idea that we ought to take care of our bodies and not act in ways that are reckless and endanger our health" (p. 41).

There is an apparent need for religious institutions and their leaders to play a more prominent role in promoting community health and wellness and to serve as role models for their congregations. The credibility of pastors, priests, rabbis, imams, and other religious leaders will be further enhanced if their messages of health and wellness given in their sermons and programs are reflected in their own behavioral patterns. In other words, religious and spiritual leaders have to walk the walk, not just talk the talk.

Health Themes Addressed by Religious and Spiritual Leaders

Perhaps the strongest influence of a religious leader on the thoughts, emotions, and actions of attendees of religious services occurs when their attention is focused on the leader's words—the sermon. Health-related themes that extol the virtues of maintaining a healthy lifestyle need to be communicated more frequently and passionately, citing religious or spiritual text to reinforce main issues. For example, in the New Testament of the Christian Bible, the apostle Paul reminds his readers

that their bodies are a dwelling place of the Holy Spirit, thereby bridging the gap between spiritual and physical dualism that may be keeping people of faith locked into unhealthy behavioral patterns. Paul contends that what we do with our bodies matters not only on a physical level but also on a spiritual level.

Religious leaders can also cite scripture to remind us that we are not owners but rather managers, or stewards, of our bodies. Maintaining healthy habits is a matter of personal stewardship. When we begin to perceive our bodies in a manner that is consistent with God's view, we begin to make decisions that affect our physical health that honors a higher power (i.e., God). Thus, maintaining unhealthy habits that lead to obesity and poor physical conditioning is a failure of that stewardship responsibility.

Another health theme found in religion is gluttony. The Gluttony in Religion highlight box lists examples of this theme from various religious texts that both religious leaders and health professionals may use with people of faith to address the association between healthy habits and spirituality or religion.

Scripture and Bodily Health

Virtually all religions devote portions of their holy texts to promote quality of life and good health. Christian scripture, particularly the New Testament of the Bible, for instance, is replete with passages that extol the virtues of living a healthy lifestyle. It is these passages that warrant attention by health professionals in their work with Christian clients who value faith in a higher power. One of the most powerful passages in the New Testament about maintaining healthy habits is found in I Corinthians 6:19-20: "Do you not know that your body is a temple of the Holy Spirit, who is in you, whom you have received from God? You are not your own; you were bought at a price. Therefore, honor God with your body." Text of this nature might be inappropriate for clients who do not maintain a religious or spiritual mind-set, but clients of faith might be very responsive to health-based text derived from scripture (Koenig, 2007).

GLUTTONY IN RELIGION

Many statements in religious texts and customs address gluttony, linking behavior with faith and healthy lifestyle choices. Gluttony is the outworking of greed and a lack of self-control. With over 150 religions worldwide, these are just a few examples of the role of religion in maintaining healthy habits.

- From the Koran: "Eat of the good things we have provided for your sustenance, but commit no excess therein, lest my wrath should justly descend on you, and those upon whom descends my wrath do perish indeed" (20:81).

- From the Old Testament of the Bible: "Do not join those who drink too much wine or gorge themselves on meat, for drunkards and gluttons become poor, and drowsiness clothes them in rags" (Proverbs 23:20-21), and "It is not good to eat too much honey, nor is it honorable to seek one's own honor. Like a city whose walls are broken down is a man who lacks self-control" (Proverbs 25:27-28).

- In the Hindu tradition, *health* means the continued maintenance of the body under normal and even abnormal environmental conditions. Hindu religious teachings on healthy living and ethical considerations are highly spiritual. One Hindu tradition, hatha yoga, is conducive to good health and prevents or addresses disease via the regulation of muscular action. The holistic approach to health in Hinduism calls attention to such causes of ill health as climatic extremes, bacterial attacks, nutritional deviance, stress, and other forms of what is called *emotional imbalance*. Good health is a function of the person's decision to cultivate habits that are conducive to physical and spiritual well-being. The concept of preventive medicine is based on the tenet that attaining good health is a religious duty, and corresponding injunctions are found in abundance in Hindu scriptures.

- From the Tao Te Ching (46): "There is no greater calamity than indulging in greed."

Physical Cures for Gluttony

- Eat smaller portions.
- Reduce fat in your daily caloric intake.
- Stop late-night eating.
- Increase physical activity.

Spiritual Cures for Gluttony

- Change your perspective: When you see as God sees, you will do as he says.
- Overeating is a spiritual problem.
- Realize that the body is a theater. God runs his film through our bodies. What's showing in your theater?

Keys to Changing Behavior

- Treat your body as a temple (temple represents respect).
- Realize that you are not the owner of your temple; you rent, not own, your temple.
- Remember that your body was created by God, for God, and to honor God.

Keys to Maintaining Healthy Habits

- Don't lose sight of the goal.
- Talk back to the spoiled child living inside you.
- Moderation is an inside job.

As another example, Jewish people must hold themselves accountable for following 613 commandments described in the Torah (Levin, 2001). These commandments are written in both positive terms ("Thou shalt") and negative terms ("Thou shalt not"). All Jewish people are held to the same standard in their devotion and accountability to God.

As discussed earlier, notable among these teachings and cautionary words are warnings against gluttony, which is disdained in many faiths. According to Colbert (2002), for example, the sin of gluttony is a strong contributing factor to poor health. The Bible, which condemns overindulgence in many things, including food, says in Proverbs 23:20-21, "Do not be among those who drink too much wine, or with those who gorge themselves on meat. For the drunkard and the glutton will become poor, and grogginess will clothe them in rags." Here, as in other verses, gluttony is placed in the same category as other sinful behavior (Cline and Ferraro, 2006).

SELECTED BIBLICAL PASSAGES THAT PROMOTE A HEALTHY LIFESTYLE

More than 56 passages in the Bible, including both Old (Tanakh) and New Testaments, extoll the importance of a healthy lifestyle.

- "Don't you know that you are God's temple and that God's Spirit lives in you? If anyone destroys God's temple, God will destroy him. For God's temple is sacred, and you are that temple" (I Corinthians 3:16-17).

- "Everything is permissible—but not everything is beneficial" (I Corinthians 10:23).

- "Let us purify ourselves from everything that contaminates body and spirit, perfecting holiness out of reverence for God" (II Corinthians 7:1).

- "How much more so am I required to scrub and scour myself, having been created in the image and likeness of God, as it is written 'For

in the image of God He made human beings'" (Genesis 9:6; Leviticus Rabbah 34:3).

- "So whether you eat or drink, or whatever you do, do it all for the glory of God" (I Corinthians 10:31).

- "Do you not know that your body is the temple of the Holy Spirit, who is in you, whom you have received from God? You are not your own. For you were bought at a price; therefore honor God with your body and in your spirit, which are God's" (I Corinthians 6:19-20).

- "It is not good to eat too much honey, nor is it honorable to seek one's own honor. Like a city whose walls are broken down is a man who lacks self-control" (Proverbs 25:27-28).

- "The good man eats to live while the evil man lives to eat" (Proverbs 13:25).

Are religiously affiliated people healthier than their nonreligious counterparts? Levin (2001) concludes from his review of this literature that "on average, people who report a religious identify are more likely to follow the dictates of their religion than people who report no affiliation at all" (p. 33). Levin continues, "Commitment to health-promoting religious doctrines encourages healthy practices that prevent illness and enhance physical and emotional health and overall well-being" (p. 33). It is the commitment to a religious text that makes such people more likely to follow the healthy habits dictated by their faith.

CONTRADICTIONS BETWEEN RELIGIOUS PRACTICE AND UNHEALTHY LIVING

Is it possible that a strong religious faith, also called *spiritual health* (Holt and McClure, 2006), may actually impede a person's sense of control and responsibility instead of promoting them in maintaining healthy habits? To what

extent do religious practices and beliefs dictate a person's health-related behavior patterns? Are people of faith healthier if they surrender control of their lives to a higher power such as the Lord or Allah compared with people who take control of their long-term health and destiny? Do firmly held religious beliefs and practices result in people taking responsibility for their health, or do these individuals surrender self-control to a higher power and ignore the findings of medical research or the advice of physicians?

Although one line of thought is that a higher power controls our destiny, which may already be determined, another perspective is that each of us has been bestowed with the free will to lead a healthy life. Young and Koopsen (2005), for instance, assert that there is a moral code to be obeyed through religious texts. It is their contention that human beings are made in the image of God, and he has given us free will to either accept or reject him. This same free will gives us the responsibility, they contend, to live a life that balances surrendering to God, in which God controls our destiny, with taking responsibility for what we can control—our health, our behavior, and our beliefs. To these authors, it is hypocritical to profess one's devotion to God yet maintain unhealthy habits that will lead to illness, disease, lack of energy, and a shortened life. The authors quote Philippians 4:13, "I can do all this through him who gives me strength," to indicate that each of us is responsible for our own quality of life with the spiritual support of a higher power, not that the higher power is responsible for keeping us healthy.

Another approach to the relationship between taking personal responsibility for one's health and perceiving a higher power as in charge of our health is what Gall and colleagues (2005) refer to as *surrender style*. The authors speculate that unhealthy behavior patterns among religious practitioners could be due to their surrendering style, which "involves an active decision to release personal control to God over those aspects of a situation that fall outside of one's control" (p. 92). Therefore, the person believes that "God is now in charge of the situation" (p. 92). This disposition promotes spiritual well-being and a deepened sense of faith, especially under stressful conditions.

Gall et al. (2005) do not suggest that surrender style gives a person license to engage in a carelessly unhealthy lifestyle because, after all, God is in control. However, it is plausible that for some people, a strong religious surrender style provides the incentive to maintain behavior patterns that medical science would consider unhealthy, such as lack of exercise and poor dietary habits. Surrender style, that is, the lack of perceived self-control, may explain a person's relatively passive attitude toward taking responsibility for a healthy lifestyle. Low self-control is often associated with severe weight gain and other unhealthy behavior patterns (Kennett and Ackerman, 1995). Perhaps the most credible source of information for engaging in healthy behavior patterns is the religious leader, as discussed earlier. New treatments and interventions are needed by religious leaders in promoting

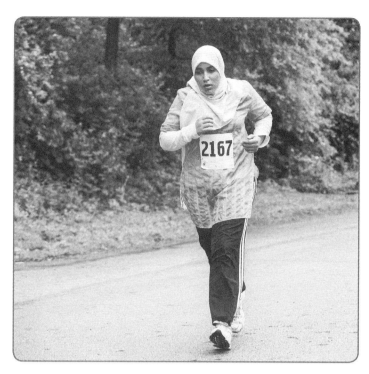

Expression of spiritual beliefs reduces stress and therefore improves physical, mental, and emotional health.

healthy behavior patterns among people of faith.

HEALTH BENEFITS OF RELIGIOUSNESS AND SPIRITUALITY

The results of numerous studies have reported favorable effects of religious practice on health (Atchley, 1997; Ferraro and Albrecht-Jensen, 1991). The likely reasons for these benefits include the use of prayer and religious behaviors and thoughts to cope with stress; reduced use of addictive drugs, nicotine, and alcohol; and elevated mood state. In addition to improved physical health, there is also an improvement in spiritual and mental health (Holt and McClure, 2006).

Spector (1996) contends that nearly every religion attempts to govern behavior concerning health, disease, and death. Some beliefs require certain health behaviors, while others forbid certain behaviors. Many doctrines or teachings of faith offer moral and practical guidance about how to attain and maintain physical health and well-being. As Levin (2001) concludes, "Studies suggest that commitment to religion, expressed as affiliation with or membership in a denomination or particular church, mosque, synagogue, or other religious institution, may have a protective effect against subsequent illness. Just as with refraining from cigarettes or alcohol or overeating, religious affiliation may prevent or delay pathogenic (illness-making) changes and have long-term benefits for physical and mental functioning and health" (p. 23). Health professionals should consider religious and spiritual beliefs, texts, and leaders as sources of information and inspiration to promote healthy habits among selected clients.

It is apparent, then, that the greatest challenge to health professionals for helping others reduce or prevent unhealthy habits, at least among people who have a strong faith and engage in religious or spiritual practices, is to determine the balance between two thought processes: on one hand surrendering one's life to a higher power while on the other hand maintaining free will for living a life consistent with one's values, health, and longevity. As Omartian (1996) contends, "The biggest problem with excess weight is not whether God still loves you. He does, and so do other people. Nor is the biggest problem whether you look good in your clothes. The most important thing is whether you're going to be incapacitated by fat-related diseases and die prematurely" (pp. 89-90). Omartian's messages resonate across many beliefs, philosophies, and religious institutions.

PRAYER AND MEDITATION

Prayer is a behavior pattern that influences mental and physical health and feelings of well-being (Levin, 2001). Without question, many people engage in acknowledging a higher power to express gratitude for their good health, wishes for performance success, hopes for the future, requests to heal the sick, and so on. Prayer is recognized in this text as a source of comfort, security, hope, gratitude, appreciation, and a sense of purpose about being consistent with one's values, particularly faith. The time, location, and content of this ritual are almost always self-determined, and the perceived outcomes of prayer are highly individualized. Sometimes prayer is reserved for attending religious services or is carried out at a certain time and place (e.g., each night before going to sleep).

FROM RESEARCH TO REAL WORLD

I asked the chief executive officer of a corporate wellness center in Orlando, Florida, why his two-and-a-half-day wellness program does not address faith as an integral part of one's belief system or include content about the role of religion and spirituality in maintaining a healthy lifestyle. He responded that it was important that the program remain secular and not impose faith as a value or a strategy to remove unhealthy habits and promote a healthy lifestyle. Ironically, most of his company's clients consider faith to be among their most important values, according to their staff.

Koenig (2007, 2008) has a different view of why health professionals and medical practitioners should include faith as one of several strategies to be addressed with clients or patients. He offers a list of dos and don'ts related to the application of spirituality in client care. See Koenig (2007) for information on the health-related habits of various religions and implications for health care professionals. Koenig (2008) suggests that health care providers consider including the following strategies in promoting a healthy lifestyle.

Do This

• *Consider patient religiosity.* Many patients are either religious or spiritual, with a vast majority believing in a higher power, and many of them would like to have some component of faith included in their health care. Religious needs should be recognized and addressed by their health care providers. Koenig (2008) reports that a common patient complaint on surveys following hospitalization is the failure to meet spiritual and emotional needs.

• *Religion influences patients' ability to cope with illness.* The ability to cope with illness or poor health provides additional incentive for people to take control of their lives, improve self-care, adhere to planned medical treatment, and replace unhealthy habits with more desirable ones.

• *Religious beliefs and practices may influence medical outcomes.* Stress has an adverse effect on the success of medical treatments and can compromise the immune system. Expression of religious or spiritual beliefs reduces stress and therefore improves physical, mental, and emotional health.

• *Patients are often isolated from other sources of religious help.* If patients are hospitalized or experience a medical event away from their faith community or religious leader, they are more likely to feel alone. In addition, clergy may not be able to visit all patients or may be limited in the frequency of such visits. Feeling isolated from spiritual support that meets the patient's needs will inhibit recovery.

• *Religious beliefs and rituals may conflict with or influence patients' medical decisions.* Particularly in response to serious illness or injury, clinicians need to know how people's beliefs and related rituals influence the type of care that they want and expect.

• *Religious beliefs influence patient health care in the community after they leave the hospital or doctor's office.* Health care providers need to know what type of support is available to clients when they leave the health care or exercise facility. Are clients isolated, or do they have a social support network? Could that network be faith-based? To meet the needs of people of faith, practitioners should become aware of exercise facilities, equipment, and reduced membership costs offered by local fitness clubs for religious institutions or local organizations.

Don't Do This

• *Prescribe religion.* According to Koenig (2008), "Health professionals should not prescribe religion to non-religious patients or actively proselytize" (p. 169) without the client's expressed desire. It is unethical to coerce someone or induce guilt about a particular belief system or behavior pattern, particularly when the person is ill or either physically or emotionally weak.

• *Record the patient's spiritual history.* If patients or clients are not religious and feel uncomfortable or resist questioning about their religious background or practice, discontinue this line of questioning immediately. In most secular settings the client's personal beliefs should not even be addressed.

• *Pray with patients.* Medical and health practitioners should avoid praying with their patients unless the patient asks and the practitioner is comfortable with it. This is an especially relevant issue if the patient's religion differs from that of the practitioner.

• *Provide spiritual counseling.* Health professionals without religious training should not usually provide spiritual counsel or advice to patients. Spiritual needs can be complex and interact with psychological and social issues. This is the role of spiritual or religious leaders.

• *Argue about religious and spiritual issues.* Health practitioners should not argue with patients or clients about religious or spiritual beliefs, even if those beliefs conflict with medical or health care. Some religions, for example, require adherents to wear certain attire or avoid members of the opposite sex in health or exercise settings.

SUMMARY

The vast majority of people around the world believe in a higher power, often referred to as *God*, and that prayer influences health and well-being (Koenig, 2007). Perhaps not surprisingly, therefore, religious and spiritual institutions possess enormous influence on the behavior of their members. To date, religious and spiritual leaders have not taken a leadership role in improving community physical and mental health despite their enormous credibility with and influence on community members and congregants. In addition, religious leaders should be more proactive and assertive in citing their spiritual or religious texts to extol the virtues of living a healthy lifestyle that is consistent with their deepest, most important values, including faith.

Health care professionals play a special role in working with religious and spiritual leaders and their institutions and congregants to express the need, often sanctioned by spiritual texts, to develop and maintain a healthy lifestyle. Another part of their role is to apply spiritual and religious texts and beliefs when interacting with clients whose most important values include faith. To gain credibility in communicating these messages, it is essential that health care professionals also demonstrate healthy habits and maintain the type of lifestyle that they promote.

In describing God's expectations that humans live a healthy life, Byl (2008) explains that "God gives you the knowledge and power generally to keep you well and to make yourself well when you are ill" (p. 9). Thus, a person of faith must ask, "What am I doing with the power of knowledge and good health that has been bestowed upon me? Am I using my knowledge to live a life that will provide me with the energy to show my devotion to a higher power? Or am I abusing my temple by the use of self-destructive, unhealthy habits?" Religious texts clearly indicate that "preserving your physical wellness is a part of abundant living, of glorifying God with all that you are, and of redeeming this world for God" (Byl, 2008, p. 9). Byl and Moroze (2008) assert that "if God has a mission, then it is helpful for His people to have a mission. If you want to honor God, then your mission needs to be consistent with God's and empowered by Him. A mission needs to be something that resonates deep within you." (p. 15). A person of faith should ask, "What kind of daily choices do I make, as opposed to choices I should make, that honor God and create a sense of meaning and purpose in my life?"

Fitness psychology includes a spiritual component, because all of us find life more meaningful and fulfilling when we live a life that is consistent with our deepest values, particularly if one of those values is faith. As Koenig (2008) recommends, "Integrating spirituality into patient care should be a priority. Because so many medical patients have spiritual needs, spiritual conflicts, or derive comfort from religious beliefs and traditions, this makes a strong argument for training health professionals to assess, respect, and make accommodations for patients' spiritual beliefs and practices" (p. 172).

Values usually drive our behavior; they reflect what we consider to be most important. Common values for most people include health, family, integrity, happiness, knowledge, and faith. Too often, however, our unhealthy habits, leading to poor fitness, obesity, and premature disease, are inconsistent with our most important values. The purposes of this chapter were to examine the role of religious and spiritual beliefs in maintaining a healthy lifestyle, the ways in which physical and mental health professionals can apply faith-based content in consulting with patients and clients of faith, and how religious and spiritual beliefs, texts, and programs can provide greater incentive to initiate and maintain healthy habits. Health professionals should also consider soliciting contributions from religious and spiritual leaders in the community in delivering messages, establishing programs, and providing counsel to community organizations regarding the close relationship between religious and spiritual beliefs and lifestyle choices.

This chapter represents one more part of the health professional's arsenal of strategies in attempts to motivate changes in health behavior. As Koenig (2007) asserts, "Religious beliefs are common among patients, help them to cope, can influence medical decisions . . . often impact mental and physical health outcomes . . . and may affect the kind of support and care patients receive."

STUDENT ACTIVITY

God Locus of Health Control Scale

The God Locus of Health Control (GLHC) scale (Wallston et al., 1999), found in form 7.1, should be administered only if the person agrees to it. The scale does not impose religion or assume a person's religious or spiritual beliefs; it is a measure that determines the extent to which people believe that God is the locus (i.e., source) of control over their current and future health status. Religious beliefs, however, are highly personal, and it is anticipated that some people will oppose answering these questions. This cannot be a required activity.

Higher scores represent a stronger belief in God as the source of control over one's health status, both present and future. The response scale is a 6-point Likert scale ranging from 1 (strongly disagree) to 6 (strongly agree). Scoring consists of adding the total number of points and determining if

- clients perceive that a higher power, such as God, controls their health;
- clients believe their free will controls their health and well-being;
- clients' views about who controls their health and well-being also influence their health-related behavior, or the extent to which they feel responsible for maintaining a healthy lifestyle; and
- clients' religious or spiritual beliefs influence their health-related actions, such as engaging in regular physical activity and proper diet and nutrition.

How does the health care provider use this information with clients or patients? As one example, people with strong religious or spiritual convictions can be informed of how religious texts promote physical and mental well-being. Health care providers must not impose religious text or content in providing services, however, and they must not assume the client's receptivity to a religious component.

In his book *Spirituality in Patient Care*, Koenig (2007) contends that health professionals should be interested in identifying and addressing the spiritual needs of their patients or clients. To Koenig, each patient's religious and spiritual beliefs should be part of the assessment (intake) process. He suggests, for instance, that the patient's personal care provider (e.g., physician, nurse), medical center chaplain, and other religious leaders play a central role in promoting a spiritual component of health-related services.

With respect to promoting exercise through the patient's or client's spiritual side, the book *Christian Paths to Health and Wellness*, edited by Walters and Byl (2008), is an excellent reference. Although aimed at a Christian audience, the book provides a valid model for delivering fitness educational material juxtaposed with religious texts. For example, sections about God's mission (p. 15) and making God's purposes your purposes (pp. 15-16) remind readers that maintaining a healthy lifestyle is part of being a steward to their vessel.

Omartian (1996) nicely associates scripture with a spiritual commitment to serving a higher power through healthy habits. "The main reason to exercise is for your health," she asserts. "Without good health you cannot do all the Lord has for you to do and you cannot be all the Lord wants you to be" (p. 117). She also states, "Do not ask the Lord to guide your footsteps if you are unwilling to move your feet" (p. 104). The effectiveness of these messages, of course, is based on clients' free will and self-motivation to act in a manner that is consistent with their faith-based values and spiritual beliefs. Health care providers, therefore, should determine their client's readiness and openness to these faith-based messages. The GLHC scale provides one source of information for making this determination.

Another way in which health care professionals may use this information is to work with religious leaders to incorporate health behavior change in their religious institutions. In one recent article, Anshel and Smith (2013) suggest ways in which religious leaders can provide programs that promote exercise and other healthy habits among their members. There are several planned strategies that religious leaders can use to promote good health among congregation members. Their primary strategy is to provide the congregation with scripture, such as preaching expository sermons—a verse-by-verse study of religious text. It is also advisable that the religious leader become a vocal proponent of living a life consistent with appropriate values such as faith, health, family, generosity, and integrity.

Program Strategies of Religious Leaders to Promote Healthy Habits Among Congregants

- Sponsor wellness programs and services in conjunction with local fitness and sport facilities (clubs, YMCA, schools).
- Designate part of the religious institution as a fitness facility, including exercise equipment.
- Sponsor exercise and health-related programs or organizations.
- Hire health-related experts (e.g., personal trainer, registered dietitian, spiritual counselor, health psychologist) to provide instruction and to overcome exercise resistance and barriers to adopting a healthier lifestyle.
- Schedule seminars or workshops that are directly linked to a wellness program and connect religious texts to living a healthy lifestyle.

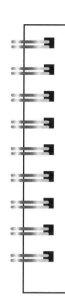

- Sponsor counseling seminars that address serious mental health concerns such as eating disorders, low self-esteem, depression, lack of perceived control over one's life that reflects an absence of free will, and related self-destructive behavior patterns and beliefs.
- Include more sermon material that extols the virtues of a healthy lifestyle, particularly if evidence is provided by religious texts.
- Establish a mentoring program that includes role models of congregants who have been successful in developing and maintaining a healthy lifestyle and who can mentor other congregants who seek improved fitness, nutrition, and other healthy habits.

FORM 7.1   GOD LOCUS OF HEALTH CONTROL (GLHC) SCALE

Please indicate the extent to which you agree with each of the following items, ranging from 1 (strongly disagree) to 6 (strongly agree).

1	2	3	4	5	6
Strongly disagree	Moderately disagree	Disagree	Agree	Moderately agree	Strongly agree

Items

____ 1. If my (health/condition) worsens, it is up to God to determine whether I will feel better again.

____ 2. Most things that affect my (health/condition) happen because of God.

____ 3. God is directly responsible for my (health/condition) getting better or worse.

____ 4. Whatever happens to my (health/condition) is God's will.

____ 5. Whether or not my (health/condition) improves is up to God.

____ 6. God is in control of my (health/condition).

Total score: _____

Adapted from K.A. Wallston et al., 1999, "Does God determine your health? The God locus of health control scale," *Cognitive Therapy and Research* 23: 131-142. With kind permission from Springer Science+Business Media.

From M. Anshel, 2014, *Applied Health Fitness Psychology.* (Champaign, IL: Human Kinetics).

REFERENCES

Anshel, M.H., and Smith, M. (2013). The role of religious leaders in promoting healthy habits in religious institutions. *Journal of Religion and Health, 52,* 1-14.

Atchley, R.C. (1997). The subjective importance of being religious and its effect on health and morale 14 years later. *Journal of Aging Studies, 11,* 131-141.

Aten, J.D., McMinn, M.R., and Worthington, E.L. (Eds.). (2011). *Spiritually-oriented interventions for counseling and psychotherapy.* Washington, DC: American Psychological Association.

Byl, J. (2008). Valuing wellness. In P. Walters and J. Byl (Eds.), *Christian paths to health and wellness* (pp. 3-12). Champaign, IL: Human Kinetics.

Byl, J., and Moroze, D.E. (2008). God's purpose and your life's mission. In P. Walters and J. Byl (Eds.), *Christian paths to health and wellness* (pp. 13-28). Champaign, IL: Human Kinetics.

Cline, K.M.C., and Ferraro, K.F. (2006). Does religion increase the prevalence and incidence of obesity in adulthood? *Journal for the Scientific Study of Religion, 45,* 269-281.

Colbert, D. (2002). *What would Jesus eat? The ultimate program for eating well, feeling great, and living longer.* Nashville: Thomas Nelson.

Ferraro, K.F., and Albrecht-Jensen, C.M. (1991). Does religion influence adult health? *Journal for the Scientific Study of Religion, 30,* 193-202.

Gall, T.L., Charbonneau, C., Clarke, N.H., Grant, K., Joseph, A., and Shouldice, L. (2005). Understanding the nature and role of spirituality in relation to coping and health: A conceptual framework. *Canadian Psychology, 46,* 88-104.

Holt, C.L., and McClure, S.M. (2006). Perceptions of the religion-health connection among African American church members. *Qualitative Health Research, 16,* 268-281.

Huff, R.M., and Kline, M.V. (2007). Health promotion in the context of culture. In M.V. Kline and R.M. Huff (Eds.), *Health promotion in multicultural populations* (2nd ed., pp. 3-22). Los Angeles: Sage.

Huff, R.M., and Yasharpour, S. (2007). Cross-cultural concepts of health and disease. In M.V. Kline and R.M. Huff (Eds.), *Health promotion in multicultural populations* (2nd ed., pp. 23-39). Los Angeles: Sage.

Kennett, D.J., and Ackerman, M. (1995). Importance of learned resourcefulness to weight loss and early success during maintenance: Preliminary evidence. *Patient Education and Counseling, 25,* 197-203.

Kline, M.V., and Huff, R.M. (2007). *Health promotion in multicultural populations* (2nd ed.). Los Angeles: Sage.

Koenig, H.G. (1999). *The healing power of faith.* New York: Simon and Schuster.

Koenig, H.G. (2007). *Spirituality in patient care: Why, how, when, and what.* West Conshohocken, PA: Templeton Foundation Press.

Koenig, H.G. (2008). *Medicine, religion, and health: Where science and spirituality meet.* West Conshohocken, PA: Templeton Foundation Press.

Levin, J. (2001). *God, faith, and health: Exploring the spirituality-healing connection.* New York: Wiley.

Murray, R.H., and Rubel, A.J. (1992). Sounding board: Physicians and healers—unwitting partners in health care delivery. *New England Journal of Medicine, 326,* 61-64.

Omartian, S. (1996). *Greater health God's way.* Eugene, OR: Harvest House.

Pargament, K.I. (1997). *The psychology of religion and coping.* New York: Guilford.

Purnell, L.D., and Paulanka, B.J. (1998). *Transcultural health care: A culturally competent approach.* Philadelphia: Davis.

Spector, R.E. (1996). *Cultural diversity in health and illness* (4th ed.). Stamford, CT: Appleton and Lange.

Wallston, K.A., Malcarne, V.L., Flores, L., Hansdottir, I., Smith, C.A., Stein, M.J., Weisman, M.H., and Clements, P.J. (1999). Does God determine your health? The God Locus of Health Control Scale. *Cognitive Therapy and Research, 23,* 131-142.

Walters, P., and Byl, J. (Eds.). (2008). *Christian paths to health and wellness.* Champaign, IL: Human Kinetics.

Young, C., and Koopsen, C. (2005). *Spirituality, health, and healing.* Sudbury, MA: Jones and Bartlett.

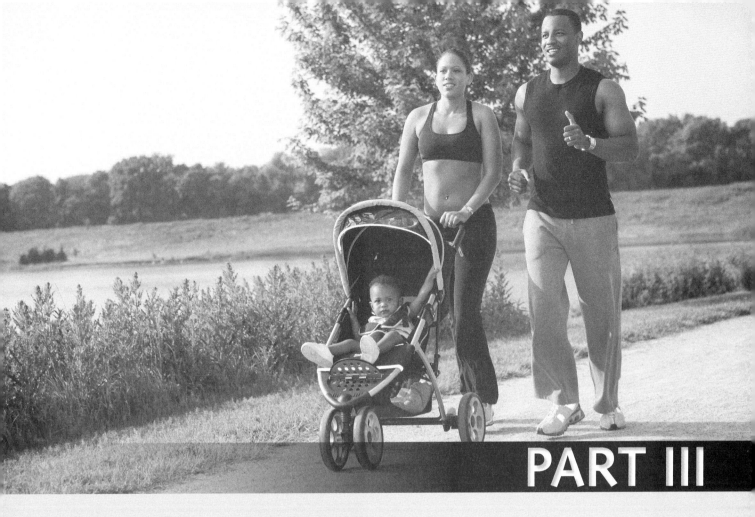

PART III

STRATEGIES FOR HEALTH BEHAVIOR INTERVENTIONS

To this point, the book has addressed the problems associated with societies that do not promote a physically active lifestyle and instead make it easy to overeat and remain sedentary. In part III, the focus is on helping clients continue their journey in developing a lifelong habit of regular exercise.

Chapter 8 addresses the differences between exercise adherence and compliance as well as ways to promote adherence. Chapter 9 covers an area that has received almost no attention by researchers—the use of cognitive and behavioral strategies to improve exercise performance and outcomes. Chapter 10 discusses fitness goal setting, indicating that it contains strong motivational properties for many people who want to use goals as an incentive to achieve and improve their perception of competence. For this latter group, goals provide evidence that the exerciser has improved, or achieved. This evidence boosts a sense of accomplishment and creates enormous satisfaction, which in turn is highly motivating and promotes exercise adherence.

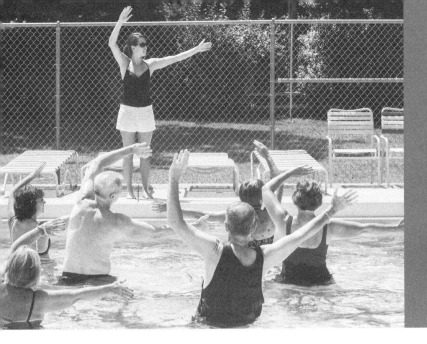

CHAPTER 8

Exercise Adherence and Compliance

> *The difference in winning and losing is most often . . . not quitting.*
>
> Walt Disney (1901-1966), animator and film producer

CHAPTER OBJECTIVES

After reading this chapter, you should be able to:

- know the differences between adherence and compliance when it comes to exercise or any other health behavior;

- identify the types of exercise adherence and compliance;

- be familiar with the ways adherence and compliance are measured;

- explain the reasons why some people begin and maintain an exercise program while others drop out; and

- describe the cognitive and behavioral strategies that health care workers can use to promote exercise adherence and compliance.

This chapter begins by asking a few questions about all-too-common human behavior. Why do most people start something and then quit? Why do so many begin new programs, attempt new habits, and initiate new behavioral patterns, including exercise, and then fail to maintain them? Why is building new rituals so difficult? Reasons abound. First, we would have to consider the person's motive to begin the new habit in the first place. Why did the person start a new exercise program, and even more important, why did he decide to quit? What good is initiating a new exercise habit if the person drops out in a matter of weeks or months? How can professionals and consultants in the areas of physical and mental health promote adherence to healthy habits, such as exercising, eating a nutritious diet, and getting enough sleep? In attempting to answer these questions, we'll first take a look at reasons for and perceived barriers to exercise participation, and then we'll examine exercise adherence and compliance.

REASONS FOR EXERCISE PARTICIPATION

The vast majority of people in Western cultures lead sedentary lives. The sedentary person has the most to gain from improving health and preventing disease, even if activity levels rise modestly. Health professionals should be equally concerned about initiating and adhering to physical activity programs, especially for the completely sedentary population.

Research on the effectiveness of interventions for developing and maintaining involvement in an exercise program has received extensive attention over the years. Some of these earlier studies have been limited to formal exercise programs that occur at specific settings and times, such as prescheduled exercise classes or other formal, structured physical activity programs (Dishman and Buckworth, 1996). At times researchers have examined the effects of interventions (e.g., social support, scheduling, online reminders) on participants' adherence to the designated program (Dawson, Tracey, and Berry, 2008). The results of these studies have been uneven, with some—but not all—results indicating significantly better adherence rates due to the interventions.

One limitation of these adherence studies is that requiring novice exercisers to attend a previously scheduled class at a given location and time may not accommodate their personal preferences for exercise type (e.g., cardiorespiratory, strength, flexibility), location (e.g., fitness facility, home, outdoors, indoors), time (e.g., early morning, lunchtime, dinnertime, evening), and proximity to home or work. The result has sometimes been high program dropout rates and poor studies with low sample sizes and disappointing results (Buckworth and Dishman, 2002; King, 1994). More recently, however, researchers have examined the effectiveness of exercise interventions using various forms of physical activity (e.g., resistance training, walking, bicycling) at home, at work, and in the community (Chenoweth, 2007).

One approach to improving exercise adherence, that is, a person's conscious decision to maintain an exercise program, is to determine the person's reasons for exercising and to create programs and opportunities that are compatible with those reasons. Markland and Ingledew (1997), for instance, validated an instrument called the *Exercise Motivation Inventory* that measures a person's motives for exercising. Through statistical analyses, their inventory derived 12 sources of exercise motivation:

1. Reducing stress (e.g., "To release tension")
2. Managing weight (e.g., "To stay slim")
3. Feeling better, or revitalization (e.g., "Because it makes me feel good")
4. Social recognition (e.g., "To gain recognition for my accomplishments")
5. Enjoyment (e.g., "Because I enjoy the feeling of exerting myself")
6. Challenge (e.g., "To help me explore the limits of my body")
7. Social affiliation (e.g., "To spend time with friends")

8. Competition (e.g., "Because I enjoy competing")

9. Following medical practitioner's advice (e.g., "My doctor advised me to exercise")

10. Avoiding poor health (e.g., "To avoid heart disease or other diseases")

11. Improving health (e.g., "To help me live a longer, healthier life")

12. Improving physical appearance (e.g., "To have a good body and a nice appearance")

Given this extensive list of reasons for exercising, what are the primary reasons for stopping? The person was motivated to begin a program, so what factors contributed to the decision to quit? This issue is a primary intervention area of health professionals and forms the main focus of this chapter. Researchers refer to the reasons for nonparticipation—either not starting in the first place or quitting—as *exercise barriers*. When health professionals become aware of an exerciser's barriers, they can use interventions and strategies to help prevent or overcome these barriers.

PERCEIVED EXERCISE BARRIERS

Exercise barriers, addressed in chapter 4, play a significant role in predicting whether people will engage in behaviors that are more likely to lead to improving health and managing disease. That is, the fewer reasons people offer to explain their lack of healthy behavior patterns, the more likely it is that they will have healthy habits. Barriers to engaging in regular exercise and other forms of physical activity are referred to as *perceived* because they reflect a person's reasons for not exercising. These reasons, such as "I don't have enough time" or "No one will exercise with me," may or may not reflect reality. Given the high number of people in many countries who are overweight and obese, made worse by a sedentary lifestyle, it is understandable that researchers have found no shortage of reasons why people do not engage in regular exercise or stop exercising after initiating an exercise routine.

Barriers have been categorized as either objective (e.g., inaccessible facilities for people with physical disabilities, disease, injury, lack of an exercise facility) or perceived (e.g., lack of time, high cost of a fitness club membership, anxiety about entering an exercise facility). In addition, barriers have also been categorized as internal, interpersonal, and environmental (Timmerman, 2007). Personal barriers such as physical fatigue or family responsibilities are associated with reduced leisure-time physical activity and increased sedentary behaviors (e.g., more time devoted to driving a car, playing computer games, or watching television).

Most studies that list perceived exercise barriers include the following: lack of time; pain, discomfort, or injury; fear of injury; unavailable exercise equipment or facility; lack of knowledge about exercise technique; finding exercise unpleasant; lack of confidence; feeling intimidated; no exercise partner; lack of support from others; history of giving up; too expensive; and no close access to a facility (Brinthaupt, Kang, and Anshel, 2010; Buckworth and Dishman, 1999). See figure 8.1 for more examples of barriers.

Perhaps the two most common psychobehavioral exercise barriers are lack of time and lack of enjoyment (Brinthaupt et al., 2010). In their review of this literature, Brinthaupt et al. concluded that lack of time is one of the most difficult barriers to overcome. The authors refer to lack of time as a *super barrier* in that it affects many other factors related to exercise. For example, lack of time goes beyond actual exercise time. It also may include travel time to and from an exercise facility; time needed to perform other valued activities related to work, leisure, family, and hobbies; and time needed to conduct other daily routines that require changing one's personal schedule (Kruger, Yore, Bauer, and Kohl, 2007). The lack of pleasure due to high physical exertion and discomfort is another barrier, particularly if the exerciser is overweight, is inexperienced in executing proper exercise technique, and lacks motivation and energy to overcome physical fatigue (Salmon, Owen, Crawford, Bauman, and Sallis, 2003). An unpleasant exercise

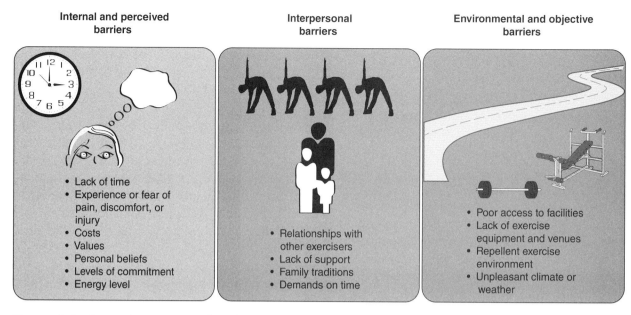

Figure 8.1 Internal, interpersonal, and environmental barriers to exercise adherence.

environment only exacerbates the reasons not to continue to exercise.

The goals of every practitioner and researcher in the areas of physical health, fitness, and mental health are to reduce the frequency and intensity of exercise barriers, to overcome these barriers, to strongly encourage people to initiate and maintain a regimen of regular exercise, and to help people develop an active, healthy lifestyle. The process by which a person maintains participation in a preplanned exercise program is called *exercise adherence*.

DEFINING ADHERENCE AND COMPLIANCE

Definitions of *adherence* and *compliance* have differed in the areas of health and exercise psychology. *Compliance* is a term often used interchangeably with *adherence*, but many writers contend that these two concepts are distinct. In addition, separating *adherence* from *compliance* has become increasingly difficult in recent years.

King (1994) defines *adherence* as "the level of participation achieved in a behavioral regimen once the individual has agreed to undertake it" (p. 186). This definition of exercise change

represents increasing exercise participation by people who are already somewhat active or are in the stages of becoming more active. *Compliance* is often defined as "the degree to which an individual follows a specific recommendation" (Bowen, Helmes, and Lease, 2001, p. 26) or "the extent to which a person's behavior (in terms of taking medication, following a diet, modifying habits [such as exercise], or attending clinics) coincides with medical or health advice" (Haynes, 2001, p. 4).

Haynes (2001) points out that the term *adherence* is preferred because *compliance* "implies subservience on the part of the patient, or constitutes blaming the patient for noncompliance" (p. 4). Thus, adherence is a concept that reflects people's self-determined actions, that is, their decision to maintain participation in an exercise program that they selected on their own volition, whereas compliance reflects the decision to maintain participation in a program that was prescribed or required by others. Nonadherence is a function of one's decision to terminate involvement in an activity, whereas noncompliance consists of acting in a manner that is contrary to given advice, recommendations, or requirements (e.g., "I will not take the medication my doctor prescribed").

Rand and Weeks (1998), using the terms *adherence* and *compliance* interchangeably, define them as "the degree to which patient behaviors coincide with the clinical recommendations of health care providers" (p. 115). Following the recommendations of others is closer to the traditional use of *compliance*, whereas *adherence* is a self-determined decision (e.g., "I am deciding to exercise on my own volition in the absence of being prompted or required by someone else to exercise."). The authors also indicate that there is no gold standard to describe satisfactory or poor adherence for all health behaviors. They assert that appropriate adherence must be operationally defined based on the situation and desired outcomes. For instance, a novice exerciser might find the traditional aerobic exercise of three times per week somewhat challenging in terms of time available to exercise, level of discomfort, time needed for recovery, and developing a positive attitude, or sense of enjoyment, toward aerobic exercise. Twice per week might be sufficient to generate a habit of aerobic training in the early stages of improving fitness and developing an exercise habit. Practitioners would do well to work with novice exercisers slowly and not push them too hard to establish desirable exercise intensity, frequency, and duration too soon in their fitness program. Developing an exercise ethic, that is, a strong belief in regular exercise and a more active lifestyle, takes time.

Researchers of adherence realize that adherence and compliance have multiple dimensions and definitions. Clinicians and researchers often categorize individuals as *adherers* or *nonadherers*; however, adherence is not a dichotomous variable. Unlike the concept of program dropout or nonparticipant, which is a yes-or-no variable, adherence rarely reflects a person who did or did not adhere to the researcher's or clinician's expectations. Instead, adherence is often assessed as a matter of degree. Appropriate adherence must be situationally defined. In their review of the literature, Rand and Weeks (1998) categorize adherence according to the extent to which a person engages in the targeted (criterion) task.

- *Appropriate adherence.* This type of adherence refers to a person who performs expected behavior over time. For example, someone who is asked to eat several small meals per day instead of skipping some meals or eating excessively at mealtime will carry out that prescribed dietary regimen daily.

- *Erratic adherence.* Sometimes called *partial compliance*, this is when a person follows a prescribed program or takes medication as required some days but withdraws or changes the required behavior other times. For instance, certain activities are necessary in the presence of certain symptoms (e.g., using antihistamines during allergy season, taking antibiotics following a surgical procedure, following a stretching protocol in response to an injury) but are not needed when the symptoms are no longer detected. As Rand and Weeks (1998) note, "Erratic adherence may also reflect forgetfulness, stress, changed schedules . . . or some other barriers to full adherence" (p. 116).

Nonadherence and *noncompliance* have also been defined and categorized in the literature. Table 8.1 provides various types and examples of exercise compliance.

COMPLIANCE AND ADHERENCE IN AN EXERCISE SETTING

- *Compliance:* A physician or personal trainer prescribes a specific exercise routine to an individual who then follows that prescription, or a client follows the nutritional advice prescribed by a registered dietitian. In both examples, the prescription is based on client test data.

- *Adherence:* The client initiates and maintains an exercise routine that is communicated by a specialist and is intended to meet the client's needs (e.g., lose weight, improve lipids profile) and reach predetermined goals (e.g., improved aerobic fitness, increased HDL cholesterol).

- *Noncompliance.* Reflects a person's chronic underuse of a substance or treatment—for example, an individual who is prescribed at least two (preferably three) resistance training sessions per week to build muscular strength, but trains only one session per week.

- *Erratic noncompliance.* This behavior is characterized by the individual's perceptions of being too busy, forgetful, stressed, or experiencing some acute problem.

- *Unwitting noncompliance.* This form of not completing a prescribed or expected protocol might include misunderstanding of the task or instructions, incorrect use of exercise techniques, inability to travel to an exercise facility, injury or pain, and lack of social support.

- *Intentional noncompliance.* This type of noncompliance is indicative of improved well-being, fear of injury or reoccurring symptoms, dislike of exercising, refusal to adapt to a new lifestyle, physical or psychological discomfort from exercise, or denial of exercise benefits.

It is the responsibility of every researcher, clinician, or educator to determine evidence of adherence or nonadherence (e.g., attendance rates and other explanations or interpretations of a person's thoughts or behaviors) so that

- results of studies can be explained and future exercise interventions can be improved.

- changes in the intervention can be considered to improve adherence rates (perhaps the prescribed activity was too difficult or did not take certain factors into account, such as transportation, program costs, or fitness and health status of participants); and

- treatment effectiveness can be determined over time, both in the short term (e.g., during the treatment period or within 60 days after the program) and long term (e.g., more than 60 days, perhaps six months or a year after the program).

MEASURING ADHERENCE

It is apparent that people who agree to engage in a given activity and then discontinue their involvement in that activity are not adhering. Sadly, this problem is all too common when it comes to health behavior. Dieting and exercise are two of the more typical types of programs that people start and then stop. However, the determination of adherence and compliance (or nonadherence and noncompliance) often differs among studies. Do we consider people to be exercise dropouts if they were prescribed

Table 8.1 Behavioral Examples of Exercise Noncompliance

Type of compliance	Behavioral example
Noncompliance Person chronically underuses an exercise program.	Person is given an exercise prescription but fails to initiate a program, completes only part of the program, or begins the program and then quits.
Erratic noncompliance Person claims to be too busy, forgetful, or stressed or experiences a sudden problem.	Person fails to incorporate exercise as part of a daily routine, is physically uncomfortable performing physical activity, or considers exercise to be one more thing to do rather than a stress reliever.
Unwitting noncompliance Person does not complete a prescribed or expected protocol.	Person misunderstands the task or instructions; exercises incorrectly, often resulting in poor outcomes (e.g., no weight loss, minimum fitness gains); is unable to travel to an exercise facility; experiences injury or pain; cannot afford fitness equipment or club membership; or lacks social support.
Intentional noncompliance Person no longer feels the need to exercise, fears injury or discomfort, dislikes exercise, refuses to change lifestyle, or denies exercise benefits.	Person resists starting or maintaining an exercise program despite suggestions from a medical or fitness specialist and generates reasons for not exercising.

a cardiorespiratory fitness program based on three 30-minute sessions per week but can attend only twice per week? Or, if they become injured and must discontinue exercise until they heal, have they dropped out? Certainly, the motives and explanations for stopping involvement in an activity depend on both situational and personal factors. If people quit their exercise program due to boredom, that's an issue that requires a different reaction and adherence strategy than if they quit exercising due to a factor beyond their control, such as illness, injury, lack of transportation to the exercise venue, bad weather, or lack of proper coaching. Haynes (2001) recommends using three means to detect adherence:

1. *Tracking appointment attendance:* Assuming there is a planned program the participants are expected to attend, Haynes suggests watching for people who fail to attend prearranged appointments or programs. In addition, people who are partial, or irregular, attendees are less likely to be adhering to their program.

2. *Detecting nonresponders:* Nonadherence is the most frequent explanation for lack of improved fitness or any other expected outcome. It is also important, however, to be sure that the individual is engaging in the proper exercise procedures under the most desirable conditions (e.g., using the correct resistance in weight training, running or walking according to a prescribed plan, feeling comfortable and motivated during exercise, having adequate water before and during exercise).

3. *Asking nonresponders about their adherence:* It is appropriate to simply ask people if they are attending exercise sessions and following through with their planned program (diet, exercise, rehabilitation) in the prescribed manner. This procedure, however, has to be carried out in a non-threatening, sensitive manner so that people do not feel defensive or anxious about telling the truth.

Adherence can be ascertained using the following options:

- Attendance at predetermined events (e.g., exercise classes, appointments, meetings)
- Self-reports (i.e., the person reports adherence to the program)
- Record keeping, in which the person completes an attendance chart and monitors progress (e.g., changes in resting heart rate, body weight, running speed, endurance time, or body weight)
- Tests (e.g., lipids profile, aerobic or strength fitness testing)
- Number of contacts with staff or coaches
- Number of appointments kept
- Interviews with others with whom the person usually keeps in contact (e.g., peers, family members, other professionals, other program attendees)
- Electronic methods of recording behavior, including the use of computers (Internet), smartphones, and text messages
- Pedometers (recording step counts)
- Accelerometers (recording step counts and speed)
- Heart rate monitors

Social Media and Fitness

Chenoweth (2007) coined the term *e-health technology* to reflect the phenomenon of using the Internet as a source of health information and behavior. He defines it as "the application of Internet and other related technologies to improve the access, efficiency, effectiveness, and quality of clinical and business practices used by organizations, practitioners, and consumers to improve and maintain the health status of individuals and organizations" (p. 97).

The continued evolution of communication technology in recent years has direct implications for promoting fitness. Mailed fliers and newsletters intended to provide consumers with the most current information about health-related research have been replaced by online communication and websites. Information updates are now instantaneous. This phenomenon is collectively called *social media*, or "the ability to use electronic means to connect to other individuals of similar interests based on one's own criteria" (Biscontini, 2012, p. 12). According to Biscontini, social media has become the most affordable and commonplace marketing tool for fitness professionals. The most popular forms of electronic communication, all free, include Facebook, Twitter, YouTube, and LinkedIn.

- *Facebook.* Facebook can be used to facilitate relationships between fitness coaches and clients and to show that the coach is more than a teacher and trainer. This vehicle promotes the coach's personality and helps clients to feel more comfortable with their coach and to know the coach as a person. Biscontini (2012) quotes one fitness coach who claims that Facebook helps clients feel valued and allows fitness professionals to show they care about them beyond the gym. Sample Facebook content includes photos of clients before and after experiencing an exercise program, information about proper techniques, testimonials from clients about what worked for them to meet fitness goals, educational materials, and advertising services. Use of photos markedly increases the read rate.

- *Twitter.* Twitter is similar in some ways to Facebook, but posts are limited to 140 characters. Biscontini contends that "Facebook currently reaches more people, but people tend to believe tweets as more newsworthy because of their immediacy" (p. 13). He suggests using free programs to link both accounts so your postings appear in both places.

- *LinkedIn.* LinkedIn helps people who do not have their own websites to connect in the professional job market. LinkedIn is becoming an effective one-stop shop for decision makers when looking for the right person for the job. Users have a current profile page that can lead readers to a personal website, Facebook, and Twitter, where more material and information are available.

Practical tips for using social media more effectively include the following:

- Attach a photograph or video clip to every set of words; photos stimulate more comments than text-based posts.

- To maintain credibility among readers, avoid changing your relationship status often.

- Use teasers; for instance, tease about an upcoming event over time or keep track of someone's progress in reaching a training or weight-control goal.

- For Facebook posts, make sure you are friends with all personal contacts or companies that you are going to mention before making the post.

Electronic Devices and Fitness

The proliferation of electronic devices has prompted researchers to examine the effects of these devices on exercise behavior, particularly with respect to adherence. If exercisers are reminded to exercise through texts, phone calls, apps, computers, or other software, particularly if the communication source is their fitness coach or other health professional, are they more likely to adhere to their exercise program? Results of several recent studies are promising in this respect.

In one study, for instance, Lombard, Lombard, and Winnett (1995) found that people who received weekly phone calls to touch base walked more often than people who received calls every three weeks or no calls at all. Phone calls, the authors concluded, form a source of emotional and social support, and they hold people accountable to their earlier agreement to exercise regularly.

In a more recent study, Richardson and her colleagues (2010) examined the effect of online community features of an Internet walking program on participant adherence and average daily step counts. In particular, the researchers measured changes in fitness and exercise adherence in response to various forms of social support communicated to participants on the Internet, such as information about exercise progress and motivational messages. They found that the group receiving online correspondence and performance feedback, as opposed to no messages, resulted in significantly less attrition (i.e., dropouts). Average daily step counts for both groups significantly

---

USING TECHNOLOGY TO ENCOURAGE EXERCISE ADHERENCE

If you are a fitness or health care professional, generate a group e-mail of clients so that you can contact them all at one time with

- a reminder to exercise or increase physical activity that day;
- specific hints to take the stairs, get up and walk, and other ways to increase their daily physical activity; or

- educational information about healthy habits.

Also, consider consulting with clients through fitness clubs, rehabilitation or medical centers, and other health-related businesses and apply your knowledge through the company client or patient e-mail system and other forms of electronic communication, if allowed.

---

improved from pretest to posttest, however, and the two groups were statistically similar. The results of this study confirm that using electronic devices can improve exercise adherence, perhaps due to providing additional social support and feedback on performance that promote achievement and competence.

Carr and his colleagues (2009) studied the effect of a 16-week Internet-delivered program intended to increase the amount of daily physical activity and both short-term and long-term exercise adherence among 32 sedentary overweight adults. Using a pedometer to measure steps per day, the results indicated significantly increased physical activity, improved cholesterol profile, and reduced percent body fat as measured immediately after the intervention. Results of long-term adherence (i.e., eight months later), however, revealed a relapse among the participants, with physical activity reverting back to baseline (preintervention) levels. In this study, at least, the Internet did not help produce a permanent lifestyle change in physical activity habits.

Other studies have examined the effect of Internet exercise programs on changes in fitness and selected health measures based on increased rates of physical activity. In a German workplace study conducted with overweight, sedentary factory employees, Krcmar, Halle, and Leimeister (2010) found that structured, Internet-delivered exercise recommendations were not superior to unstructured, Internet-delivered exercise recommendations over a 12-week intervention.

The investigators attribute these results partly to high dropout rates in both groups; only 77 of 140 initial participants completed the study. There were significant gains in fitness over the 12-week program, but no measure of long-term adherence was reported.

In a Canadian study, Dawson et al. (2008) compared group-based and Internet-based physical activity interventions. They found that the Internet intervention attracted more participants, but the group-based participants showed significant improvement in fitness, exercise self-efficacy (i.e., building self-confidence about exercise performance and desirable outcomes), and exercise adherence. The Internet group, however, did improve in life satisfaction after the intervention. The researchers concluded that although the Internet reaches far more people than traditional approaches to improving physical activity levels, the changes may not be as positive as face-to-face interventions. "The internet," they assert, "offers possibilities for a group that require specifically tailored interventions" (p. 542). Far more research is needed in producing high-quality Internet interventions that markedly improve fitness, level of physical activity, and other health behaviors.

DEVELOPING AN EXERCISE HABIT

Habits develop when people schedule behaviors at specific times and on a regular (i.e., daily, weekly) basis (Loehr and Schwartz,

2003). Loehr and Schwartz use the term *positive ritual* if the intention of a habit is to improve health, energy, well-being, and quality of life. Specifically, the authors describe a positive ritual as "a behavior that becomes automatic over time—fueled by some deeply held value" (p. 14). A ritual, used interchangeably with the term *habit*, is a carefully defined, highly structured behavior. To Loehr and Schwartz, "The power of rituals is that they insure that we use as little conscious energy as possible where it is not absolutely necessary, leaving us free to strategically focus other energy available to us in creative, enriching ways" (p. 14).

For instance, a person who has planned a 30- to 45-minute workout should develop a set of rituals that will create optimal benefits from the session. The rituals are planned and executed before (e.g., water intake, light aerobic work, mild stretching), during (e.g., interval training, resistance and aerobic exercises,

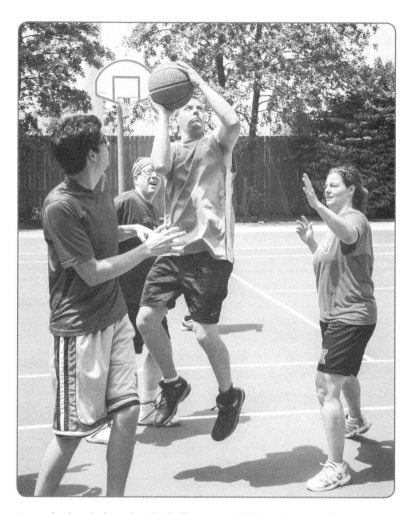

A regular lunch-hour basketball game with friends and colleagues can make exercise an enjoyable habit.

preplanned sequence of activities), and immediately following (e.g., water intake, more extensive stretching, shower) the session.

Developing a habit, especially when it comes to replacing unhealthy behaviors with more desirable routines, is enhanced when the new habit is attached to a value and linked to a specific time and place (Anshel, 2008). Thus, the habit of engaging in regular exercise is promoted when exercise is anchored by values such as health (e.g., "I need good health to be successful and have energy"), family (e.g., "I need to be a good example to my children and maintain my health to live a long, productive life"), and faith (e.g., "I recall scriptural passages that pronounce the benefits of a healthy lifestyle, which is sanctioned by a spiritual power"), among many others. Exercise habits

are more likely to form when the session is planned, let's say, during the lunch hour on three days a week. Because these sessions are planned in advance, they are more likely to be fulfilled. Inviting at least one other person to exercise together, a strategy called *social support*, enhances adherence and habit development.

Changing a person's habits is difficult. Reasons abound but include psychological comfort (e.g., bad habits may reduce stress, create feelings of familiarity, and require less mental effort), social convenience (e.g., doing what others also do), and convenience (e.g., addictions to certain behavior patterns, adapting to life's demands expediently and cheaply). Understandably, changing bad habits is challenging and rarely permanent. Merely warning a person about the long-term consequences of persisting with an unhealthy habit or simply providing educational materials have not been shown to induce permanent changes or sometimes even short-term changes in self-destructive habits.

This section offers a unique approach to addressing health behavior change if the client sincerely wants to overcome a bad habit. It includes two components, or processes: (1) completing four steps, or actions, in the proper sequence to provide a structure for directing client behavior and (2) using interview strategies in the consultation process—that is, asking clients certain questions to induce commitment and motivation to making long-term changes in selected unhealthy behaviors.

Four Steps for Directing Behavior Change

So, what is the process of developing and maintaining habits that are in our clients' best interests and are consistent with their deepest values? There are four steps to replacing unhealthy behavior patterns with healthy ones. The first is to acknowledge that habits begin with two personal dispositions: feeling in control of one's life and taking responsibility for one's health and quality of life. Both perceptions are necessary to progress in replacing negative habits with positive alternatives. Justifications for not exercising, not eating properly, and maintaining other self-destructive, unhealthy lifestyle behaviors result in a sense of helplessness, and negative habits persist. Failure to change behavior consists of a list of excuses (e.g., "I just can't find the time to exercise," "I must have my bowl of ice cream before bedtime").

The second step is to develop a 24-hour chart that allows the health care worker to help clients schedule their healthy habits. Examples include times for eating small meals and healthy snacks (frequent eating increases metabolism and leads to weight loss), time to recover from nonstop work, time for at least 30 minutes of exercise, time for presleep rituals (within 2 hours of bedtime), reflection time or prayer, and other habits that increase energy and improve quality of life.

The third step in health behavior change is to help clients recruit social support from various sources. Examples include finding a partner, such as a friend, family member, coach, mentor, or religious leader, who will support the client's effort to reduce or eliminate some undesirable habits. Ideally, the most influential sources of social support will hold the client accountable for changing behaviors and perhaps even assist the client in carrying out an action plan and offer support to engage in regular exercise, eat healthier food, or provide reminders about the importance of remaining vigilant in leading a healthier lifestyle.

The fourth and final step is to develop an action plan consisting of scheduling new routines that will replace the negative habits. Examples include reducing the intake of sweets, such as replacing pastry with fruit for a snack or dessert; avoiding late-night eating, especially just before bedtime; replacing at least some carbonated drinks with water or juice; and engaging in regular exercise, even if it's just walking after a meal. Inserting each new ritual into a specific time frame and location will improve adherence to it, so specificity of the action plan is essential. For instance, at what time and where will the client exercise three times a week? When are meals being consumed and how will the client ensure that portions are small? What activities are scheduled for recovering from the relentless demands of the client's time? When are fun activities scheduled?

Consultation Strategies for Inducing Behavior Change

The second stage of changing unhealthy client behaviors is consultation content, which consists of asking a series of questions and addressing objectives. Table 8.2 provides a few guidelines for interviewing clients in a way that will facilitate building rituals toward health behavior change.

Table 8.2 Interview Prompts for Building Health Behavior Rituals

Consultation sequence for replacing unhealthy habits	Questions for clients
Building rapport and trust	"What do you want to be able to change and why?" "Can you give me a bit of background that might help explain why this is important to you?" "Can you take me through a typical day in which this issue comes up?"
Reviewing the benefits of the unhealthy habit	"All of us do things every day we know are not good for us. What are the benefits of the habit you want to change?"
Reviewing reasons for changing the unhealthy habit	"In what ways do you see this behavioral tendency as unpleasant or undesirable?" "Why change?"
Reviewing short-term costs and long-term consequences	"What are the possible dangers, costs, or consequences of continuing this habit?" "Do you find these consequences acceptable? Are they something you can live with and feel you won't be harmed?" "Do you detect danger to your health or happiness, or is everything OK?"
Determining what is not acceptable	"What will it take in the way of information, test scores, or advice from experts that might prompt you to change and to replace your current habit with one that is better for your health?"
Determining values	"Let me ask you about what's really important to you. These are called *values*, your core beliefs about what is most important. Here is a list of values. Please pick out the five most important ones."
Identifying disconnects	"Among the five you selected, can you see any inconsistency, or disconnect, between a particular value and the health behavior you want to change? That is, do you see a lack of compatibility between any of your most important values and an unhealthy behavior you want to change?" "What are the consequences of this disconnect?" "Are these consequences acceptable to you? If not, are you ready to work toward replacing the unhealthy habit with a healthier, more desirable one?"
Developing an action plan	At this stage the health coach develops a schedule in conjunction with the client that provides a few new routines that incorporate the client's values. The schedule should include time for going to bed and waking up, presleep rituals, proper eating patterns, exercise, recovery breaks during the day, rituals for coming home from work, spending time with family members, and more.

STEPS TO ACHIEVING EXERCISE ADHERENCE

Mental and physical health care professionals, fitness coaches, and researchers agree that change must come from within; no one can force another person to change. To maintain healthy habits, fulfill our mission that gives us purpose in life, and reach our potential in our professional and personal lives, we need to be fully engaged, which requires energy, commitment, and self-motivation, and we must change our life stories when they need serious editing. Exercise, then, is not an end—a goal in itself—but a means to an end, that is, an important vehicle that forms the energy source of good health. The challenge, therefore, in overcoming a culture that relishes a sedentary lifestyle is to help people not only begin a program of regular physical activity but also to adhere to it.

Based on their review of related literature, Buckworth and Dishman (2002) concluded that "without intervention, there is a 50-50 chance that someone who has started an exercise program will stop within six months" (p. 229). The most common reasons for dropping out of an exercise program include failure to meet expectations, lack of enjoyment, injury, and lack of time. Adherence to an exercise regimen is more likely if health professionals help clients and patients follow a few important guidelines, including the following.

Have Realistic Expectations and Be Patient

Too many people quit exercise programs when their expectations, often unrealistic, are not met (e.g., losing a great deal of weight in a month, being able to keep up with the fitness instructor, eliminating excessive fat from the tummy or thighs). It is imperative to remind exercisers, particularly novices, that reaching desirable fitness outcomes, such as losing weight, improving musculature, and other known benefits, takes time. It took them years of physical self-abuse and inactivity to get into their current unfit condition, and it will take time to overcome those years of unhealthy habits. However, it does not take much time to simply improve both strength and aerobic fitness. This is because muscles were made to move; they become stronger and more efficient when stressed. Exercise is natural and advantageous thanks to our genetic predisposition to remain physically active.

It is important to remind clients not to expect significant improvements in fitness, weight loss, musculature, mental health, anxiety, or other desirable outcomes too soon. A sedentary lifestyle means that exercise is a struggle at the start. They should not be impatient about experiencing the benefits of physical activity. Over time, usually within six weeks, exercise will improve their fitness level, self-esteem, and even mental health. Novice exercisers can expect to take at least six to eight weeks of properly performed exercise to detect the benefits of a long-term commitment to exercise. At the same time, their body weight may not decrease dramatically (see the next point). Patience, not quitting, is the proper response.

Do Not Focus on Body Weight

The scale does not always tell the truth, especially after clients begin an exercise program. It fails to disclose how much of their weight is fat and how much is muscle. Because muscle weighs more than fat, and muscle is gained through exercise, their body weight may or may not change. But their fitness has improved dramatically and they are much healthier. Therefore, their body weight may remain the same even if there is a noticeable change in clothing size accompanied by feeling thinner and having more energy. The scale, which reflects weight loss, can certainly be a motivator to continue an exercise program. However, a more likely and more accurate indicator of improved fitness outcome is percent body fat, usually obtained from a skinfold test. Percent body fat measures how much of one's weight is fat and how much is muscle, or what is called *lean body weight*.

Improving health should be the main reason for exercise. Results of a meta-analysis conducted by Blair and Brodney (1999) indicated that people who are overweight or obese experience similar physical and mental benefits from exercise as people who are healthy weights.

Receive Instruction on Exercise Technique

Proper exercise technique must be learned. Clients should invest in a personal trainer and learn to exercise correctly. This way, they will exercise more efficiently and will improve their fitness more quickly. Proper warm-ups and cool-downs, sufficient water intake before and during the exercise session, and postexercise stretching are other strategies that a personal coach will communicate and help monitor.

Optimal benefits from exercise occur from two main types of training, cardiorespiratory (aerobic work) and strength. Both types have enormous benefits for mental and physical health. Aerobic exercise, in particular, leads to improved self-esteem, reduced anxiety and depression, and heightened tolerance to stress. In addition, stretching improves joint flexibility and helps reduce injury and discomfort.

Schedule Exercise Times and Places

Health professionals often hear this common excuse and perceived barrier for not exercising—"I don't have enough time." Notice that researchers have labeled this a *perceived* barrier, meaning that reasons for not exercising, including lack of time, are excuses based on the clients' interpretation of their situation and are not necessarily supported by reality.

There are ways to get around the "I don't have enough time" excuse, however. We require only three hours of exercise per week. That means that less than 2% of the week is needed to obtain the minimal benefits of an exercise program. It is important to plan exercise sessions in advance to ensure we make time for them. This includes getting exercise gear ready for use the night before (store it in the car, leave it by the door, or rent a locker at the gym).

Joining a fitness club is advantageous because most people rarely feel motivated to exercise at home. This is because home is associated with relaxation and rarely is associated with vigorous physical activity; thus, exercise equipment sits unused in so many homes. If financial resources allow, it might be better to join a fitness club, where the atmosphere is motivating and clients can exercise with friends (an important source of social support) and use high-quality equipment. If exercising at home, it is best to keep equipment easily accessible (e.g. in front of the TV or sound system) and schedule exercise (e.g. during the TV news).

Create a Social Support Network

As reviewed in chapter 6, some people enjoy exercising with others, while others prefer to exercise alone. For some people, considerable recognition and approval from others is central to their motivation to exercise or to do anything else. Exercising with a friend and obtaining encouragement from someone whose opinion and friendship are valued are examples of a concept called *social support*. Social support can be either direct (e.g., exercising with a partner) or indirect (e.g., speaking encouraging words, providing transportation, paying someone's fitness club membership, purchasing fitness equipment for the home). Exercisers need to surround themselves with people who express positive statements and encouragement to maintain adherence to an exercise program. Social support, according to Buckworth and Dishman (2002), includes "formal or informal comfort, assistance, and/or information from individuals or groups and can vary in frequency, durability, and intensity" (p. 203).

Feel a Sense of Achievement

Two of the most important sources of motivation are feeling competent in performing the task and feeling a sense of achievement from that competence. Health care professionals should prioritize the development of these feelings in clients because they are strongly associated with intrinsic motivation, as discussed in chapter 2. The concepts of perceived competence, need achievement, and intrinsic motivation, although covered earlier, will be revisited here because of their close association with exercise adherence.

Central to exercise motivation, particularly intrinsic motivation, is the exerciser's sense of satisfaction, achievement, and competence in performing, completing, and maintaining exercise sessions. The use of numbers, such as changes in exercise time (speed), resistance (weight training), repetitions, frequency, distance, and fitness test scores, can all indicate improved performance. These are strong sources of long-term exercise adherence.

People differ in the extent to which they are motivated in situations that are challenging and competitive and in which the likelihood of success is somewhat uncertain. A personality trait called *need achievement* helps determine a person's level of motivation to be in achievement settings, such as competitive sport and other activities that create excitement and challenge.

Similarly, the motivation to persist in an activity is increased by a feeling called *perceived competence*. Perceived competence reflects people's interpretations of their current level of skill, either in general (e.g., "I'm a pretty good runner") or in a specific situation (e.g., "I feel pretty confident about keeping up with my aerobics instructor"). It is related to the belief in one's ability to effectively complete a task (Alderman, Beighle, and Pangrazi, 2006), and it is a significant factor in deciding to regularly engage in exercise. As Alderman et al. contend, "The willingness to try new experiences and continue to participate in physical activity often depends on an [individual's] perception of her or his ability level, or perceived competence" (p. 42). In their review of related literature, the authors found a strong relationship between perceived competence and participation, enjoyment, and performance quality in competitive sport. Reinboth, Duda, and Ntoumanis (2004) found similar links between perceived competence and involvement in exercise. Level of perceived competence may more clearly be associated with performance success than any other component of motivation, particularly intrinsic motivation.

Perceived competence is an inherent component of intrinsic motivation; we become more attracted to an activity when we perform it well. If our perceived competence decreases, we tend to quit, and that is exactly what leads to dropping out in sport and exercise settings. One effective and objective way to increase a person's perceived competence is to use quantitative data that reflect improvement. Examples include changes in exercise time (speed); amount of weight lifted (resistance); number of repetitions; exercise frequency; running, jogging, or walking distance; and changes in fitness tests and percent body fat to indicate improvement over time. As indicated earlier, it is imperative for health professionals to provide instruction, feedback, and other forms of information to clients and patients that encour-

age feelings of competence (e.g., "Your form has improved greatly in that exercise") and achievement (e.g., "Great job in jogging nonstop around the track. You couldn't jog even half a lap when you started three months ago.").

MENTAL BARRIERS TO EXERCISE ADHERENCE

Exercise is challenging, no question about it. People who have spent years leading a sedentary lifestyle cannot expect to strengthen muscles, make new demands on the heart and lungs, lose weight, and reach performance goals in just a few weeks. However, it will not take a great deal of time to feel better and adjust to new physical demands they place on themselves. They simply need patience. Without it, they will quit. They will lack adherence, and this is exactly the problem with at least half the people who initiate exercise programs. Our high-achieving, impatient culture, made worse by personality traits such as negative perfectionism, high trait anxiety, and pessimism about the future, often does not allow us to set reasonable goals and to develop strategies to reach those goals.

Emotions, thoughts, and feelings drive behavior in one of two directions: positive, toward achieving success and developing a better, healthier, more energetic lifestyle, or negative, toward maintaining unhealthy habits, being overweight, lacking energy, and living a life inconsistent with one's values about what is important. Improving a client's lifestyle takes effort—and a plan. Health and fitness professionals need to revisit the client's values, connect each value to a new routine that will create and maintain a more active lifestyle, and improve physical and mental health. Adherence to a program of regular exercise, the theme of this chapter, is of paramount importance in doing everything in our power to take control of our destiny. In the words of former British prime minister Sir Winston Churchill, "Continuous effort—not strength or intelligence—is the key to unlocking our potential" (qtd. in Cook, 1993).

A person's decision to discontinue an exercise habit often has a psychological explanation. Here are some of the more common conditions that can lead to dropping out of an exercise program. Hopefully, health professionals can develop and apply effective responses to these excuses that will change the client's mind about quitting.

Anxiety

Anxiety consists of feelings of worry or threat about the future, as discussed in chapter 5. Anxious thoughts cause worry and distract the exerciser from the task at hand—and waste energy. Sources of exercise anxiety include worry about meeting goals, physical appearance, being accepted by others (even strangers at a fitness club), and using time to exercise instead of doing something else ("I could be watching TV or finishing a report instead of going to the gym"). Ironically, exercise actually reduces both short-term (acute) and long-term (chronic) anxiety. Exercise is what the doctor ordered for improved mental health, including reduced anxiety (deMoor et al., 2006). Health professionals should strongly consider exercise as one behavioral strategy for helping their clients manage anxiety, particularly if clients are given social support in their new exercise program.

Depression

Most people experience unhappiness and negative emotions; this is normal. Ongoing, deeply negative mood states, however, may be a more serious mood disorder referred to as *clinical depression* (APA, 2000). Depression is a mood disorder that ranges from mild to severe and can be due to a medical condition, substance use, or psychopathology (mental illness). A sedentary lifestyle may induce or promote depression, but exercise has been shown to reduce it in over 70 studies across various age groups and for both genders (Leith, 1998).

One factor that influences the effect of exercise on depression is whether the person has selected and is enjoying the type of physical activity. A second factor is whether the exercise is of sufficient intensity, frequency, and duration to improve fitness outcomes and lead to psychological benefits. Taking a quiet, slow walk through the park, although pleasant and relaxing, may not be sufficient to reduce depression (Brosse, Sheets, Lett, and Blumenthal, 2002). Buckworth and Dishman (2002), in support of recommendations from ACSM, suggest the following exercise guidelines for people with depression who are otherwise healthy: three to five days a week (frequency) for 20 to 60 minutes each session (duration) at 55% to 90% of maximal heart rate (intensity). Certified fitness coaches should aim to meet these standards when prescribing exercise for depressed clients.

Negativity

It is impossible to remain motivated and on task if self-talk is negative, such as, "I don't like this," "I feel terrible," or "I'm tired." Replacing those thoughts with positive statements that are optimistic and enthusiastic induces more effort and energy. Examples include, "I can do this," "I feel good," "Just three more minutes to go," and "Hang in there." To quote an anonymous writer, "You cannot be unhappy and enthusiastic at the same time."

Negative and antagonistic feelings and emotions can impair the development of an exercise habit, especially for novice performers. The problem with negative thinking is that it results in low effort and sets up the individual to fail. This process is similar to the self-fulfilling prophecy; one's performance level will be consistent with one's expectations.

Examples of negative thinking that serve as barriers to exercise success include lack of confidence (e.g., "I don't think I can do this"), intimidation (e.g., "I don't belong in this fitness facility," "People are laughing at me"), pessimism (e.g., "I'll never lose weight," "Exercise will never be enjoyable"), self-criticism (e.g., "I can't run even one lap of that track, so why even try?", "Exercise is not for me; I'll always be weak"), impatience (e.g., "I've been exercising for three weeks and still run out of steam when jogging"), and irrational thinking (e.g.,

"I've always been heavy; why change now?", "People just have to accept me the way I am," "My spouse thinks my weight and appearance are just fine").

There are several implications for health care professionals when it comes to addressing mental health. First, consultants should not attempt to diagnose or treat mental illness unless they are licensed psychologists or have other appropriate credentials related to this area. There are serious legal implications of providing treatment to a person who did not request it, was not diagnosed correctly, or did not receive the proper treatment. The key term that reflects the proper thing to do if mental illness is suspected is *referral*; that is, health care professionals must refer clients to a licensed mental health professional for diagnosis and treatment if mental illness, such as depression, chronic anxiety, or another condition, is suspected.

A second implication for dealing with psychological barriers to maintaining healthy habits, particularly related to exercise and nutrition, is the need to schedule meetings between the client and qualified health coaches, such as a certified personal trainer and a registered dietitian. Exercise and nutrition both influence mental health and should not be ignored when attempting to change client health behavior. Relationships with local experts in these areas should be established before referral in order to become familiar with the expert's background, skills, location, types of services rendered, and personal qualities. Sometimes clients prefer a male or female coach or can meet the consultant only on certain days at certain times. It is essential that the health care professional try to coordinate the client's needs and preferences with the coach's characteristics.

Perfectionism

Perfectionism is a trait reflecting a person's disposition toward "setting excessively high standards of performance in conjunction with a tendency to make overly critical self-evaluations" (Frost, Marten, Lahart, and Rosenblate,

1990, p. 450). It is usually studied as a trait measure—stable and cross-situational—not a state (situational) measure (Antony and Swinson, 2009).

Perfectionism has both positive and negative features. The positive aspects of perfectionism include setting and attempting to achieve high personal standards, striving to achieve lofty but realistic goals often leading to success, and being conscientious and self-confident (Flett, Hewitt, Blankstein, and Mosher, 1991). Negative features, not uncommon among people who go overboard in attempting to achieve goals, include feeling deep concern about making mistakes, which leads to heightened anxiety; having doubts about one's actions; setting excessively high standards; having difficulty recognizing success; and overemphasizing precision, neatness, order, and organization. People who fit these behavior and thought patterns are referred to by clinical psychologists as *neurotic perfectionists*. They have a propensity to engage in self-destructive behaviors, excessive self-criticism, failure to recognize achievement and competence, and feelings of "It's not good enough" (Antony and Swinson, 2009; Adderholdt-Elliott, 1987).

Neurotic perfectionists set unattainable goals and might engage in overtraining or exercise addiction. Their self-talk is based on messages they received when they were young, reminding themselves that "It's not good enough" and "I can do better." Their expectations of others are also excessive. Perfectionists need to learn how to set reasonable goals and to recognize their own achievements and those of others, especially in exercise settings. They need to have indicators of success and to acknowledge when they have reached those indicators.

Implications for working with clients who reveal perfectionistic thinking include referral to a mental health professional so that its sources can be identified and treated. Perfectionism can play a role in attempts at self-improvement; however, when standards and goals are excessively high, when self-expectations for achievement are unrealistic, and when the person expects others to meet these same excessive standards, often at the expense of alienating others, then this condition becomes an obstacle to happiness, confidence, and mental health.

Another implication for working with perfectionistic clients is the need to help them set realistic but challenging goals that are measurable and observable, to help them detect times when they have met their performance expectations, and to verbally and directly recognize their accomplishments. One important strategy that validates positive feedback and gives the consultant credibility is to base feedback on numbers—perhaps fit-

ness test results, blood test results, improved exercise performance (e.g., increased resistance in weight training, faster jogging times, reduced body-fat percentage), or some other measure that quantifies improved physical performance.

Finally, perfectionists often need to change their irrational thinking by being reminded of their accomplishments, favorably comparing their competence level with others, and being more realistic about their self-expectations. Perfectionism, particularly when excessive (also referred to by mental health professionals as *irrational*, *maladaptive*, or *neurotic*), has specific sources, such as parents, sport coaches,

FROM RESEARCH TO REAL WORLD

George and colleagues (2012) conducted an extensive review of past research on the effectiveness of interventions aimed at improving exercise behavior among adult males (over age 18). Their review included 14 studies that focused on physical activity only and 9 studies that combined physical activity and nutrition. They found that 10 of the 14 physical-activity-only intervention studies and 4 of the 9 combined intervention studies demonstrated significant increases in physical activity. Following are the intervention elements that were primarily responsible for increased physical activity and fitness levels.

• *Face-to-face tailored advice.* Facilitating both physical activity and dietary changes for positive health outcomes occurred when fitness staff offered individualized advice in person.

• *Internet-based interventions.* The review by George et al. (2012) also examined the effectiveness of Internet-based interventions. They found that interventions "using the Internet to promote healthy lifestyle behaviors have the potential to facilitate changes" (p. 296). Use of self-monitoring, social interac-

tion, daily step counting with a pedometer, and competition (i.e., comparing teams on fitness performance measures) markedly improved fitness during the intervention.

• *Additional recommendations for effective interventions.* The authors suggested several strategies that facilitated various measures of fitness. Lectures on health and lifestyle choices were not beneficial; however, more effective strategies were encouraging participants to make physical activity part of their regular daily or weekly routine; using individualized (rather than group) programs; recognizing successes (even small ones), such as meeting a goal for the first time; and frequently using the advice of health professionals. As George et al. (2012) stated with respect to the importance of advice coming from professionals, "If advice and information is to be respected and taken into account by men, it needs to be seen as emanating from a reliable source" (p. 297). This review included male adults only, and a similar review of exercise intervention studies for female participants is needed. It is apparent that innovative approaches are needed to encourage regular physical activity as a lifestyle choice.

or teachers, and this may be pointed out as an issue that is nothing to be ashamed about and that might require professional consultation to address it.

WEINER'S ATTRIBUTION MODEL APPLIED TO EXERCISE ADHERENCE

Weiner's models have strong implications for promoting physical activity, particularly in exercise settings. The model predicts, for instance, that exercisers will quit their program if they

- experience consistent failure in their exercise program or they perceive that the outcomes of their exercise are unsuccessful (i.e., not meeting personal goals), no matter what others think;

- feel unhappy about their exercise outcomes rather than viewing their lack of success or fitness as a temporary condition (e.g., "I should have lost more weight by now");

- feel responsible for not being successful in reaching their goals; and

- perceive this problem or disappointment as relatively long term (e.g., "I won't ever lose weight," "My obesity is genetic," "I'll never feel good about exercising").

Exercise adherence, or persistence, is possible, however, if exercisers view at least some aspects of their exercise experiences as successful (e.g., improving their exercise performance even if they did not reach a personal goal, being able to keep up with the instructor). This is why fitness coaches, exercise leaders, and exercise partners have to find something positive to say about the exerciser's performance (e.g., "You are doing more repetitions than two weeks ago," "You are jogging nonstop at least two minutes longer than when we started last month").

Positive feelings can still follow unsuccessful outcomes if performers conclude that they have benefited from the experience (e.g., "I didn't exercise as well as I would have liked, but at least I broke a sweat and burned a few calories," "I didn't jog very far but I feel good anyway") or that they were unable to control the outcome (e.g., "I'll never be able to keep up with these younger, fitter exercisers at the club, but I am improving"). In this way, Weiner's new model provides flexibility in explaining and predicting future performance based on a variety of emotions and thought processes inherent in exercise situations.

Weiner (1985) found that causal attributions are more likely when a goal is not attained or when an outcome is unexpected. Following these guidelines, exercisers who are suddenly injured, have an unexpected unpleasant experience at a fitness facility, or are unhappy about their performance are more likely to attempt to explain these events (i.e., make causal attributions) than exercisers who have pleasant experiences. This is because providing reasons for unpleasant events is comforting and justifies continued participation, creating a sense of optimism and hopefulness (Alloy, Abamson, Metalshy, and Hartlage, 1988). In addition, perceived success that is attributed to internal causes (e.g., high ability, high effort) results in feelings of pride. Perceived failure, on the other hand, induces guilt and sometimes anger (McAuley and Duncan, 1989).

In summary, Weiner's model posits that people are motivated to explain the reasons for performance outcomes, which has high motivational value. People who engage in regular exercise or other forms of physical activity are likely motivated by their perceived competence, feelings of achievement, and successful outcomes, as opposed to people who are exercise dropouts or who prefer a sedentary lifestyle and are not motivated to engage in regular physical activity. Researchers, practitioners, and educators have their work cut out for them in changing a person's lifestyle from inactive to active and increasing the person's self-awareness about the benefits of regular physical activity and the consequences of a sedentary lifestyle for health, happiness, and quality of life (see table 8.3).

Table 8.3 Practitioner Strategies for Encouraging Motivational Causal Attributions

Prediction of model	Strategies
Quitting exercise due to perceived failure	Provide positive information that reflects increased competence, good effort, and improvement. Set realistic goals or no goals at all.
Feeling unhappy about exercise outcomes	Provide clients with reasonable and realistic expectations. Inform clients that improved fitness, weight loss, and other desirable outcomes take time, effort, and long-term commitment.
Feeling responsible for being unsuccessful in reaching performance and health goals	Clients need reassurance that they are not to blame for unmet goals. They must control only what is controllable—their own behavior—and stay with the program. Emphasize the importance and benefits of adherence.
Perceiving the problem or disappointment as long term	Exercisers must view their early fitness experiences as successful. There must be some degree of measurable improvement and reduced perceived exertion. The experience must not remain unpleasant. Continually teach proper exercise techniques and use social support (e.g., exercising with coaches or friends) to improve the client's mood and sense of belonging to the program and the facilities.

SUMMARY

Researchers and practitioners have attempted to improve the effectiveness of interventions that result in starting and maintaining an exercise program. Many of these studies and programs have been fraught with limitations. Better interventions that promote exercise participation and other forms of physical activity are needed. People have many reasons for wanting to begin and adhere to exercise programs (e.g., weight management, social recognition, enjoyment, social affiliation, improved health, improved appearance). There are also several obstacles to exercise participation (e.g., not enough time, pain or injury, lack of nearby facilities and equipment, high costs of a fitness club membership and exercise footwear and clothing) that must be addressed by health care professionals.

The term used to describe the decision to maintain participation in an exercise program, *adherence*, is defined as the level of participation achieved in a behavioral regimen once the individual has agreed to undertake it. *Compliance*, a similar concept, is often defined as the degree to which an individual follows a specific recommendation or the extent to which

a person's behavior coincides with medical or health advice. Popular use of online programs and social media and the ubiquitous use of smartphones make electronic devices another source of information and consultation in promoting client health.

There are two components of health behavior change that include four steps. These components consist of a structure for directing client behavior and interview strategies in the consultation process (i.e., what health care professionals need to ask their clients to induce commitment to behavior changes). Finally, there are mental barriers to exercise adherence that may require the expertise of a mental health professional who is clinically trained to help people deal with conditions such as chronic anxiety, depression, irrational thinking, and excessive perfectionism, each of which may impede the confidence and energy needed to maintain an exercise program and other healthy habits. Health care professionals need to refer clients to mental health professionals with the proper credentials for diagnosis and treatment to improve client motivation and adherence to prescribed cognitive-behavioral interventions.

STUDENT ACTIVITY

Exercise Commitment Checklist

How can you increase your clients' commitment to increasing daily physical activity and leading a more active lifestyle? One approach is to record their level of commitment using the following checklist. Either record your own scores on the checklist or administer it to another person who agrees to act as your client for the purposes of this activity. This first set of scores will serve as the pretest. Then administer a three-week intervention in which you try to improve your own scores or the scores of your client. If you (or the client) score low on any item, try to address the reason and work toward improving the item score within three weeks. Then retake the checklist after three weeks to see if the scores have improved. If you or the client do not want to improve the low scores on any item, there is one last task: Identify the short-term costs and long-term consequences of maintaining this low score. If you find the costs and consequences acceptable, then leave it alone and move on to improving the other items.

FORM 8.1   EXERCISE COMMITMENT CHECKLIST

Name: _____ Date: _____

Rate yourself on each statement indicating the extent to which you feel committed to improve your health and fitness through regular exercise.

Level of Commitment

1	2	3	4	5
Very low	Somewhat low	Moderate	Somewhat high	Very high

____ 1. I am willing to sacrifice other things to improve my fitness.

____ 2. I really want to improve my health.

____ 3. Some of my deepest values and beliefs include remaining healthy for my family and friends.

____ 4. I give 100% when I exercise.

____ 5. I have a scheduled exercise plan for the week.

____ 6. I take personal responsibility for my health, fitness, and well-being.

____ 7. I can make the time and effort to maintain an exercise program, even when I am tired.

____ 8. I am determined to reach my exercise goals.

____ 9. I am open to exercise instruction to improve my technique.

____ 10. I exercise at least three times per week.

____ 11. I acknowledge that I must do more than casual walking to gain exercise benefits.

____ 12. I am improving my aerobic fitness.

____ 13. I am improving my muscular strength.

____ 14. When I feel fatigued during exercise I continue to give 100%.

____ 15. I get myself psyched up before and during exercise.

____ 16. I am in the process of reaching my fitness goals.

____ **Total**

> 72-80 = extremely committed (90-100%).
> 56-71 = somewhat committed (be careful): on the way toward dropping out.
> <56 = red zone (uncommitted): likely to drop out.

From M. Anshel, 2014, *Applied Health Fitness Psychology*. (Champaign, IL: Human Kinetics).

REFERENCES

Adderholdt-Elliott, M. (1987). *Perfectionism: What's bad about being too good?* Minneapolis: Free Spirit Publishing.

Alderman, B.L., Beighle, A., Pangrazi, R.P. (2006). Enhancing motivation in physical education. *Journal of Physical Education, Recreation & Dance, 77,* 41-51.

Alloy, L.B., Abamson, L.Y., Metalshy, G.I., and Hartlage, S. (1988). The hopelessness theory of depression: Attributional aspects. *British Journal of Clinical Psychology, 27,* 5-21.

American Psychiatric Association (APA). (2000). *Diagnostic and statistical manual of mental disorders* (4th ed.). Arlington, VA: Author.

Anshel, M.H. (2008). The disconnected values model: Intervention strategies for health behavior change. *Journal of Clinical Sport Psychology, 2,* 357-380.

Antony, M.M., and Swinson, R.P. (2009). *When perfect isn't good enough*: Strategies for coping with perfectionism (2nd ed.). Oakland, CA: New Harbinger.

Biscontini, L. (2012, May/June). Building fitness relationships: The encyclopedia of social media. *American Fitness, 30,* 12-14.

Blair, S.N., and Brodney, S. (1999). Effects of physical inactivity and obesity on morbidity and mortality: Current evidence and research issues. *Medicine and Science in Sports and Exercise, 31* (11 supplement), S646-662.

Bowen, D.J., Helmes, A., and Lease, E. (2001). Predicting compliance: How are we doing? In L.E. Burke, and I.S. Ockene (Eds.), *Compliance in healthcare and research* (pp. 25-41). Armonk, NY: Futura.

Brinthaupt, T.M., Kang, M., and Anshel, M.H. (2010). A delivery model for overcoming psychobehavioral barriers to exercise. *Psychology of Sport and Exercise, 11,* 259-266.

Brosse, A.L., Sheets, E.S., Lett, H.S., and Blumenthal, J.A. (2002). Exercise and the treatment of clinical depression in adults: Recent findings and future directions. *Sports Medicine, 32,* 741-760.

Buckworth, J., and Dishman, R.K. (1999). Determinants of physical activity: Research to application. *Lifestyle Medicine,* 1016-1027.

Buckworth, J., and Dishman, R.K. (2002). *Exercise psychology.* Champaign, IL: Human Kinetics.

Carr, L.J., Bartee, R.T., Dorozynski, C.M., Broomfield, J.F., Smith, M.L., and Smith, D.T. (2009). Eight-month follow-up of physical activity and central adiposity: Results from an Internet-delivered randomized control trial intervention. *Journal of Physical Activity and Health, 6,* 444-455.

Chenoweth, D.H. (2007). *Worksite health promotion* (2nd ed.). Champaign, IL: Human Kinetics.

Cook, J. (1993). *Book of positive quotations.* Minneapolis, MN: Fairview Press.

Dawson, K.A., Tracey, J., and Berry, T. (2008). Evaluation of workplace group and Internet-based physical activity interventions on psychological variables associated with exercise behavior change. *Journal of Sports Science and Medicine, 7,* 537-543.

deMoor, M.H.M., Beem, A.L., Stubbe, J.H., Boomsma, D.I., and deGeus, E.J.C. (2006). Regular exercise, anxiety, depression and personality: A population-based study. *Preventive Medicine, 42,* 273-279.

Dishman, R.K., and Buckworth, J. (1996). Increasing physical activity: A quantitative synthesis. *Medicine and Science in Sports and Exercise, 28,* 706-719.

Flett, G.L., Hewitt, P.L., Blankstein, K.R., and Mosher, S.W. (1991). Perfectionism, self-actualization, and personal adjustment. *Journal of Social Behavior and Personality, 6,* 147-160.

Frost, R.O., Marten, P., Lahart, C., and Rosenblate, R. (1990). The dimensions of perfectionism. *Cognitive Therapy and Research, 14,* 449-468.

George, E.S., Kolt, G.S., Duncan, M.J., Caperchione, C.M., Mummery, W.K., Vandelanotte, C., Taylor, P., and Noakes, M. (2012). A review of the effectiveness of physical activity interventions for adult males. *Sports Medicine, 42,* 281-300.

Haynes, R.B. (2001). Improving patient adherence: State of the art, with a special focus on medication taking for cardiovascular disorders. In L.E. Burke and I.S. Ockene (Eds.), *Compliance in healthcare and research* (pp. 3-21). Armonk, NY: Futura.

King, A.C. (1994). Clinical and community interventions to promote and support physical activity participation. In R.K. Dishman (Ed.), *Advances in exercise psychology* (pp. 183-212). Champaign, IL: Human Kinetics.

Krcmar, H., Halle, M., and Leimeister, J.M. (2010). An Internet-delivered exercise intervention for workplace health promotion in overweight sedentary employees: A randomized trial. *Preventive Medicine, 51,* 234-239.

Kruger, J., Yore, M.M., Bauer, D.R., and Kohl III, H.W. (2007). Selected barriers and incentives for worksite health promotion services and policies. *American Journal of Health Promotion, 21,* 439-447.

Leith, L.M. (1998). *Exercising your way to mental health.* Morgantown, WV: Fitness Information Technology.

Loehr, J., and Schwartz, T. (2003). *The power of full engagement: Managing energy, not time, is the key to high performance and personal renewal.* New York: Free Press.

Lombard, D.N., Lombard, T.N., and Winnett, R.A. (1995). Walking to meet health guidelines: The effect of prompting frequency and prompt structure. *Health Psychology, 14,* 164-170.

Markland, D., and Ingledew, D.K. (1997). The measurement of exercise motives: Factorial validity and invariance across gender of a revised Exercise Motivations Inventory. *British Journal of Health Psychology, 2,* 361-376.

McAuley, E., and Duncan, E.T. (1989). Causal attributions and affective reactions to disconforming outcomes in motor performance. *Journal of Sport and Exercise Psychology, 11,* 187-200.

Rand, C.S., and Weeks, K. (1998). Measuring adherence with medication regimens in clinical care and research. In S.A. Shumaker, E.B. Schron, J.K. Ockene, and W.L. Mcbee (Eds.), *The handbook of health behavior change* (2nd ed., pp. 114-132). New York: Springer.

Reinboth, M., Duda, J.L., and Ntoumanis, N. (2004). Dimensions of coaching behavior, need satisfaction, and the psychological and physical welfare of young athletes. *Motivation and Emotion, 28,* 297-313.

Richardson, C.R., Buis, L.R., Janney, A.W., Goodrich, D.E., Sen, A., Hess, M.L., et al. (2010). An online community improves adherence in an Internet-mediated walking program. Part 1: Results of a randomized controlled trial. *Journal of Medical Internet Research, 12,* e71. doi:10.2196/jmir.1338

Salmon, J., Owen, N., Crawford, D., Bauman, A., and Sallis, J.F. (2003). Physical activity and sedentary behavior: A population-based study of barriers, enjoyment, and preference. *Health Psychology, 22,* 178-188.

Timmerman, G.M. (2007). Addressing barriers to health promotion in underserved women. *Family and Community Health, Supplement, 1,* S34-S42.

Weiner, B. (1985). An attributional theory of achievement motivation and emotion. *Psychological Review, 92,* 548-573.

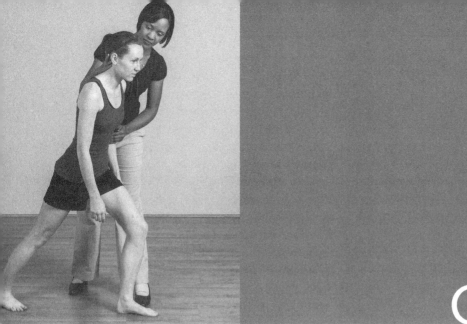

CHAPTER 9

Cognitive and Behavioral Strategies

> Believe in yourself and there will come a day when others will have no choice but to believe with you.

> Oscar Wilde (1854-1900), writer and poet

CHAPTER OBJECTIVES

After reading this chapter, you should be able to:

- explain the differences among strategies, interventions, and programs that improve health behavior, particularly related to fitness, and

- become familiar with types of cognitive and behavioral strategies and programs that are intended to improve exercise performance.

This chapter addresses the nuts and bolts of helping people develop and maintain a healthy lifestyle, with a particular emphasis on improved fitness. It addresses the array of cognitive and behavioral strategies, interventions, and programs that favorably influence client motivation, emotions, thoughts, and performance. These are evidence-based strategies, meaning that they have been shown to be effective in the research literature published in scholarly journals and books for both academic and applied reader markets. While researchers and practitioners differ on what constitutes a proven technique (i.e., researchers typically demand more scientific proof of effective outcomes), it remains clear that one size does not fit all. What may be effective for one exerciser or for one type of situation may not be effective for other exercisers and situations. It is also important that health professionals not provide too many techniques at one time. It is easy for exercisers to become overwhelmed when they are asked to learn, think about, and apply too many things at once. Introducing new techniques slowly until one or two are integrated into the client's repertoire of strategies is key.

INTERVENTIONS, TREATMENTS, AND STRATEGIES

Starting and maintaining an exercise program requires conscious planning of location, time, and performance content. This process is called an *intervention*. Interventions include one or more strategies, categorized as cognitive or behavioral, that are intended to change some predetermined outcome (Singer and Anshel, 2006). The primary goal of an intervention is to encourage sedentary or irregularly active people to adopt regular exercise habits and to keep physically active people exercising on a regular basis (Buckworth and Dishman, 2002). Interventions guide what needs to be changed and which strategies should be used.

Interventions are a global concept that includes all types of strategies, treatments,

and mental skills programs that are intended to improve performance outcomes. Singer and Anshel (2006) define an *intervention* as "the process by which sport psychologists attempt to influence the thoughts, emotions, or performance quality of sports competitors and teams" (p. 63). Health coaches and practitioners, then, are people who intervene by positioning themselves between the client and the environment or situation in which they function in order to provide information and instruction to clients about the proper use of mental or behavioral strategies. Thus, health coaches are outsiders who come between performers and the environment to enhance physical performance quality and outcome. Of course, practitioners must first determine the client's concerns, needs, goals, and limitations before prescribing an intervention.

What makes an intervention effective? Numerous studies have tested the effectiveness of specific cognitive or behavioral strategies and interventions on exercise participation and adherence. Many effective strategies, such as cues to action (i.e., stimuli in the environment that prompt exercise participation), self-monitoring (i.e., keeping records of progress, including ratings of perceived exertion and activity logs), goal setting, music, personalized performance coaching (i.e., personal training), social support, and positive instructional feedback to improve self-efficacy and develop exercise skills have been shown to improve performance in sport (Anshel, 2012) and exercise (Anshel, 2005).

Despite being used interchangeably in the literature, treatments and interventions are not the same. A *treatment* is a specific procedure, or action, that is intended to elicit a predictable outcome. An *intervention*, however, consists of a series of treatments, or a program, that is performed over a longer period of time and may consist of several forms of treatment. A treatment may be given under different circumstances or by different people using slight variations. A sample treatment might consist of providing instruction on the use of coping strategies in response to chronic or acute stress. A coping-skills intervention, on the other hand, would require the individual to learn and apply multiple treatments.

For example, in a recent study, Anshel, Umscheid, and Brinthaupt (2013) examined the effect of combining a wellness program with coping skills, as opposed to a program using coping skills alone, on perceived stress and perceived energy levels among emergency dispatchers. The results indicated that combining both treatments—learning proper coping skills and engaging in exercise and nutrition coaching—resulted in less perceived stress and more energy than using coping skills alone. Thus, an exercise program is a treatment. Combining exercise with other lifestyle habits that promote health (e.g., nutrition coaching, stress management, other lifestyle changes that improve mental well-being) is an intervention.

Strategies are self-initiated, conscious processes designed to enhance a specific outcome or to achieve a goal. If the strategy consists of the person's thoughts or emotions, it's called a *cognitive strategy*. A cognitive strategy is a mental technique used to improve cognition, that is, the processing of visual, auditory, and tactual input, or to favorably influence the performer's emotions, such as reducing anxiety, improving attentional focusing, maintaining concentration, and coping with stress (Anshel, 2005). With respect to physical activity, cognitive strategies are intended to improve performance quality and outcomes. Examples of cognitive strategies include positive self-talk, anticipation, precueing and cueing, psyching up, coping skills, relaxation techniques, and visualization (also called *mental imagery*).

Along these lines, another approach to the study of mental skills in enhancing physical performance is psychological skills training (PST). According to Vealey (1988), PST involves "techniques and strategies designed to teach or enhance mental skills that facilitate performance and a positive approach to sport competition" (p. 319). The premise of PST is that people need to apply mental skills and strategies to meet the demands of and overcome adversity associated with various forms of physical performance (e.g., sport, exercise, rehabilitation).

Vealey differentiates between *psychological skills* and *methods*: "Skills are qualities to be attained, as opposed to methods which are procedures or techniques . . . to develop skills" (p. 326). Mental skills are divided into foundation skills (e.g., self-awareness, self-confidence), performance skills (e.g., optimal mental and physical arousal, optimal attention), and facilitative skills (e.g., lifestyle management, interpersonal skills). Methods are categorized as foundation methods (e.g., physical practice, education) and PST methods (e.g., goal setting, imagery, relaxation). A similar structure can be applied when describing ways to facilitate meeting the demands of physical activities, including exercise. Here's an example related to applied fitness psychology.

Foundation skill 1: "I am self-aware that I am overweight and, as a result, lack energy and do not feel good about myself. I understand there are long-term consequences for remaining overweight over a long time period, including spending most of my money on health care and not seeing my child graduate."

Foundation skill 2: "I am confident that if I remain patient and insert an exercise workout into my daily schedule (or at least three days a week) that I will become fitter, lose weight, and feel better."

Performance skill 1: I use positive self-talk and psyching up in combination to be mentally ready just prior to engaging in my workout.

Performance skill 2: I use vivid imagery or visualization to mentally practice a few exercises (aerobic or resistance training) and to associate positive feelings while mentally performing each exercise.

A primary role of health practitioners is to help clients select and correctly use the strategies that best meet their needs. Table 9.1 lists some common cognitive strategies and, later in this chapter, table 9.2 lists examples of behavioral strategies that are intended to improve exercise performance. These strategies are described according to the conditions in which they might be most effective and when used in combination as part of a mental skills program. The remainder of this chapter reviews the use of cognitive and behavioral interventions according to their purpose and intended outcomes, ultimately for the goal of enhancing performance.

COGNITIVE STRATEGIES

This section concerns the use of cognitive strategies, also called *mental skills*, that favorably influence exercise performance and fitness or attitudes about exercise and fitness. Most of these have been established in the sport psychology literature and used successfully in sport settings, and they have a direct impact on exercise performance.

The key objective in using a cognitive strategy to manage discomfort is to promote self-control, that is, to know when to monitor feelings of discomfort and when to ignore those feelings. Some conditions warrant a combination of attending and ignoring feelings of discomfort, while other conditions require going in one direction or the other. Typically, however, pain is debilitating and unpleasant, often requiring the performer's attention. The performer, therefore, needs to develop mental skills to manage the discomfort.

Positive Self-Talk

Exercisers want to engage in self-statements that are uplifting and motivating, termed *positive self-talk*. The result will be more effort and intensity, better concentration, and greater enjoyment of the task. The purposes of self-talk vary. When the technique is used to gain or to maintain self-confidence, focusing inwardly and thinking about one's strengths rather than about one's opponent can generate a sense of self-control and responsibility for the outcome of a contest. Positive self-talk is an effective way to maintain self-confidence (Vealey, 2001), and it is a universal practice among successful performers in sport and other venues of physical performance.

Table 9.1 Cognitive Strategies to Improve Exercise Performance and Adherence

Cognitive strategies	Function
Positive self-talk	Covert (self) statements that confirm one's readiness to perform successfully (e.g., "I am ready")
Relaxation	The reduction or complete absence of muscular activity in the voluntary muscles; comes in various forms, including progressive relaxation and autogenic training
Mental imagery or visualization	Thoughts that form mental representations of physical performance
Bizarre imagery	A mental representation of unrealistic events such as medication that dissolves a virus or tumor
Thought stopping	Saying "Stop!" to oneself to cease negative thoughts and emotions
Psyching up	Thinking about the task at hand to increase excitation, energy, and feelings of challenge, engagement, and connectedness to the task
Association	Conscious attempt to link mind (focused attention) and body (muscles used for exertion)
Dissociation	Disconnecting attentional focus from physical exertion and instead focusing on external stimuli
Mental toughness	Dealing effectively with external demands through emotional resiliency; remaining in mental control in overcoming adversity
Mindfulness	Thinking and acting in the present moment in a less reactive and judgmental manner
Accurate causal attributions	Explaining success as due to internal causes (i.e., high ability or effort) while explaining failure as due to external causes (e.g., difficult task, superior racing opponent, bad luck)

Another reason to engage in positive self-talk is to analyze physical skills and movements. Some athletes use positive self-talk in a postrace analysis by asking themselves, "Did this work?" "Did we do this?" "Did we forget about it?" A key word in this strategy is *positive*. Self-statements such as "Concentrate on the task," "I can do this," and "I'm feeling better" offer strong motivation, confidence, encouragement, and favorable future expectations to handle the physical demands associated with exercise and other forms of vigorous physical activity. Other examples of self-talk in exercise settings include "Let's do it," "I feel good," and "Stay with it." The use of single words or phrases that influence mood is also effective, such as "Go," "Focus," and "Get it!" The exerciser needs to develop a script that consists of specific things to say and to predetermine the time and conditions under which they will use the script (e.g., before aerobic activity or weight training). Positive self-talk builds confidence and, in turn, increases effort and exertion (Vealey, 2001). A few more examples include "I can do this; I've prepared and I'm ready," "I'm looking forward to working out," and "Two more reps—that's it!"

Relaxation

Relaxation is the reduction or complete absence of muscular activity in voluntary muscles. Various forms of relaxation have proven popular because they help reduce anxiety and stress. Each type of relaxation strategy serves a specific purpose. Examples include progressive relaxation, autogenic training, biofeedback, imagery, centering, and hypnosis. Though full descriptions of these techniques go beyond the scope of this chapter, they all serve similar purposes in reducing muscular tension, lowering arousal level, and improving emotional status.

However, relaxation is not always appropriate in response to unpleasant thoughts, emotions, and muscle tension. Some people find that reaching a relaxed state is undesirable, ineffective, and even stressful in itself. In addition, sometimes increased emotional arousal

or heightened concentration is warranted. Along these lines, some people might find behavioral strategies such as light exercise, reading, watching TV or a film, or engaging in conversation to be more relaxing than the use of specific relaxation techniques. If used correctly, however, relaxation training is a valid and proven means of preventing or reducing muscular tension and anxiety while improving concentration and self-confidence.

Mental Imagery

Imagery, also called *visualization*, consists of thoughts that form mental representations of physical performance. It is used for several reasons and to meet various types of goals (Martin, Moritz, and Hall, 1999). Imagery may be used to rehearse and learn new exercise skills and strategies, build self-confidence, develop automated routines during physical activity, and manage discomfort or pain. Imagery begins, then, with thinking about its purpose, followed by taking a few minutes to relax, close the eyes, and imagine performing the skill or activity successfully.

The use of visualization, or mental imagery, is not only a common and effective technique in sport performance but also in exercise settings. It can be used for numerous purposes, such as gaining confidence, learning new exercise routines, reducing tension and anxiety before exercising, increasing excitation and psychological readiness, overcoming mental and physical fatigue, and increasing motivation. Obtaining desirable outcomes from imagery requires following specific guidelines and procedures. As outlined by Hall (2001) and Martin et al. (1999), exercisers should find a time and a place void of visual or auditory distractions. Next, they think through the environmental features, specific exercises, and sensations and feelings experienced during the exercise routine in a highly desirable, positive manner. Then they mentally rehearse the activity being performed in perfect form and with a desirable outcome.

Before starting the imagery experience, the exerciser should take a minute or two to relax because relaxation improves the vividness of the image. Find a quiet time and location for the client to relax and concentrate. Then follow a script that mentally takes your client through the situation in a pleasant manner that meets performance expectations. Clients must always imagine success, never failure; that is the blueprint you want them to create.

Bizarre Imagery

The purpose of bizarre imagery is to increase exercise motivation and to distract the person from the challenges of physical exertion. Whereas normal imagery is a mental representation of real-life situations, bizarre imagery is a mental representation of unrealistic events. For example, cancer patients are sometimes asked to imagine their tumors shrinking as they receive chemotherapy. Cardiac or pulmonary patients might imagine rapid changes in the circulatory system that are medically impossible during an exercise bout. An overweight person might imagine fat dissolving or arteries widening while exercising.

Thought Stopping

A common dilemma in exercise is engaging in self-statements that reveal unpleasant feelings about the task at hand. Unpleasant feelings, especially if they continue during exercise, may lead to demotivation, reduced effort, and even dropping out of further participation. In response to negative feelings, exercisers should say to themselves, "Stop!" The negative thoughts go away because the command to stop acts as a verbal cue to cease further unpleasant thoughts and instead focus on a more positive and uplifting message. Thoughts go from irrational to rational.

Psyching Up

For some activities, such as the exertion of physical exercise that often requires high arousal and energy, the performer's thought processes must be upbeat and active. A cognitive technique called *psyching up* consists of thinking about the task at hand and having thoughts of excitation, challenge, engagement, connection, and high energy. Psyching up can

be experienced in either physical or mental form. Physically, the person can engage in tasks that require more energy and increased physiological responses such as heart rate, respiration rate, and muscle tension. Mentally, psyching up usually consists of thoughts that increase confidence, motivation, arousal, and concentration. Examples of psyching up include thinking, "Let's do it!" and "I'm ready."

Association

Sometimes association is used by exercisers or rehabilitation patients to confront rather than avoid or ignore thoughts of discomfort— as long as a physician has given approval to engage in physical activity, of course. Conscious attempts to link the mind and body are called *association*. For example, association is used as a weightlifting technique in which the lifter's attentional focus is internal, that is, on the muscles executing the lift. Lifting weights is often a required task in rehabilitation programs. To overpower the feelings of discomfort, exercisers use self-statements such as, "I will get through this," "Ignore my body and concentrate on the task at hand," or "Focus," or they can use pain as a cue to become psyched up.

Dissociation

Health fitness psychology is a field that promotes the strong links among thoughts, emotions, and physical performance, but a primary goal of managing discomfort is to do the opposite—to ignore it through distraction by an external stimulus. This involves a cognitive strategy called *dissociation*, which attempts to disconnect one's focus from physical exertion and move it instead to external stimuli. Instead of focusing on the discomfort of tired legs during a workout, for example, the person focuses on some external stimulus, such as music, the workout instructor, or another environmental cue not linked to physical exertion. Other examples that might involve dissociation include distance running and exercise rehabilitation that requires uncomfortable movements. When people focus their attention on an external stimulus (e.g., a ball in play, an opponent or teammate), they are ignoring their own sensations, including pain and discomfort.

Mental Toughness

The concept of mental toughness has received greater attention in the sport psychology literature in recent years (e.g., Jones, Hanton, and Connaughton, 2007). *Mental toughness* is traditionally defined as having a natural or developed psychological edge that enables the person to deal effectively with external demands. The result is performing more consistently while remaining determined, focused, confident, and in control, particularly under pressure. In addition, mentally tough people demonstrate emotional resiliency by bouncing back from physical and mental challenges related to exercise, fitness improvement, and the physical demands of rehabilitation.

Mental toughness in exercise settings consists of eight dimensions:

1. Managing one's physical and emotional arousal, that is, when to become psyched up and when to be more subdued in meeting performance demands

2. Being fully engaged and focused on the exercise task at hand

3. Overcoming initial feelings of physical fatigue and maintaining exertion

4. Perceiving exercise as a challenge rather than as a threat

5. Acknowledging the benefits of maintaining an exercise habit

6. Remembering one's performance and outcome goals and using them as motivation for exercise adherence

7. Interpreting physical exertion as desirable and a means to improve one's physical conditioning and health

8. Acknowledging the long-term benefits of maintaining an exercise habit

How does one teach mental toughness? Because it is dispositional and part of one's character, it is challenging to influence a person's general perceptions and feelings. Fitness coaches can, however, instruct exercisers to

deal with adversity, accept facts about physical conditioning, associate exertion with improvement, to perceive difficult or stressful situations as challenges rather than as threats and sources of trouble and anxiety, and stand up to exercise barriers (e.g., "Don't accept defeat in your mission to lose weight, improve your energy, and develop a healthier lifestyle, and respond to failure with even more determination and give 100% toward reaching your goals."). Mental toughness in the sport psychology literature is often applied in physical training and rehabilitation settings, so it should be compatible in exercise and fitness settings as a way to reach one's ideal performance state.

Mindfulness

Mindfulness is a state of complete attention on the present (Petrillo, de Kaufman, Glass, and Arnkoff, 2009). When you're mindful, you observe your thoughts and feelings from a distance—from the outside looking in—without judging them as positive or negative. Instead of letting life pass you by, mindfulness means living in the moment and awakening to experience (Grossman, Niemann, Schmidt, and Walach, 2004). There has been an increase in the number of published studies on mindfulness in recent years, and the current body of scientific literature on the effects of mindfulness practices on a person's thoughts, emotions, and performance has been impressive. Studies suggest that mindfulness is useful in the treatment of pain, stress, anxiety, depressive relapse, disordered eating, and addiction. Mindfulness practice also improves the immune system, and it alters activation symmetries in the prefrontal cortex, a change previously associated with an increase in positive affect and a faster recovery from negative experiences (McCracken, Gauntlett-Gilbert, and Vowles, 2007).

Accurate Causal Attributions

Exercisers, particularly novices, will be physically challenged to complete one or more exercises, working through the significant increase in effort, sweating, and fatigue. If exercisers give 100% effort toward meeting fitness goals and they improve their exercise performance, they should interpret their exercise attempts as successful and then attribute this success to high effort. This is called making *high-effort causal attributions*. Linking effort to success has great motivation value because it is related to the performer's feelings of self-control and competence. Low performance quality should rarely be attributed to low ability ("I just can't do it because I am not good enough"). On the other hand, a few people might find it difficult to move in a coordinated manner during an aerobics class or might accurately conclude that their fitness level is simply too low to meet a performance goal. However, if they have given optimal effort and their fitness is improving, that is, the exercises seem less difficult to complete, they can view these outcomes in a positive manner (i.e., "I'm not quite there, yet, but I'm making progress; I'm getting better"). See Anshel (2012) for guidelines for making effective causal attributions in response to perceived success and perceived failure that should promote motivation.

BEHAVIORAL STRATEGIES

A behavioral strategy consists of actions that are intended to improve performance. Sample behavioral strategies include the use of music; light exercise, often used to reduce stress or anxiety; goal setting; social support; self-monitoring; and record keeping. Both cognitive and behavioral strategies improve the athlete's emotions, increase the speed or efficiency of information processing (e.g., anticipation of stimuli, positive self-expectations, decision making), and ultimately optimize performance. Table 9.2 lists sample behavioral strategies that may be used in exercise settings, and each strategy is discussed in greater depth in the following sections.

Individual Coaching

For many people, starting an exercise program is stressful. Novice exercisers are often filled with anxiety about many unknowns:

- Will I be able to exercise without pain?
- Will I hurt myself?
- I have not exercised since I was a kid; I don't know what to do or how to do it.
- Will I look awkward to others who see me?
- Will others who are fitter, thinner, or younger laugh at me?
- Will I have time to continue my exercise program?
- I hated exercising in high school. Why am I doing this now?

The novice brings thoughts of previous exercise attempts and fears about injury, fatigue, and how the body will respond to new physical demands. Heightened self-consciousness, doubts about meeting performance goals, and not being taught the correct way to exercise only worsen these initial feelings of doubt and pessimism.

Any novice exerciser who visits a fitness program or facility needs to be welcomed, comforted, and informed. The program should have preset routines that help new participants feel at ease upon entering the facility, secure a set of preexercise routines (e.g., locker room use, availability of services, towels, and programs), and feel comfortable starting a particular program. Instruction on exercise technique should always be offered at the start of participation so that the exerciser doesn't experience a debilitating injury.

Someone on staff, particularly a fitness or membership coach, should address new members' concerns and how the staff might help reduce them. Examples include establishing a program of teaching proper exercise techniques, helping members set realistic goals, and promoting secure and comfortable feelings in an environment filled with uncertainties, intimidation, and physical and emotional challenges. Novice exercisers need to feel they fit in and not be self-conscious about their lack of prior training and their current physical appearance. The failure to personally and professionally connect with clients will almost certainly lead to their dropping out of the program.

Table 9.2 Behavioral Strategies to Improve Exercise Performance and Adherence

Strategy	Examples
Individual coaching (fitness, nutrition, time management, stress management)	Working with a trained and skilled professional to improve health, fitness, and quality of life
Psychological (mental health) services	Working with a licensed mental health professional to examine psychological factors (e.g., low self-esteem, depression, irrational thinking) that might impede exercise adherence and reaching desirable health-related goals
Educational materials	Information, usually in written or verbal form (e.g., newsletters, guest speakers), about improving health, fitness, energy, and quality of life
Club or organization memberships	A group of individuals with similar interests in health, fitness, and exercise meeting regularly to provide social support, develop friendships, and conduct programs that improve knowledge
Social support (direct and indirect)	Exercising with another person (direct) or being encouraged to exercise and to engage in other healthy habits from someone else (indirect); fulfills a need to feel connected to others during exercise
Modeling	Observing others perform an exercise task so as to learn and properly perform the viewed task
Environmental features	Providing any type of material to exercisers that encourages physical activity or improves knowledge or exercise performance (e.g., posters, newsletters, water fountains, massage services, well-maintained furniture and exercise equipment)
Physical location	Attending exercise facilities within 3 mi (5 km) of the person's home or work for improved exercise adherence
Music	Moving in synchronization to music to improve physical endurance, momentum, and exercise performance
Pedometers	Wearing a motion sensor that assesses the number of steps taken (usually measured per day) in order to increase the person's daily physical activity
Scheduling	Planning routines, habits, rituals, and events to avoid forgetting them; exercise needs to be planned as part of a person's daily schedule
Time of day	Exercising at the preferred time of day and days of the week
Social engineering	Going to a specific time and place to achieve a particular goal (e.g., exercising at the club when attendance is low, such as midafternoon)
Perceived choice	Performing a preferred type of exercise rather than being coerced or required to perform certain undesirable exercises
Goal setting	Consciously targeting observable and desirable outcomes (e.g., performing exercises that lead to improved fitness and weight management)
Small, attainable units of progress	Detecting improvement and success to improve exercise motivation
Rewards	Receiving rewards for tangible evidence of improved exercise performance, competence, or goal achievement
Performance feedback	Receiving information about performance quality to reinforce effort and recognize competence
Exerciser checklist or self-monitoring	Following a detailed written list of tasks related to fitness preparation, exercise performance, postexercise, and lifestyle
Record keeping and attendance	Keeping written documentation to indicate fitness progress or attendance (e.g., attendance at a fitness program, entering a facility, using equipment)
Lifestyle management	Having healthy habits that include exercise, nutrition, adequate rest, and other rituals that improve health and well-being

Mental Health Services

Should a person attending a fitness club or physical rehabilitation program have access to a mental health professional? What would be the professional's role and responsibility? What issues would be addressed? How could the client be assured that all information would be strictly confidential? How can fitness club management and mental health professionals make this service available to all club exercisers but at the same time ensure that users of this service are not known to anyone other than the mental health professional? Who would pay for this service—insurance or the client? Where would this service be provided—in the facility, close to a separate entrance to the club, or at a private office away from the facility? How would this service be promoted, and what issues would be addressed? Would the mental health professional work in coordination with personal trainers in trying to help the client improve fitness, avoid dropping out, and learn to use performance-enhancing strategies? What would be the mental health professional's title? Performance consultant or counselor? Psychologist? Mental health coach? Though it is clear that clinical services are sometimes needed to address a client's psychological needs for the client to feel more comfortable in an exercise program, less certain is where and how this service should be provided.

Researchers have known for many years that exercise improves mental health by reducing anxiety and depression, elevating mood, and influencing the decision to exercise, including exercise initiation, participation, and adherence (Applegate, Rohan, and Dubbert, 1999; Stathopoulou and Powers, 2006). In one study, for example, Anshel, Brinthaupt, and Kang (2010) examined the effect of the disconnected values model on changes in selected aspects of mental health over a 10-week wellness program. Their results indicated that anxiety and depressed mood were significantly reduced, while positive well-being, self-control, perceptions of general health, and vitality all significantly increased from pre- to posttest. Less well known, however, is the extent to which mental health, particularly mental illness (called *psychopathology* by clinical and counseling psychologists), can create barriers to exercise and sabotage attempts to start and maintain an exercise program (Applegate et al., 1999).

Perhaps participants in exercise programs would prefer that issues related to mental illness be avoided and that psychological interventions focus on the following:

- Improving performance
- Building confidence
- Managing anxiety related to exercise participation, including social physique anxiety that reflects concerns about one's physical appearance
- Teaching clients how to use exercise for stress reduction
- Providing intervention information to improve client motivation
- Helping clients set and achieve challenging goals
- Teaching mental skills that enhance exercise performance (psyching up, imagery, and others discussed earlier in this chapter)
- Providing social support
- Linking the strengths of each personal trainer with the unique needs of each client
- Addressing disordered eating and other obstacles to proper dieting and problem eating
- Acting as the liaison for participants who need to communicate with club staff, management, or someone to whom they can turn for advice

Nevertheless, as Anshel et al. (2010) concluded, it is apparent that mental health concerns, such as clinical depression, chronic anxiety, low self-esteem, and concerns about body image, can become impediments to starting and maintaining regular exercise. Obtaining psychological services remains an important behavioral strategy to promote physical and mental health and well-being.

Educational Materials

The written word is a powerful tool in helping people understand the value of what they do—in this case, exercise. Although it is best to avoid complicated, difficult-to-understand research journal articles when providing information to the public, other sources such as magazine articles, segments of books, and even materials created by staff provide exercisers with a better understanding of and justification for their exercise habits and techniques. Monthly newsletters with featured articles that address various exercises, techniques, and findings from recent studies also have great motivational value.

Organization Memberships

Group membership and affiliation are natural, normal needs of humans. Groups provide comfort and security and meet social needs. The more people feel emotionally attached to an exercise program, facility, or fitness group, the more likely they are to maintain their involvement. Running clubs, groups who meet for weekly lectures or other functions, banquets that recognize fitness achievement, exercise-related events (e.g., weekend jogging or biking), company- or individual-sponsored contests (e.g., the John Smith Annual Run), outdoor activity clubs, annual guest speakers, award events, health-related conferences or seminars, and exhibitions (e.g., powerlifting, aerobic dance) are sample behavioral strategies that create excitement and motivation to exercise.

Social Support

The role of social support has been discussed in chapter 6, and the influence of others in promoting exercise adherence and fitness outcomes has been well established in the literature. Although some exercisers are happy to be left alone and to exercise in isolation, most novice performers need to feel connected to others during their routines. As indicated earlier, this process is called *social support*. The need for social support is especially important when the individual lacks confidence, is uncertain about exercise technique, welcomes the companionship of others for motivational purposes, needs assistance in carrying out an exercise routine correctly, prefers the company of others, or finds that being accountable to another person, such as a coach, provides an incentive to adhere to the program. Staff members should introduce themselves to participants, try to increase the social component of group exercise programs, instruct participants on exercise equipment, and develop exercise protocols. For people who exercise at home, family or friends should clearly and enthusiastically express support for their exercise habit.

Secondary, indirect forms of social support consist of ways to facilitate the exerciser's habit, such as driving the person to the exercise venue, giving a fitness club membership as a gift, encouraging the person to maintain an exercise program or habit, and supervising or monitoring the exerciser's responsibilities (e.g., babysitting, performing work-related tasks, recording a favorite TV program). As Sarafino (1994) contends, "People are more likely to start and stick with an exercise program if these efforts have the support and encouragement of family and friends" (p. 267).

Modeling

Sometimes exercisers feel intimidated by younger, fitter, perhaps thinner exercisers, leading to self-consciousness and discomfort in a public facility. To help novices not feel intimidated, why not ask them to observe the performance of a fit exerciser or even a leader of fitness classes? Perhaps the novice can find the performance of a highly fit person motivating and use the fit person as a model of exercise technique.

Environmental Features

Another behavioral strategy concerns arranging the exercise environment so that it is exciting, intimate, and motivating. In full agreement with Chenoweth (2002), facilities should include colorful walls; up-to-date, clean equipment that works properly; and perhaps pleasant and upbeat music, all of which contribute to an enthusiastic and exciting atmosphere. Broken equipment should be fixed as soon as possible, particularly if participants rely on the equipment as part of their mental well-being during exercise (e.g., televisions, music, water fountains). Broken equipment communicates insensitivity ("We want your membership money but do not care about providing a valuable service that you want") and poor management ("We are not in touch with program needs"), and it reduces the credibility of the facility by not providing high-quality equipment to promote fitness.

Workout areas, showers, locker rooms, and all floors should be cleaned at least daily. Soap and shampoo in shower areas should be checked and filled at least twice daily, and towels (if provided by the club) and garbage should be picked up and placed in containers routinely. There should be separate facilities for confidential meetings with members, such as to discuss a member's health or feelings, membership information, personal training instruction, or even mental health counseling. In addition, important information about the club should be easily accessible at the front counter, such as reprints of fitness-related articles and other educational materials, business cards of staff (including the club's manager), scheduled special programs, and general club information (e.g., hours of operation, membership costs). Perhaps most important, however, is the type of atmosphere that staff members create with their friendliness, sincerity in helping others, dress, and professional conduct.

Physical Location

Previous studies have shown that exercise adherence is far more likely if the exercise facility is located within 3 miles (5 km) of home or work (Goldstein, 2001). It is important, therefore, that clients need not travel too far outside their normal commute or from home or work to use an exercise facility. Employees may be more likely to use exercise facilities that are located at or near the workplace, such as a fitness room filled with high-quality, well-maintained equipment and preferably staffed with an exercise coach.

What about exercising at home? There is a reason home exercise equipment often goes unused and sits in basements and garages. We tend to associate home with relaxation, recreation, entertainment, and recovery from life's storms. We do not link home with hard physical exertion. In addition, the home environment offers many distractions that often prevent the establishment of an exercise habit. It is not surprising, therefore, that many people tend to purchase exercise equipment with the best of intentions and then stop using it. Instead, they should exercise in a high-energy atmosphere that increases their incentive and commitment to exercise regularly.

Music

It is well known, according to scientific studies (e.g., Anshel and Marisi, 1978), reviews of literature (Karageorghis and Priest, 2010; Karageorghis and Terry, 1997), and my own empirical observations as a former fitness director, that music can increase a person's arousal level and improve exercise endurance. One explanation of the benefits of music on physical performance is the dissociation effect, in which the performer focuses on the music while bodily sensations are ignored or at least receive far less attention. Another explanation is that music increases somatic and cognitive arousal, thereby producing more adrenalin and helping exercisers excel in activities that depend on faster reactions and movement speed. Slower, more relaxing music will ostensibly prove more beneficial for less intense sports such as golf, archery, and bowling.

It is not surprising that music is almost always playing in exercise facilities; it improves mood and the incentive to remain active. Some exercisers prefer their own music and wear headphones. Music has the advantage of distracting the exerciser from the challenges of physical exertion, which produces fatigue, higher heart rate, and sweating. Music should also improve exercisers' moods if they enjoy the musical selection (Karageorghis and Terry, 1997).

Health professionals want to make sure that any music used is compatible with the preferences of most facility and program users. They should also ensure that the music is clear (e.g., recorded properly, played on proper equipment). No music at all is preferable to undesirable musical selections or poor-quality sound.

Pedometers

A pedometer is a body-worn motion sensor that assesses physical activity, specifically the number of steps taken per day. It has been used to encourage physical activity. According to Kang, Marshall, Barreira, and Lee (2009) in their extensive review of the literature on pedometer exercise, "Taking 10,000 steps/day appears to be a reasonable goal of daily activity for healthy adults. Individuals who accumulate 10,000 steps/day are more likely to meet the physical activity guidelines by engaging in the amount of activity promoted by the Centers for Disease Control and Prevention (and other government agencies)" (p. 648). Based on their meta-analysis of research in this area, the authors concluded that "the use of pedometers has a moderate and positive effect on the increase of PA (physical activity) in intervention studies" (p. 652).

In addition to pedometers, exercise interventions might include devices such as accelerometers (which include speed of movement in addition to number of steps) and heart rate monitors that use heart rate to measure exercise intensity and achieve a cardiovascular effect in approaching the exerciser's target heart rate. Each of these devices provides information that has motivational value to maintain an active lifestyle.

Scheduling

Routines, schedules, habits, and rituals bring some degree of order to what would otherwise be a chaotic life. We need structure in our lives in order to achieve our goals and to be productive. Attempting to replace a person's unhealthy habits with more desirable ones is enormously difficult, partly because change is uncomfortable and risky. But the chance of exercising or performing some other task on a regular basis is far greater if it is planned in advance. Plans that are more detailed are more likely to be carried out (Loehr and Schwartz, 2003). Clients and their coaches should select days of the week and the most convenient time of day that is most likely to result in vigorous exercise. Speaking of time of day, however, it is best not to exercise aerobically within two hours of bedtime (see the following section).

Time of Day

Exercise leaders and physiologists are often asked, "When is the best time of day to exercise?" Not surprisingly, people differ on the time of day they prefer for exercise. Some people enjoy working out first thing in the morning, while others wake up and the first thing on their mind is getting a cup of coffee—fast! Time preferences for exercise are influenced by convenience (e.g., "I have more time to exercise after work," "I prefer to get my workout out of the way before work"), body chemistry ("I feel more awake and ready to perform later in the day"), personality ("I love to wake up early, get pumped up, and breathe the cool morning air"), availability of social support such as someone to exercise with or a fitness coach, timing of job demands, and convenience and availability of fitness facilities and equipment (Applegate et al., 1999).

According to O'Connor and Davis (1992), who confirmed the findings of several earlier Swedish studies, whether we choose to exercise during the day or night does not influence the benefits received. In other words, it does not matter. Early morning exercise is as physiologically effective as nighttime exercise. There is one exception to that rule, however: Researchers have found that it is best *not* to engage in aerobic exercise within two hours of going to sleep. Studies indicate that for most individuals high-intensity aerobic exercise close to bedtime will reduce time spent in deep sleep. However, people who possess high aerobic fitness recover from aerobic exercise faster than people who are less fit, so the rule about exercising close to bedtime is more relevant for people with lower aerobic fitness. The bottom line is this: People should exercise at a time of day that is convenient and compatible with their adherence to a lifestyle that incorporates regular exercise.

Social Engineering

The concept of social engineering comes from the stress management literature and refers to people consciously placing themselves in situations, conditions, or environments that reduce or control sources of stress. Examples include driving down a less traveled road or going to a social event at a less crowded time. In fitness settings, exercisers can carry out specific strategies to physically change their environment to make exercise more pleasant. For example, they can avoid a crowded exercise facility by choosing a less busy time to work out. The highest volume of exercisers during the week is the dinner hour, so entering the facility in the early morning, midmorning, or midafternoon might be more compatible with the person's need to avoid a heavy crowd. It is highly likely the equipment will be more readily available during these off hours and staff will be more available to provide instruction. In addition, fewer people in attendance means less likelihood of being observed by others, which may be important to people who are highly self-conscious.

Perceived Choice

One reason people drop out of exercise classes is because they do not enjoy the type of exercise they are being asked to do. To use a cliché, one size does not fit all. It is true that aerobic exercise is needed to improve cardiorespiratory fitness. It is also true that cardiorespiratory exercise is the best way to burn the most calories when attempting to lose or control weight. It is possible, however, for exercise leaders to provide clients with options that are best suited to their individual needs and

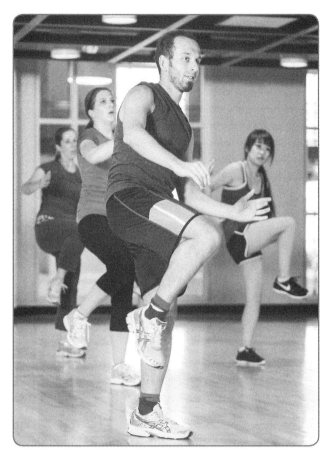

Fitness professionals should encourage clients to find an exercise environment that is enjoyable and then use behavioral strategies such as music, scheduling, coaching, and goal setting to help them achieve their goals.

wishes. Not everyone enjoys using treadmills, for instance, and many people loathe jogging, especially those who are overweight and unfit.

Perceived choice is about providing clients with exercise alternatives that are compatible with their needs and, even more important, with their preferences. Clients need to develop a habit of increased physical activity, and if they prefer swimming or brisk walking to jogging, then staff members need to develop programs using those exercise choices. After clients have developed a set of routines and an exercise habit, perhaps they are more open to using other types of exercise. This issue is especially important for people who have lower-limb discomfort, are overweight or obese, or have limited experience. Many people dislike treadmills and other types of exercise that place considerable pressure on lower limbs or a sore back. The best approach to promote exercise adherence and making exercise a lifestyle habit is to give exercisers choices about the types of activities they can perform that will have similar health and fitness benefits. Tasks should be relatively easy and not too intense at first; slowly increase task difficulty and intensity as the client becomes more comfortable.

Goal Setting

Setting goals is a significant motivator when it comes to improved performance, particularly with respect to exercise and fitness. Failure to properly set and meet goals and expectations is a primary reason for quitting exercise programs, particularly within the first six months of starting a program. This is why it is so important to help people have realistic expectations about exercise outcomes and to understand the need to be patient in overcoming years of leading a sedentary lifestyle. Meeting short-term, performance-based (process) goals that are moderately challenging will improve confidence and encourage people to stick with the program. Failure to meet exercise and fitness goals often leads to disappointment, perceived failure in achieving expected outcomes, and quitting the exercise program.

Sample goals in exercise settings include the following: "I will complete 20 minutes nonstop on the treadmill at a speed of 3 miles per hour and an elevation of 1," "I will complete three sets of eight repetitions lifting 40 pounds," and "I will reach my training heart rate during five work–rest interval training sessions, each of which consists of running for 3 minutes and then walking for 30 seconds." Notice that these goals are performance (process) goals rather than outcome (product) goals (e.g., "I will lose 3 pounds," "I will lose 2% body fat"), which are long-term goals and not under the exerciser's control.

Attainable Units of Progress

As indicated earlier, building intrinsic motivation (chapter 4) is strongly linked to the perception of competence. A person requires information that reflects feelings of achievement in a particular task or toward meeting a specific goal. The best way to boost intrinsic motivation in exercise settings is to provide the exerciser with information that reflects improvement and competence. This process is not likely to occur quickly; instead, there can be a series of experiences and information installments that create perceptions of competence over time. The person must detect these incremental improvements, however small, which involves providing the exerciser with small, attainable units that reinforce the perception of moving toward achieving outcome goals. This is why using a relatively small unit of time (minutes, for example) is more likely to reflect competent performance than measuring performance by relatively larger units (such as distance in miles).

Rewards

According to positive social reinforcement theory, rewards have information value about competence (Anshel, 2012). A reward, such as a T-shirt or some other form of recognition, reflects the achievement of a certain level of competence (e.g., 500-mile club) or group affiliation (e.g., YMCA running club), enhancing a sense of accomplishment or group identification. Both outcomes markedly improve participation satisfaction and adherence. In order to build intrinsic motivation, that is, feelings of satisfaction, enjoyment, and competence, it is best to link the reward directly to a desirable performance outcome or achievement rather than as a response to participation that the person expects.

Performance Feedback

Performance feedback is inherent to learning and to improved performance. Proper exercise technique and protocol require information feedback. General performance feedback is also needed as a motivational strategy. Acknowledging improvement increases exercisers' perceived competence, thereby raising their confidence, which often results in long-term adherence. All information feedback, whether positive or critical, should reflect observable and measurable behavior (e.g., "That was a great effort at completing those repetitions") rather than more abstract content (e.g., "You're looking better," "Nice going"). In addition, giving feedback intermittently (i.e., regularly but not constantly) is more effective than giving it all the time. The key point is that exercisers need to hear and observe positive messages about their performance or about outcomes derived from their efforts.

Self-Monitoring

The use of exercise techniques and scheduling is a science that consists of specific skills and strategies to obtain the benefits of exercise. For example, researchers have known for decades that improving cardiorespiratory fitness requires aerobic exercise, which consists of raising the heart rate to a formula-based level at least three times per week on alternate days for a minimum of 30 minutes per session. In addition, starting a new exercise program is intimidating and stressful both mentally and physically. Perhaps it is not surprising that so many people quit three to six months after starting a new program. The exercise novice needs help, and plenty of it. A self-monitoring checklist provides the information exercisers need to obtain optimal results and to reach personal fitness goals.

Self-monitoring consists of listing the thoughts, emotions, and actions that should be part of the person's exercise-related protocol. It is not a test; there is no right or wrong answer. Rather, the checklist provides a set of guidelines for making exercise as pleasant and performed as correctly and efficiently as possible. Thus, a score of 5 is always desirable. Items that are scored 1 through 3 require the performer's attention in attempting to raise those scores. The goal in completing this checklist, which is located in chapter 3, is to increase the total score for each segment.

For the novice exerciser, fitness coaches should review the checklist once per week and then less often after the first month. Eventually, perhaps after six weeks of regular

monitoring, the checklist will serve as an occasional reminder of rituals before and during exercise sessions. With time, exercise rituals will become habits, and the issue of quitting versus adherence will not be as relevant. So, maintaining the checklist is more important in earlier stages of developing exercise routines, and it eventually becomes less important with time and experience.

In addition, selected items on the checklist may be irrelevant to some people. For example, some individuals would rather exercise alone than with others, so the item that addresses exercising in a group setting can be eliminated from the checklist. Any other item that is contrary to the exerciser's needs and preferences can also be eliminated, as long as omitting it will not induce quitting or injury.

Record Keeping and Attendance

For most exercisers, keeping records is an important method for showing achievement and success. It is normal to feel motivated in response to improvement and competence, an issue that is at the heart of intrinsic motivation (see chapter 4). Exercise leaders and other health care specialists should work with clients to record baseline measures of various dimensions of fitness and other measures that can change over a reasonable time period (usually within three to four months) and then monitor the client's progress by maintaining those records. The perception of improvement as shown by test scores leads to a sense of accomplishment and satisfaction. It confirms to clients that their efforts to improve their fitness and reach other desirable goals have been successful.

Performance data should be recorded, updated, and monitored in quantitative form, reflecting numbers rather than, or in addition to, general comments such as "Nancy did a good job today" or "John is feeling better about his exercise progress." Examples of data include duration of aerobic activity; amount of resistance lifted; number of repetitions of an activity; degrees of flexibility (stretching); changes in percent body fat; number of laps, minutes, or distance jogged; and even frequency of attending the fitness venue or a particular program. "Seeing on paper how far they have progressed can be very reinforcing," Sarafino (1994, p. 267) contends.

It is important to keep tabs on the exerciser's attendance not only to determine exercise adherence but also to acknowledge as soon as possible any pattern of absenteeism that might indicate dropping out. Although it is possible that absent clients are deciding to exercise in places other than the designated location, absences provide the first warning sign of quitting. Contacting an absent client communicates a sense of caring and professionalism that clients will appreciate, and commitment to an ongoing exercise program is strongly tied to meeting exercise goals and developing a lifestyle of increased physical activity. Regular attendance after a segment of time, let's say over the summer or the calendar year, might warrant recognition at an annual awards banquet or some other form of acknowledgment.

Lifestyle Management

The benefits of exercise do not happen in a vacuum. To obtain these benefits, exercise should be incorporated into a person's lifestyle as one of many routines that influence energy, work productivity, general physical and mental health, and quality of life. Lifestyle management is perhaps the most important behavioral strategy of all. It includes a series of healthy habits involving exercise, nutrition, rest, and other rituals that improve health and well-being.

EXERCISE PROGRAMS AND INTERVENTIONS

Programs may consist of several strategies and components that a person carries out to produce an effective outcome. Two such programs are called *motivational interviewing* (Rollnick, Miller, and Butler, 2008) and the *disconnected values model* (Anshel, 2008). There are several other fitness-related programs in

the applied literature; these are simply two examples that illustrate the value of using complete programs.

Before providing guidelines for selecting an effective health behavior intervention, it is important to remember the definitions of terms reviewed earlier in this chapter. A *treatment* is a specific procedure, or action, that is intended to elicit a predictable outcome. An *intervention* consists of a series of treatments, or programs, that are performed over a longer period of time and may consist of several forms of treatment. As described later, the disconnected values model is an intervention. Finally, an action plan is a treatment and forms the last segment of many interventions.

The following components should be included when selecting exercise interventions, according to Goldstein (2001) and Anshel (2008):

- Multiple treatments that influence behavior change in an exerciser (e.g., providing instruction on benefits of proper nutrition for exercise performance and energy, using mental health therapy to change attitudes toward emotional eating, teaching self-regulation strategies)
- Cognitive and behavioral strategies that improve psychological readiness, confidence, and exercise performance
- Sustaining power, meaning the intervention can be practiced independently by the exerciser and become a long-term (lifestyle) habit
- Observable and measureable outcomes from the intervention
- Client choice of exercise types, location, and schedule
- Development of a firm and positive relationship between the client and health professional

Motivational Interviewing

Motivational interviewing is an intervention framework that has received increased attention for changing health behavior in recent years. It is a client-centered method to improve intrinsic motivation to develop healthy habits by performing three essential functions:

1. Collaborating with the client to create a safe, supportive, and nonjudgmental environment within which to initiate the client's behavior change

2. Exploring with the client reasons for and against behavior change, the goal of which is to resolve ambivalence

3. Developing the client's sense of autonomy (responsibility) for changing behavior

Thus, it is the client, not the counselor or coach, who must decide if, how, and when change will occur.

Although originally developed to help people overcome addictions to alcohol and drugs, motivational interviewing has also been shown to be effective for increasing exercise and other forms of physical activity (Martins and McNeil, 2009). As explained by Miller and Rollnick (2002), motivational interviewing is best described by four premises:

1. Motivational interviewing is client centered, focusing on the client's concerns and perspectives. It does not focus on teaching new skills, reshaping cognitions, or reexamining the past. The focus is on the person's current concerns as well as on any misalignments between the person's past experiences and personal values (core beliefs about what is important).

2. Motivational interviewing focuses on specific changes in behavior. The client and interviewer exchange views about the most desirable and realistic changes, and the interviewer addresses possible barriers to change (i.e., what are the obstacles that might prevent change from occurring?).

3. Motivational interviewing is a method of communication—a collaborative technique—that evokes natural change. It is not coercive. Changes must be in the person's best interest and relevant to the person's values and concerns.

4. The focus of motivational interviewing is to elicit intrinsic motivation for change;

change is not imposed. The goal is to increase the person's motivation to initiate behavior change and improve adherence to new, desirable behaviors.

Motivational interviewing consists of three stages: collaboration, evocation, and autonomy.

• *Collaboration:* The counselor provides an atmosphere that is conducive rather than coercive to change by providing awareness and acceptance of the client's reality that may have previously been unnoticed by the client.

• *Evocation:* This stage resides within the client; intrinsic motivation for change is improved by drawing on the client's own perceptions, goals, and values. The counselor assumes that the client has important knowledge, insights, and skills necessary for change.

• *Autonomy:* The client's capacity for self-direction is affirmed; the counselor provides options for informed choice rather than instructing the client on what to do.

See Rollnick, Miller, and Butler (1999) for ways in which motivational interviewing has been applied to change health behavior.

Disconnected Values Model

The disconnected values model consists of cognitive and behavioral strategies that contrast people's beliefs, called *values*, with their unhealthy habits. Based on inconsistencies between behavioral patterns and values, it generates an action plan that allows people to carry out new behaviors that replace negative, unhealthy habits. The focus of this model is to give a framework for practitioners (e.g., licensed psychologists, sport and exercise psychology consultants, mental health professionals, physical fitness trainers, performance coaches) to provide clients with the incentive to develop a long-term exercise habit. Figure 9.1 illustrates the model (Anshel, 2008).

The disconnected values model is intended for young and middle-aged adults (rather than children, adolescents, and the elderly) for three reasons. First, the model was conceptualized and practiced with an adult population. Second, unlike adults, children

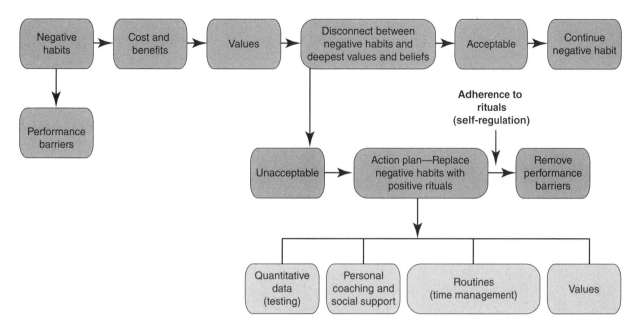

Figure 9.1 Overview of the disconnected values model.

Adapted, by permission, from M.H. Anshel, 2008, "The disconnected values model: Intervention strategies for health behavior change," *Journal of Clinical Sport Psychology* 2: 357-380.

and adolescents do not tend to contemplate the costs and long-term problems associated with health-inhibiting behaviors, and their values differ markedly from those of adults. Third, age groups differ in their most important values, and therefore in the personal needs and sources of motivation that drive behavior—both healthy and unhealthy. For example, limitations in physical health or unique sociocultural conditioning may inhibit exercise behavior, particularly among the elderly. In addition, adolescent age groups will see less relevance or personal interest in maintaining healthy behavior patterns, as opposed to their adult counterparts.

Not surprisingly, motives for exercising also differ as a function of age. For instance, changes in body weight and improved musculature would be a primary exercise motive for younger age groups. Exercise as a means of social interaction is far more common among the elderly, and restrictions on physical activity due to taking medication are also more common among older adults. Finally, age groups have unique barriers to exercise habits. The elderly, for instance, are more likely to

consider transportation or medication a barrier to regular exercise, while this is less likely among the younger adult population. Thus, the disconnected values model is intended for the adult population (not including elderly adults).

The disconnected values model is based on interactions between the practitioner and the client. These interactions include receiving information (e.g., facing the truth about who you are and how you live), self-reflecting (e.g., acknowledging the costs and long-term consequences of a sedentary lifestyle), determining personal goals (e.g., knowing what you want or need), and identifying strategies to reach those goals (e.g., generating an action plan that replaces negative habits with positive ones).

Negative Habits

The disconnected values model begins by acknowledging the existence of negative habits, which are thoughts, emotions, or tasks people experience regularly that they agree are not in their best interests yet remain under their control. Despite their ability to prevent or stop these negative habits, they continue to experience them. In this example, not exercising and poor nutrition are negative habits that need changing.

Humans do not maintain a habit without benefits. The primary reason a person engages in a negative habit is because the perceived benefits of the habit outweigh its costs and long-term consequences. For example, the negative habit of late-night eating (i.e., consuming food just before bedtime) has the perceived benefit of quickly satisfying hunger with food that tastes good. The costs of late-night eating include sleeping less soundly (e.g., frequent trips to the bathroom) and gaining weight. Long-term consequences include developing heart disease, obesity, and type 2 diabetes. Often, these costs and consequences are either not acknowledged or are perceived as less important than meeting the person's short-term goals. Under these conditions, the negative habit persists.

Barriers to High Performance

Barriers to high performance consist of any persistent thoughts, emotions, or actions that compromise health or happiness (Dunn, Andersen, and Jakicic, 1998). Whether these barriers are actual (e.g., injury, anger) or perceived (e.g., time constraints, discomfort, anxiety), they are almost always controllable and thus changeable. For instance, the emotional barrier of anxiety can be controlled by addressing the source of concern (e.g., irrational thinking) and developing adaptation strategies (e.g., positive self-talk, self-analysis, distraction activities) to overcome anxious thoughts. Thus, people who are uncomfortable and self-conscious about exercising among younger, fitter, thinner people at a fitness facility should focus on their exercise regimen while ignoring others in the room. People who have time constraints can develop time management strategies and obtain social support from significant others to allow for exercise time.

The root cause of barriers to high performance success in the disconnected values

model is maintaining negative habits. These psychobehavioral tendencies are labeled *negative* because they have a deleterious effect on the person's quality of life, and continued expression of the negative habits is directly linked to problems in work performance. For example, the negative physical habit of not exercising will lead to low energy and fatigue, the emotional negative habit of persistent anxiety will lead to poor decision making, and the negative physical habit of poor work–life balance results in poor relationships with family. One function of the model, therefore, is to help clients detect their negative habits and how they lead to reduced quality of life. After linking negative habits, such as lack of exercise, to reduced quality of life, the primary goal at this stage is to examine the "benefits" of maintaining the negative habits.

Determining One's Deepest Values and Beliefs

Clients are given a list of values—their beliefs about what is really important to them—and then asked to rank these values. It is likely that health and family would be ranked near the top. Perhaps integrity, happiness, honesty, character, excellence, commitment, and concern for others would be other highly rated choices.

The decision to begin and maintain an exercise program is more likely if clients acknowledge that

- the costs and long-term consequences of a negative habit are greater than the benefits,
- these costs run counter to the clients' deepest values and beliefs about what is important, and
- the discrepancy between the clients' values and negative habits is unacceptable.

Thus, behavior change is more likely to be permanent when clients conclude that life satisfaction is linked to behavior that is consistent with their values.

Establishing and Accepting the Disconnect

To help clients detect inconsistencies between their values and their negative habits, practitioners ask, "To what extent are your values consistent with your actions? If you value your health, for instance, do you have habits that are not good for you and therefore are inconsistent with your values? What about your family? Do you value your spouse, children, parents, or someone else who is important to you? If you lead a sedentary lifestyle and are not involved in an exercise program, yet one of your deepest values is to maintain good health, to what extent is your value inconsistent with your behavior? Is there a disconnect between your beliefs about good health and your unhealthy behavior patterns?"

If clients acknowledge that the negative habit of not engaging in exercise is inconsistent with their deepest beliefs about what is important to them, the follow-up questions are, "Do you see a disconnect between your values (e.g., health, high quality of life, happiness) and any negative habits (e.g., lack of exercise)? Is this disconnect acceptable?" If clients find the disconnect between the negative habit and values is acceptable even after identifying the costs and long-term consequences of this habit—and sometimes people feel that changing the negative habit is either undesirable or beyond their control—then no change in behavior is likely to occur. If this is the case, perhaps there is another disconnect between negative habits and values that the client will find unacceptable. People are far more likely to commit to behavior change and to develop and carry out an action plan if a designated disconnect is unacceptable to them.

Developing an Action Plan

The decision to initiate an exercise program, ostensibly because the disconnect between the negative habit of nonexercise and the client's values is unacceptable, is followed by developing a detailed action plan to create a habit of regular exercise during the week. Specifics include exercise type, locations, days of the week, and times of day; tests to establish a baseline of fitness and health indicators; and availability of social support and personal fitness coaching. The results of past studies indicate that specificity of timing and precision of behavior dramatically increase the probability of successfully carrying out a self-controlled action plan. The action plan is not unlike the between-shot and preshot routines of a professional golfer (Bull, Albinson, and Shambrook, 1996).

The action plan consists primarily of three factors that markedly enhance permanent commitment to regular exercise:

1. A specific time within a 24-hour period for exercise engagement

2. A set of routines that support the exercise habit (e.g., selected thoughts and behaviors before, during, and following the exercise session; exercising with a friend and promoting other forms of social support; minimizing distractions that will interfere with exercise plans)

3. Linking these specific times and routines to the person's deepest values and beliefs about what is important, resulting in removal of the existing disconnect

Clients often need rapid, short-term experiences to quickly alter their behavior. These experiences, or strategies, are called *one-time action steps*. The practitioner works with the client to develop an action plan consisting of new routines that are scheduled into the workday and week. For example, a 24-hour time sheet should incorporate components scheduled at specific times that are connected to the client's values. These normally include strategies to extend physical capacity to create more energy (Loehr and Schwartz, 2003). Some examples are presleep rituals (e.g., no food or alcohol within one hour of bedtime, planned relaxation activities, positive communication with family members), specific sleep and wake-up times, exercise sessions, meals, snacks, recovery breaks, times to connect with family and significant others, and other rituals linked to each dimension and the client's values.

FROM RESEARCH TO REAL WORLD

As discussed throughout this book, one of the primary reasons a person drops out of physical activity programs, including exercise, is a lack of social and professional support. Often, the exercise novice is asked to take on the sole responsibility of initiating an exercise program without proper instruction, testing, prescription, and confidence in a manner that will foster improved fitness and meeting other personal goals. Perhaps not surprisingly, novices frequently decide to quit further participation. The clinical delivery wellness model was developed and carried out by this author with university faculty and staff supported by a two-year internal grant at Middle Tennessee State University (2006-2008). Data from five 10-week campus wellness programs were reported in studies by Anshel and Kang (2007a, b) and Brinthaupt, Kang, and Anshel (2013).

The focus of this delivery model is the pervasive use of experts, called *coaches* in the program, to lend support to participants. All of the participants were unfit exercise novices, and four coaches were incorporated into the program. The program director was a performance coach who organized the program and provided a two-hour orientation. In addition to describing the program, the orientation also had motivational properties and created a sense of optimism, excitement, focus, and long-term commitment to the program.

The second coach was the client's personal trainer, or fitness coach. This person provided pre- and postprogram fitness testing and weekly coaching. Fitness coaches were assigned to their clients based on clients' preferences for a male or female coach and availability for regular coaching meetings.

The third coach was a registered dietitian. This coach reviewed each client's lipids profile (i.e., a blood test administered by nurses at the university student health center) for indicators of the client's dietary habits, including cholesterol and triglycerides; provided nutrition education to client groups; and met individually with clients to prescribe proper dietary habits.

The fourth coach was a licensed psychologist referred to as a *life skills coach*. Her role was not to provide psychological counseling but rather to use a psychological inventory to detect possible indicators of mental illness or thought processes that might impede the client's participation and long-term adherence. Conditions such as depression, chronic anxiety, irrational thinking, and chronic sleeplessness are red flags that suggest the person might want to consider seeing a mental health professional. This coach did not administer psychological counseling as part of the program but instead provided a professional recommendation for follow-up with a licensed mental health professional.

Taken together, this delivery model resulted in extraordinary program adherence. Postprogram participant evaluations, reported by Anshel and Kang (2007a, b), indicated that the inclusion of multiple coaches was a life-changing experience for many participants. Clearly, helping exercisers through the process of improving their fitness and changing their lifestyle requires considerable personal and psychological support. More research on the effectiveness of these delivery models is needed.

The disconnected values model serves as an intervention tool for sport and exercise consultants, performance coaches, and licensed mental health professionals. Traditionally, research and practice in exercise psychology have been concerned primarily with the psychological and behavioral factors that predict or influence exercise participation, adherence, and performance. The role of practitioners in exercise settings, however, has not been given sufficient attention by writers, practitioners, and researchers.

The disconnected values model provides an opportunity for practitioners to address a growing need in promoting physical activity to an increasingly unhealthy population. The model consists primarily of replacing one set of behaviors, deemed negative or unhealthy, with another set of behaviors that are positive or healthy. It does not include psychotherapy and other skills that require licensure as a psychologist, thus allowing practitioners with an array of skills and interests to apply it in exercise settings. However, for optimal effectiveness in applying the model, it is important that the practitioner

- possess superb communication skills;
- establish a close, trusting relationship with the client;
- engage with the client in a quiet, isolated environment;
- promise strict confidentiality of information the client provides;
- avoid judging the client's feelings and actions;
- provide support to carry out the action plan (e.g., establishing partners, identifying needed equipment or resources, suggesting existing programs or specialists); and
- monitor progress with follow-up sessions.

One implication for practitioners in applying the disconnected values model is the behavioral nature of this intervention. Determining the effectiveness of the model for helping clients improve their participation in and adherence to exercise behavior requires behavioral assessment. The examples of behavioral assessment provided in Anshel (2008) are well within the training and experience of practitioners and reflect the model. They include behavioral interviewing (e.g., identifying negative habits such as not exercising), behavioral inventories (e.g., determining selected psychological dispositions that are associated with inactivity), task-relevant behavioral checklists (e.g., self-monitoring that provides instructional feedback on performing exercise skills or executing an effective fitness program), and performance profiling (e.g., asking clients to self-examine their attitudes, perceived barriers, level of mastery, and other factors that might promote or impede future exercise participation).

THE PROBLEM OF OVERPRESCRIPTION

This chapter describes a vast array of cognitive and behavioral strategies that are intended to facilitate exercise performance, improve exercise adherence, and increase readiness and motivation to make a long-term commitment to an exercise program. Armed with this arsenal of techniques, it is not uncommon for some well-meaning coaches and other health professionals to proscribe too many new strategies within a relatively short time. The result may be client confusion and preoccupation with using all the learned strategies at one time, increasing the level of mental distraction, frustration, and stress and eventually leading to performance failure and even dropping out of exercise. This problem is called *paralysis by analysis* in the pedagogy literature, and it is recommended that specialists prescribe relatively few strategies at one time, or even just one strategy. Novice exercisers are in new territory, and they need to begin to integrate the recommended techniques with as little stress, confusion, and anxiety as possible.

It is important, therefore, to remember three things. First, skills, including cognitive and behavioral strategies, need to be learned and mastered over time. Second, exercisers can be burdened by learning too many strategies at one time. And third, exercisers differ in their need to use certain types of strategies and programs. One size does not fit all. Some mental techniques are applicable only to certain types of exercises and under specific fitness program conditions. One rule of thumb is to prescribe and teach a single technique, and then let clients take a few weeks to integrate the technique into their exercise patterns until it is seamless and feels natural to them.

APPLYING MOTIVATION THEORY

In the final analysis, the goal of every fitness program and health practitioner is to build intrinsic motivation in clients. Discussed at length in chapter 2, intrinsic motivation consists of engaging in a task for pleasure, satisfaction, and feelings of competence. It is based on Deci's (1975) cognitive evaluation theory. Changing exercise behavior is related to two main components of intrinsic motivation: self-determination (feelings of high self-control) and information (feelings of high perceived competence). Intrinsic motivation incorporates both cognitive and behavioral strategies that result in a person's long-term commitment to exercise and other healthy habits. That is the real goal of these strategies and programs.

To make a lifestyle change that incorporates physical activity, people must make their own decisions about how they live (Vansteenkiste, Soenes, and Lens, 2007). Everyone has specific needs and preferences, which is why clients should experience the following:

- A list of exercise programs to choose from
- Exercise locations that they find comfortable
- Instruction on correct exercise techniques
- Positive instructional feedback on their exercise performance to gain a sense of achievement and competence
- A support system, perhaps consisting of family, friends, or coaches who recognize the exerciser's efforts or accompany the exerciser in the journey toward improved fitness and health
- Experiences that improve their confidence, enjoyment, and sense of accomplishment and competence in performing exercise routines and reaching both short-term (i.e., each session) and long-term (i.e., over weeks and months) exercise goals

The cognitive evaluation model and other motivational theories include several interacting components that improve motivation, especially intrinsic motivation. The primary goal of fitness professionals is to encourage clients to adopt exercise as a lifestyle habit. There is no time in life when any healthy person should avoid exercise. In addition, both intrinsic and extrinsic motivation promote long-term exercise adherence. Both are valid participation motives, that is, reasons for exercising.

There are several takeaway messages for fitness professionals concerning intrinsic and extrinsic motivation to promote exercise behavior, especially for novice exercisers. First, increasing the participant's autonomy and controllability likely improves intrinsic motivation. Second, higher intrinsic motivation is associated with more positive attitudes toward exercise and long-term exercise adherence as compared with higher extrinsic motivation. This is because, according to Markland and Ingledew (2007), "when intrinsically oriented motives predominate, participation is likely to be accompanied by a sense of volition and freedom from pressure, and therefore long-term commitment is to be expected, and engagement will be accompanied by positive exercise-related cognitions and affect" (p. 24). Finally, extrinsic motivation can also be effective in promoting long-term exercise habits and exercise enjoyment. For instance, motives such as losing weight, improving appearance, or trying to please others are internally controlling but reflect extrinsic motivation (Markland and Ingledew, 2007). Extrinsic motivation can facilitate exercise behavior when the person identifies with and values the outcomes of the behavior, such as weight loss or improved physical appearance (Ryan et al., 1997).

Another theory about the influence of intrinsic and extrinsic motivation based on how we explain the outcomes of our performance is called *attribution theory*. Let's reexamine the components of motivation theory, particularly intrinsic motivation, and then include exercise-related examples for each component.

Reasons for Participation

Which is better for exercisers, task involvement or ego involvement? As Markland and Ingledew (2007) report, understanding the person's motives for engaging in exercise or another form of physical activity is a significant predictor of the person's intrinsic or extrinsic motivation, which in turn predicts exercise adherence. For task-involved exercisers, intrinsic motivation increases because exercise is experienced as an end in itself. Motivation is derived from the intrinsic enjoyment, satisfaction, sense of achievement, and even fun that occur during exercise. For ego-involved exercisers, however, self-worth is based on performance, such as completing a certain exercise task in meeting an internally set goal or standard, and failing to meet that standard is a possible threat to self-esteem. Ego involvement results in attempts to meet a performance standard rather than focusing on achieving a certain task, and the result is less intrinsic motivation. To paraphrase Frederick and Ryan (1995), people who find relatively little enjoyment in exercise and think that its value lies only in losing weight or improving appearance are unlikely to induce task involvement, therefore undermining their long-term exercise participation.

Example: A novice exerciser wants to learn exercise techniques and perform each exercise flawlessly to obtain optimal results. There is no interest in comparing exercise performance outcomes against a standard or being evaluated by fitness testing or by another person. However, even if the exerciser is being evaluated, intrinsic motivation will not decrease if the exerciser views such evaluations as having low functional significance.

Thus, the main motivational issue an exerciser should address is not "Could I keep up with the instructor?" or "Did I beat my previous best?" but rather, "Did I enjoy myself?" or "Do I feel the benefits of exercising regularly?" If the response is "No, I did not enjoy myself," then the exerciser should think about the possible reasons for these feelings. Are expectations too high for achieving short-term and long-term goals? Is the exercise too intense and should begin with less intensity? The exerciser may need encouragement from others—a form of social support—to reappraise the experience in a more favorable light. The exerciser might say, for instance, "I wish this were easier and more enjoyable, but if I remain patient and keep exercising on my schedule of at least three times per week, it will eventually get easier." Or, the exerciser might conclude that the program is, in fact, getting easier with time and the benefits (e.g., weight loss, firm muscles) are becoming apparent. Roberts (1992) contends that people in management positions, such as fitness coaches and exercise facility managers, can improve the motivational climate of a program by informing exercisers that improvement is one important criterion for success, as opposed to relying solely on exercise outcomes (e.g., number of repetitions, amount of weight lifted, speed of distance running) to improve intrinsic motivation.

Controlling Function

Are people exercising of their own volition for their own personal satisfaction—internal, self-determining factors—or due to external factors, such as pleasing others, competing, and earning prizes? Intrinsic motivation is closely associated with self-determination. Another controlling factor is task involvement—intrinsic motivation is higher for task-involved exercisers, while extrinsic motivation is the primary motivational source for ego-involved exercisers. At least in the early stages of getting fit, ego involvement is less likely to be enjoyable and more likely to increase anxiety (perceived threat about appearing unfit or looking overweight in fitness clothing compared with younger, fitter exercisers).

Example: Intrinsic motivation is not possible if a person feels coerced into exercising; the individual must want to exercise. The novice exerciser—or friends or family members of one—should emphasize the fun aspect of physical activity and the value of staying in top physical condition. Ideally, all forms of physical activity should be viewed as enjoyable and imperative for better health and well-being. The exerciser should feel confident in handling the demands of physical exertion; the human body was meant to remain physically active to maintain proper development and functioning.

Information Function

Perceived ability strongly influences intrinsic motivation. Not surprisingly, performing skills with competence and consistency to produce superior performance is a basic human need and strongly influences self-esteem. Feelings of competence are central to intrinsic motivation because it produces the perception of high ability. Humans rarely continue to engage in a task that they are performing poorly, or more accurately, that they *perceive* themselves as performing poorly.

> Example: One goal of fitness leaders, teachers, and parents is to offer encouraging remarks to others regardless of the actual outcome (e.g., "Keep trying—you're looking better"). Positive feedback should reflect performance effort and improvement. Feedback can actually increase intrinsic motivation if it reinforces the performer's feelings of competence and provides useful information. For instance, the exerciser's feelings of competence will increase in response to compliments or positive feedback from the fitness coach. A similar increase in intrinsic motivation can also follow negative feedback if it is accompanied by a positive message (e.g., "You still have to improve your endurance, but I see nice improvement"). However, negative feedback, especially if offered repeatedly by a credible source (e.g., parents, coaches, trainers), can reduce intrinsic motivation if the feedback produces feelings of reduced competence, resulting in reduced pleasure from the activity.

Can awards, a source of extrinsic motivation, ever be used to increase intrinsic motivation? Absolutely. Receiving an award (e.g., a trophy, certificate, or any other tangible reward for participating) is another form of feedback and is common in running groups, community recreational centers, and fitness clubs. Awards can either reduce or increase intrinsic motivation depending on how the recipient perceives the message.

Awards are intrinsic motivators if exercisers perceive them as representing improved performance or some other indicator of success. The award, then, has positive information value; the information reflects high competence and achievement (Duda, 1993). However, if a person engages in exercise primarily to receive an award or recognition rather than for its intrinsic satisfaction or pleasure, and if the exerciser expects and even depends upon receiving the award as a reason for exercising, then the award is an extrinsic motivator (Roberts, 2012).

One way to determine if people are intrinsically or extrinsically motivated to exercise is to ask them, "If there were no awards or recognition given for engaging in regular exercise, would you still want to exercise?" If the answer is "Yes," then intrinsic motivation is likely the primary incentive to participate. An answer of "No," on the other hand, would indicate that the individual's reasons for exercising are based on extrinsic motivation. One good example of exercise as an extrinsic motivator is the high importance some people place on working toward obtaining a prize or receiving recognition (e.g., the 10,000-mile running club, a T-shirt recognizing the exerciser's accomplishment, being eligible to enter a race).

Perhaps the best suggestion for using the information function to increase intrinsic motivation is to keep the message positive or, if negative or critical, to make it instructive. Fitness leaders should provide compliments in response to desirable actions, habits, or attitudes. They should also offer verbal recognition to all exercisers for their effort and improvement. The objective here is to avoid making rewards, physical changes in physique, or reliance on recognition reasons to participate and instead make rewards and other positive feedback a reflection of success.

Therefore, it is important that fitness leaders and parents of children who need to engage in more physical activity do everything they can to avoid feelings of low ability and to search for and recognize any desirable behaviors exhibited by the participant. As Duda (1993) concluded, "Individuals are less likely to perform up to their potential and maintain their involvement in achievement activities when they do not feel competent" (p. 426).

SUMMARY

Interventions consist of techniques (e.g., cognitive and behavioral strategies, treatments) that are intended to improve performance outcomes. The primary goal of exercise interventions is to encourage sedentary or irregularly active people to adopt regular exercise habits and to keep physically active people exercising on a regular basis. Whether cognitive (i.e., thoughts or emotions) or behavioral (i.e., observable actions), strategies are self-initiated, conscious processes designed to enhance a specific outcome or to achieve a goal. Sample cognitive strategies include positive self-talk, visualization, association, dissociation, and psyching up. Behavioral strategies include the use of music, social support, perceived choice (of exercise type), scheduling, self-monitoring, and record keeping. At times, strategies are combined to form program interventions that must be carried out in a predetermined and prescribed manner. Examples include motivational interviewing, the disconnected values model, and the cognitive evaluation model. Taken together, interventions, treatment programs, and strategies should be an integral part of the exerciser's arsenal of skills that facilitate exercise performance and help exercisers reach their goals.

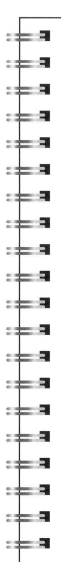

STUDENT ACTIVITY

Cognitive and Behavioral Strategies Fitness Program

Develop a 10- to 12-week fitness program with either a classmate or a real client that consists of carrying out three or four of the strategies reviewed in this chapter. Conduct a personal interview with the client, asking questions about exercise history, any physical restrictions or past medical issues that might influence the type of exercises that can be performed, preferences for types of exercises and scheduling, and willingness to work with a fitness coach. During the program, implement a selection of cognitive and behavioral strategies based on the client's needs.

Setting up your client with a fitness coach to perform a set of pretests that determine various fitness measures is also advised. Tell the client that the same tests, which are used to prescribe an appropriate fitness program, will be administered again in 12 weeks to detect improvements in these measures. Pretests might include submaximal $\dot{V}O_2$ (to measure cardiorespiratory efficiency), upper-limb and lower-limb strength, percent body fat, waist circumference, and body mass index (BMI). Also measure the client's exercise adherence, that is, the extent to which the client is engaging in exercise according to the prescription. The recommendation is a minimum of three times per week for most aerobic fitness programs and twice per week for strength training. Record adherence as the percentage of the time that clients are attending or exercising according to their prescriptions. Full adherence is 100%. Attending 8 of 20 prescribed sessions is 40%. The best measure of changes in eating habits is a lipids profile, which is a blood test that can be administered by a registered nurse or phlebotomist. Blood testing can be a bit costly, though many universities offer the service either on campus or through a local medical center at reduced cost. Each of these tests should be able to detect changes in scores in a 10- to 12-week program.

REFERENCES

Anshel, M.H. (2005). *Applied exercise psychology: A practitioner's guide to client health and fitness.* New York: Springer.

Anshel, M.H. (2008). The disconnected values model: Intervention strategies for health behavior change. *Journal of Clinical Sport Psychology, 2*, 357-380.

Anshel, M.H. (2012). *Sport psychology: From theory to practice* (5th ed.). San Francisco: Benjamin-Cummings.

Anshel, M.H., Brinthaupt, T., and Kang, M. (2010). The disconnected values model improves mental well-being and fitness in an employee wellness program. *Behavioral Medicine, 36*, 113-122.

Anshel, M.H., and Kang, M. (2007a). Effect of an intervention on replacing negative habits with positive routines for improving full engagement at work: A test of the disconnected values model. *Journal of Consulting Psychology: Practice and Research, 59*, 110-125.

Anshel, M.H., and Kang, M. (2007b). An outcome-based action study on changes in fitness, blood lipids, and exercise adherence based on the disconnected values model. *Behavioral Medicine, 33*, 85-98.

Anshel, M.H., and Marisi, D.Q. (1978). Effect of music and rhythm on physical performance. *Research Quarterly, 49*, 109-113.

Anshel, M.H., Umscheid, D., and Brinthaupt, T. (2013). Effect of a combined coping skills and wellness program on changes in perceived stress, job satisfaction, and muscular strength among police emergency dispatchers: An action study. *Journal of Police and Criminal Psychology, 28,* 1-14.

Applegate, B.W., Rohan, K.J., and Dubbert, P.M. (1999). Exercise and psychological health: Research evidence and implications for exercise professionals. *Clinical Exercise Physiology, 1,* 113-119.

Brinthaupt, T.M., Kang, M., and Anshel, M.H. (2013). Changes in exercise commitment following a values-based wellness program. *Journal of Sport Behavior, 36,* 3-22.

Buckworth, J., and Dishman, R.K. (2002). *Exercise psychology.* Champaign, IL: Human Kinetics.

Bull, S.J., Albinson, J.G., and Shambrook, C.J. (1996). *The mental game plan: Getting psyched for sport.* Eastbourne, UK: Sports Dynamics.

Chenoweth, D.H. (2002). *Evaluating worksite health promotion.* Champaign, IL: Human Kinetics.

Deci, E.L. (1975). *Intrinsic motivation.* New York: Plenum.

Duda, J.L. (1993). Goals: A social-cognitive approach to the study of achievement motivation in sport. In R.N. Singer, M. Murphey, and L.K. Tennant (Eds.), *Handbook of research in sport psychology* (pp. 421-436). New York: Macmillan.

Dunn, A.L., Andersen, R.E., and Jakicic, J.M. (1998). Lifestyle physical activity interventions: History, short- and long-term effects, and recommendations. *American Journal of Preventive Medicine, 15,* 398-412.

Fredrick, C.M., and Ryan, R.M. (1995). Self-determination in sport: A review using cognitive evaluation theory. *International Journal of Sport Psychology, 26,* 5-23.

Goldstein, A.P. (2001). *Reducing resistance: Methods for enhancing openness to change.* Champaign, IL: Research Press.

Grossman, P., Niemann, L., Schmidt, S., and Walach, H. (2004). Mindfulness-based stress reduction and health benefits: A meta-analysis. *Journal of Psychosomatic Research, 57,* 35-43.

Hall, C.R. (2001). Imagery in sport and exercise. In R.N. Singer, H.A. Hausenblas, and C.M. Janelle (Eds.), *Handbook of sport psychology* (2nd ed., pp. 529-549). New York: Wiley.

Jones, G., Hanton, S., and Connaughton, D. (2007). A framework of mental toughness in the world's best performers. *Sport Psychologist, 21,* 243-264.

Kang, M., Marshall, S.J., Barreira, T.V., and Lee, J. (2009). Effect of pedometer-based physical activity interventions: A meta-analysis. *Research Quarterly for Exercise and Sport, 80,* 648-655.

Karageorghis, C., and Priest, D.L. (2010). Music in sport and exercise: An update on research and application. *Sport Journal, 13.* www.thesportjournal.org/article/music-sport-and-exercise-update-research-and-application.

Karageorghis, C.I., and Terry, P.C. (1997). The psychophysical effects of music in sport and exercise: A review. *Journal of Sport Behavior, 20,* 54-68.

Loehr, J., and Schwartz, T. (2003). *The power of full engagement: Managing energy, not time, is the key to high performance and personal renewal.* New York: The Free Press.

Markland, D., and Ingledew, D.K. (2007). Exercise participation motives: A self-determination theory perspective. In M.S. Hagger and N.L.D. Chatzisarantis (Eds.), *Intrinsic motivation and self-determination in exercise and sport* (pp. 23-34). Champaign, IL: Human Kinetics.

Martin, K.A., Moritz, S.E. Hall, and C.R. (1999). Imagery use in sport: A literature review and applied model. *Sport Psychologist, 13,* 245-268.

Martins, R.K., and McNeil, D.W. (2009). Review of motivational interviewing in promoting health behaviors. *Clinical Psychology Review, 29,* 283-293.

McCracken, L., Gauntlett-Gilbert, J., and Vowles, K.E. (2007). The role of mindfulness in a contextual cognitive-behavioral analysis of chronic pain-related suffering and disability. *Pain, 131,* 63-69.

Miller, W.R., and Rollnick, S. (2002). *Motivational interviewing: Preparing people for change* (2nd ed.). New York: Guilford.

O'Connor, P.J., and Davis, J.C. (1992). Psychobiologic responses to exercise at different times of day. *Medicine and Science in Sports and Exercise, 24,* 714-719.

Petrillo, L.A., de Kaufman, K.A. Glass, C.R., and Arnkoff, D.B. (2009). Mindfulness for long-distance runners: An open trial using Mindful Sport Performance Enhancement (MSPE). *Journal of Clinical Sport Psychology, 3,* 129-142.

Roberts, G.C. (1992). Motivation in sport and exercise: Conceptual constraints and convergence. In G.C. Roberts (Ed.), *Motivation in sport and exercise* (pp. 3-29). Champaign, IL: Human Kinetics.

Roberts, G.C. (2012). Motivation in sport and exercise from an achievement goal theory perspective: After 30 years, where are we? In G.C. Roberts and D.C. Treasure (Eds.), *Advances in motivation in sport and exercise* (3rd ed., pp. 5-58). Champaign, IL: Human Kinetics.

Rollnick, S., Miller, W.R., and Butler, C.C. (1999). *Health behavior change: A guide for practitioners.* London: Churchill Livingstone.

Rollnick, S., Miller, W.R., and Butler, C.C. (2008). *Motivational interviewing in health care: Helping patients change behavior.* New York: Guilford.

Ryan, R.M., Frederick, C.M., Lepes, D., Rubio, N., and Sheldon, I. (1997). Intrinsic motivation and exercise adherence. *International Journal of Sport Psychology, 28*, 335-354.

Sarafino, E.P. (1994). *Health psychology: Biopsychosocial interactions* (2nd ed.). New York: Wiley.

Singer, R.N., and Anshel, M.H. (2006). An overview of interventions in sport. In J. Dosil (Ed.), *The sport psychologist's handbook* (pp. 64-88). New York: Wiley.

Stathopoulou, G., and Powers, M.B. (2006). Exercise interventions for mental health: A quantitative and qualitative review. *Clinical Psychology: Science and Practice, 13*, 179-193.

Vansteenkiste, M., Soenes, B., and Lens, W. (2007). Intrinsic versus extrinsic goal promotion in exercise and sport: Understanding the differential impacts on performance and persistence. In M.S. Hagger and N.L.D. Chatzisarantis (Eds.), *Intrinsic motivation and self-determination in exercise and sport* (pp. 167-180). Champaign, IL: Human Kinetics.

Vealey, R.S. (1988). Future directions in psychological skills training. *Sport Psychologist, 2*, 318-336.

Vealey, R.S. (2001). Understanding and enhancing self-confidence in athletes. In R.N. Singer, H.A. Hausenblas, and C.M. Janelle (Eds.), *Handbook of sport psychology* (2nd ed., pp. 550-565). New York: Wiley.

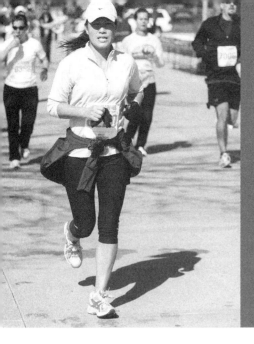

CHAPTER 10

Fitness Goal Setting and Leadership

> *Continuous effort—not strength or intelligence—is the key to unlocking our potential.*
>
> Sir Winston Churchill (1874-1965), former British prime minister

CHAPTER OBJECTIVES

After reading this chapter, you should be able to:

- describe specific strategies for improving exercise motivation to help ensure long-term adherence to an exercise habit, and
- set goals and teach proper goal-setting techniques to clients.

Goal setting has strong motivational properties and is inherent in attaining high-quality physical performance. As a motivational tool, setting goals helps focus the performer's effort and provides a means to monitor progress or performance success (Burton and Naylor, 2002). Goal setting is a science; there is a right way and a wrong way to set goals if goals are to have motivational value. Elite athletes, for instance, correctly set challenging yet realistic goals (Orlick and Partington, 1986).

Has goal setting been shown to be effective? The answer is yes and no. The case in favor of goal setting is reflected in a study by Kyllo and Landers (1995), who used a statistical technique called *meta-analysis* to analyze the results of 36 studies to obtain a generalized result. The researchers found that setting even moderate goals led to significant improvement in performing sport skills or other motor tasks. Performance was optimal when goals were

- set in absolute (observable) terms,
- short term as well as long term,
- set with the participation of the subject (e.g., athlete, exerciser),
- quantifiable (measurable), and
- made public to enhance accountability (although this can create anxiety and remove confidentiality if not done appropriately).

There is an apparent lack of similar research with respect to goal setting in exercise settings. Effective goal setting consists of the following criteria based on an extensive body of related research.

DIRECTION AND QUALITY OF BEHAVIOR

Every goal includes two basic components, direction and amount or quality of behavior. To Burton (1992), *direction* represents focusing one's behavior on a particular outcome. *Amount* or *quality* of behavior indicates a minimal standard of performance that is anticipated and desired. Thus, goals have value in motivating people to take direct action by concentrating on a particular outcome, increasing their mental and physical effort, and creating new strategies to solve problems, improve the motivation to maintain effort, and adhere to a predetermined plan of action. This is particularly powerful after a person experiences failure (Kingston and Hardy, 1997). Examples of goals that include direction and amount or quality of behavior are "I will look all ground balls into my glove that are hit to me" and "I will use a drop shot (in tennis) when I am near the net and my opponent is near the baseline."

GOALS AND PERSONALITY

The effect of goal setting is also a function of personality or disposition, a concept called *goal orientation*. More than one disposition is related to the person's need and preference for setting goals and the effectiveness of goal setting on motivation and subsequent performance level. Burton (1992) and Nicholls (1984) link the dispositions of need achievement with goal orientation. The authors contend that need achievement, goal orientation, and goal-setting style each reflect the influence of goal setting on the individual.

For example, as described earlier, people who have a need to set goals and are highly motivated to meet their goals are said to have a high goal orientation. If they perform particularly well in achievement settings, that is, they are highly motivated in competitive situations in which their competence is evaluated, they are said to have a high need to achieve and they tend to prefer achievement-oriented situations (Nicholls, 1984). Burton (1992) contends that people possess one of two goal orientations, performance and outcome.

PERFORMANCE AND OUTCOME GOALS

The critical factor responsible for motivational behaviors is perceived competence or ability, and a person's goal orientation influences the development of perceived competence and how it affects achievement behavior, such as the need to become fit and lose weight. Goal

---

SAMPLE EXERCISE PERFORMANCE GOALS

Good Performance Goals

I will relax and feel confident before the exercise class so I enjoy the experience.

I will complete three sets of 10 repetitions of biceps curls.

I will complete 20 sit-ups without stopping.

Poor Performance Goals (Not Controllable)

I will win the race.

I will reduce my percent body fat by 3% in the next 30 days.

I will finish in the top three places in this 5K race.

---

orientation becomes stronger when exercisers increase their perceived competence, master new tasks, or improve their skills (or fitness).

With a performance goal orientation, success is defined in terms of internal standards; success is a function of comparing present with previous performance. For people with this orientation, the process of achieving goals is more important than the final product, which reflects a preference for setting and reaching performance (process) goals (Kingston and Hardy, 1997).

An outcome goal orientation, on the other hand, concerns maintaining positive views of one's competence while avoiding negative judgments. This is accomplished in exercise settings by proving, validating, or documenting fitness improvements, typically through social comparisons (e.g., "I can run as far and fast as anyone else my age"). Positive social comparisons are essential in order to maintain high perceived competence. Thus, task mastery and improvement are only a means to an end (e.g., weight control, improved fitness), not ends themselves (Anshel, 2012; Duda and Whitehead, 1998).

The challenge to health care providers and coaches, such as personal trainers and registered dietitians, is to determine the exerciser's needs and preferences and then provide goal-setting strategies that meet those needs. Based on their meta-analysis of studies to determine the effectiveness of goal setting, Klein, Wesson, Hollenbeck, and Alge (1999) concluded that

- to improve motivation and enhance perceived competence, goals should be based on performance—what the person actually does—rather than a particular outcome (the end result);

- goals that relate to improving one's appearance, losing weight, or winning a competitive event (outcome goals) are not always under the exerciser's control; and

- this finding reduces the purposes of goal setting, which should be to focus the participant's effort and to increase motivation.

Not assuming responsibility for outcomes that are uncontrollable (e.g., "As a new exerciser, there is no way I can keep up with the fitness class leader") is more motivational than feeling that uncontrollable outcomes were somehow the individual's responsibility (e.g., "I should be able to be able to do everything my fitness instructor is doing"). For optimal motivation from goal setting, it is best to assume responsibility for behaviors that are under the person's direct control (Howley and Franks, 2007).

GOAL-SETTING GUIDELINES IN EXERCISE SETTINGS

Goal setting is a science that has received extensive attention from researchers over the years. However, less goal-setting research has been conducted in the area of exercise and fitness. The practice of setting goals has enormous potential for improving the performer's motivation, attentional focus, and sense of achievement and competence. Despite these advantages, goal setting can have detrimental effects on motivation and performance outcomes if it is not done correctly. Sometimes goals add pressure and anxiety to tasks that the performer otherwise views as pleasant and enjoyable. Under these conditions, goals may not prove helpful. Nevertheless, here are several guidelines for the proper use of goal-setting techniques in exercise settings.

Observable and Measurable

The science of goal setting includes detecting evidence that a performance goal has been met. This evidence is based on outcomes that are observable and preferably measureable. Performance-based goals that are observable and measurable promote perceived competence, fulfill the performer's need to achieve, and therefore improve intrinsic motivation. Thus, exercisers know if they attained a goal when the outcomes are visually observed and measured. Evidence that a goal was met helps form the basis for setting future goals.

Challenging but Realistic

While goals must be challenging, they must also be realistic and based on previous best performance. If a goal is to provide incentive, then it has to be within the exerciser's perceived reach; otherwise it will lose its value and the exerciser will not feel the level of incentive and effort necessary to reach it. Goals that the performer perceives as too easy also do not increase motivation. Factors in setting challenging but realistic goals include the exerciser's performance history, pretest data, comparison of the exerciser's performance with others who possess similar characteristics, and monitoring of the exerciser's level of commitment, available time, and other

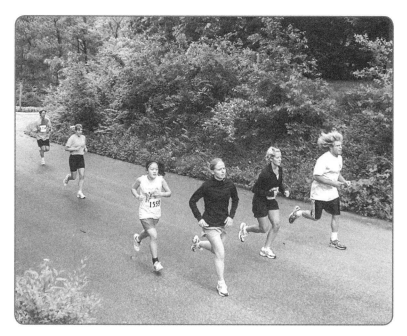

Running in a popular race may be a long-term goal, but many people will need help establishing smaller goals first, such as walking around a track.

resources to reach the goal (MacKinnon, Ritchie, Hooper, and Abernethy, 2003).

Self-Set Versus Externally Set

Is a goal set by the exerciser more motivating and effective than a goal set by an external agent, such as a fitness trainer, sport coach, friend, or partner? One of my former students was an elite collegiate swimmer who became despondent and eventually quit the team after her coach set a speed goal that the swimmer believed was unrealistically fast. Her depression about the unachievable goal resulted in her reducing her effort, feeling helpless about the situation, feeling hopeless that the situation would improve, and eventually quitting the team. If her coach had negotiated the challenging new goal with her, basing it on past performance with her input, the goal-setting strategy would have had its intended benefits and she would have felt more motivation to persist until she met the goal. She felt quitting was her only option to stop the pain of persistent failure in not meeting the externally set goal for performance speed. Goals are

---

SAMPLE SERIES OF SHORT-TERM GOALS TO MEET A SINGLE LONG-TERM GOAL

Long-Term Goal

I will be able to jog nonstop around the track 10 times (laps) after three months.

Series of Short-Term Goals

1. I will attend the fitness facility to jog a minimum of three times per week on alternate days.

2. For each workout I will perform preexercise routines in preparation for training (e.g., drink sufficient water before and during my workout, avoid meals within two hours of jogging, and wear proper exercise attire).

3. Over three weeks I will work with a personal trainer to obtain preprogram data and to obtain the proper exercise prescription and techniques for both jogging (aerobic) and strength training components of my workout.

4. I will engage in interval training on the track consisting of 10 bouts of work–rest intervals. For the first month, each work–rest bout will consist of jogging nonstop for 60 seconds followed by 15 seconds of walking. I will complete these 10 intervals three times per week.

---

more motivational when they are negotiated between the performer and the person to whom the performer is accountable.

Specific

Make goals specific to the demands of the task. Challenging goals are even more effective when they include specific details. Asking athletes to improve their performance speed by five seconds, a particularly difficult goal in all-out tasks such as swimming, is more effective than vague goals to "do your best" or "try to improve." In one study, Anshel, Weinberg, and Jackson (1992) found that setting a specific, difficult goal—an improvement of 100% on a juggling task—markedly increased subjects' intrinsic motivation and performance compared with setting easy or no goals. Examples of specific goals include "I will 'look the ball' into my hands with every catch" and "I will kick the soccer ball into the left half of the net on at least 8 out of 10 attempts."

Short Term and Long Term

Short-term goals in exercise settings, usually ranging in time from immediately to one week, are needed to reinforce the exerciser's sense of competence and success early on. Experiencing early success is crucial to a person's commitment to persist in the task that

will lead to achieving the goal. This is at least partly because of the common human needs for achievement and perceived competence. Short-term goals allow us to meet these needs.

Long-term goals, also important with respect to exercise adherence and motivation, range from several weeks to months and even years. Long-term goals allow people to evaluate the quality of their performance when compared with goals that were established early in the designated time frame. Ideally, a series of short-term goals should lead to a realistic yet challenging long-term performance goal. See Sample Series of Short-Term Goals to Meet a Single Long-Term Goal for an example of how a several short-term goals lead to a long-term goal.

STRATEGIES FOR FITNESS COACHES AND PERSONAL TRAINERS

Exercise is often performed in group settings, such as fitness classes, jogging clubs, rehabilitation clinics, or other types of interest groups. Groups have a high motivational effect on people who thrive on social support (discussed further in chapter 6), particularly a type of social support called *companionship support* (Wills and Shinar, 2000). *Social support* refers to a person's feeling of comfort, care, assistance, and information received from others. To Wills and Shinar, companionship support reflects the availability of others with whom one can exercise, such as an exercise group. Group exercise settings are preferred and highly motivational if the individual enjoys exercising in a group and the type and intensity of exercise are compatible with the person's needs and fitness level.

Fitness coaching and exercise class leadership are an art and a science. It's an art in that the fitness coach needs effective communication skills and other personal qualities (e.g., caring about exercise participants, being self-motivated to demonstrate compassion and sensitivity toward others). And it's a science because fitness coaching requires good teaching skills, a high fitness level, and extensive knowledge of fitness principles and movement techniques.

Personal Qualities of Fitness Coaches

Have you ever heard the term *bedside manner* when describing the personality and communication skills of a physician or other medical practitioner? This concept refers to the physician's ability to demonstrate compassion, empathy, sincerity, genuineness, humor, authenticity, and honesty in addition to competence. A positive bedside manner builds trust and loyalty in the doctor–patient relationship, and patients are more likely to feel confident and positive about their health status. These positive feelings in turn promote mental health and general well-being, which improve healing and overall physical health.

The characteristics associated with a good bedside manner have strong implications for exercise and fitness coaches. Although it is difficult to operationally define and quantify (i.e., give a numerical value to) positive personal qualities, most people can identify communication skills and behavior patterns that reflect professionalism and genuine concern for the exercise client's well-being. Here are some behavioral characteristics of high-quality fitness coaches that promote the

client's willingness to begin and adhere to programs that improve fitness and help the client reach short-term and long-term goals:

- Maintain your own high level of fitness and healthy physique.
- Develop fitness testing and prescription skills.
- Demonstrate correct exercise technique.
- Teach exercise skills and techniques.
- Develop an action plan, also called an *exercise prescription,* in detail and teach clients how to keep written records of their progress.
- Build client relationships to promote trust and loyalty.
- Agree with the client on future directions and actions.
- Keep records to demonstrate exercise adherence, attendance, and improvement.
- Provide recognition and approval of client effort and performance outcomes.
- Be sensitive to the client's individual needs and medical history.
- Demonstrate a caring attitude; show empathy.
- Let clients tell you their stories. Be patient and allow them to provide as much information as they feel comfortable communicating.
- Be a good listener.
- Introduce clients to others of similar ages or fitness levels who also exercise in the facility or program.
- Know that outcome is not the only thing that matters.
- Remember the self-fulfilling prophecy. If you expect more from clients—within reason and the reality of their limits—they are more likely to achieve more.
- Make exercise and the fitness environment enjoyable and fun.

Many quotations about motivation have implications for goal setting in fitness and exercise settings. For example, Sir Alexander Patterson is quoted as saying, "The secret of discipline is motivation. When a man is sufficiently motivated, discipline will take care of itself" (qtd. in Cook, 1993, p. 337). Goal setting requires discipline and persistence over time in achieving challenging goals. Because challenging goals require optimal effort to successfully achieve them, only long-term motivation will bring the exerciser enormous satisfaction; meeting easy goals does not bring the same level of satisfaction. Meeting challenging goals requires optimism and an attitude of "I can do that if I try hard enough."

A related quote, from former major league baseball pitcher Catfish Hunter, is "Winning isn't everything. Wanting to win is" (qtd. in Cook, 1993, p. 337). The desire to succeed is highly controllable by the exercise participant. Hunter's quote shows that motivation begins with wanting—that is, a strong desire to set and meet challenging goals for changing one's life and living a life consistent with one's values, including replacing self-destructive behavior patterns with healthier habits. One person who has enormous credibility and an important role in helping exercise participants achieve their aspirations is the fitness or exercise coach, referred to in this chapter as a *fitness coach*. The fitness coach is one type of health care professional. Fitness and health coaches are in the business of helping others want to win the battle of developing and maintaining healthy habits.

Professionalism

Fitness coaching is more than merely barking out instructions, giving fitness tests, and writing exercise prescriptions. It also includes maintaining a level of fitness and physical appearance that are commensurate with clients' expectations. Fitness coaches are also fitness models to their clients. They lose credibility if they do not live up to their instructions and motivational statements by appearing unkempt and being unable to perform the exercises they are asking others to perform. Therefore, always strive to maintain your own high level of fitness and healthy physique.

Effective fitness coaches are capable of conducting an array of fitness tests. You should develop fitness testing and prescription skills, including tests for upper- and lower-body strength, tests that measure cardiorespiratory fitness (e.g., submaximal $\dot{V}O_2$), percent body fat, and joint flexibility, among others. Test results should be used to generate an exercise prescription that is tailored to the client.

Good fitness coaches are able to show clients how to correctly perform all exercises being prescribed, including resistance exercises, floor exercises, stretches, and movements that are accompanied by music. Correct exercise technique is essential for significant improvements in fitness. Fitness coaches must receive the proper educational and training experiences from reputable mentors and certification programs. Interested readers should seek additional information about certification and educational programs by contacting local fitness clubs, university exercise science programs, national scientific organizations such as ACSM (2010), or national fitness organizations to obtain information about their certification programs, some of which are online. Most fitness clubs require national certification in order to work in their facilities. Sample national organizations in the United States include the following:

- IDEA Health and Fitness Association (www.ideafit.com)
- American Council on Exercise (www.acefitness.org)
- American Sports and Fitness Association (www.americansportandfitness.com)

Feelings of competence form the basic premise for intrinsic motivation. The single most important factor that builds perceived competence is learning and performing new skills that eventually lead to attaining short-term and long-term goals—there is no greater motivator in pursuing one's goals than success. Success, however, is planned; it does not happen accidentally. Building skills such as correct movement techniques and use of exercise equipment is essential to achievement. Fitness coaches must help their clients learn skills, identify indicators of improved performance, maintain their commitment and energy in pursuing

---

AMERICAN COLLEGE OF SPORTS MEDICINE (ACSM, 2010) STANDARDS FOR PHYSICAL ACTIVITY

Cardiorespiratory Training for Adults

Engage in moderately intense activity, such as brisk walking, five days per week for a minimum of 30 minutes per session at an intensity that noticeably increases heart rate, preferably between 60% and 85% of the person's predicted maximum.

Cardiorespiratory Training for Older Adults

Accumulate 30 to 60 minutes of moderate physical activity most days of the week.

Cardiorespiratory Training for Children and Adolescents

Gradually increase current activity levels to 90 minutes per day of physical activity.

---

goals, engage in proper physical training, and use mental strategies that build confidence and facilitate performance.

Be sure the client is informed about an action plan that takes into account specific routines that will be performed before and during the workout. Many clients may be intimidated by exercise machines, while others may be fitter, leaner, and more knowledgeable about using the equipment correctly. All clients should learn a set of rituals that lead to heightened motivation. Clients should know exactly what they should do upon entering a fitness facility so that they are not self-conscious about appearing different or inferior (which happens frequently, especially among middle-aged and older clients). The sooner everything becomes familiar and ritualized, the sooner the person will feel comfortable, confident, and motivated to continue the journey to better fitness and health.

The action plan consists of the preset routines and a schedule for carrying out these routines that is consistent with meeting goals. Participants need a structure within which to maintain their exercise efforts and aspirations. An action plan also allows clients to set and monitor reasonable expectations about meeting their goals. Fitness coaches need to prescribe an appropriate program and also create a structure for the journey ahead. Clients must be convinced of two things: the worthiness of their aspirations to improve their health and fitness and their ability to act upon and achieve them. Clients have to feel convinced

that they and their fitness coach share the same vision.

Consider prescribing to each client a self-monitoring checklist as part of the action plan. The checklist may include guidelines for the exerciser's thoughts and actions before, during, and immediately following exercise sessions. It may also include lifestyle changes to improve energy, weight management, and general health (see chapter 3 for a sample checklist).

Communication Skills

Learn and use each group member's first name. This promotes trust between the fitness coach and his or her clients. Exercisers who are addressed by their first names become less intimidated by the authority figure and feel more connected to the group. The nonverbal message is that the fitness coach, often called a personal trainer, knows and recognizes them. Trust is based on familiarity. This suggestion does not include socializing with clients; rather, it means making an effort to let clients tell their stories; allowing free expression of feelings, especially on body-related and health-related issues; discussing their hopes and desires for improving fitness and reaching other goals; discussing topics unrelated to exercise so that trust and familiarity begin to take root; and showing a genuine concern for the client not only as a client but as a person.

It is important for clients to detect improvement in at least one measure of their fitness program. Keeping records of test results, attendance, and other quantitative measures increases intrinsic motivation and a sense of achievement, both significant predictors of long-term exercise adherence (Mackinnon et al., 2003). Records identify changes in the client's status and reflect improvement and competence.

The needs for prestige, status, attention, importance, appreciation, and recognition are firmly based in human nature, and they drive motivation. These needs may even be greater for people who engage in difficult and challenging tasks, such as intense physical exercise. Fitness coaches are a primary source of meeting these needs among exercise participants. Recognition and approval should be communicated with sincerity and based on observed performance (e.g., "Your exercise form is looking much better," "I'm proud of you for showing up three times a week like we agreed"); they should not be generalized and abstract (e.g., "Way to go," "Good job").

Interpersonal Skills

Be sensitive to the client's needs and medical history. Everyone brings a unique set of psychological needs, medical history, and physical condition to the exercise venue. Some people are unable to perform certain exercises due to physical limitations or poor fitness. These individuals should not be humiliated in the presence of others if they cannot perform every repetition or demonstrate all exercises correctly. Previous medical problems and conditions may also limit client performance. Finally, people differ in their comfort with exercising in a public setting, particularly among other exercisers who may be younger, fitter, and leaner (Berger and McInman, 1993).

Psychologists have known for years that empathy (i.e., being able to identify with the emotions of others) is a learned characteristic. It is not part of our genetic heritability; it must be taught. We all differ in the extent to which we are able to demonstrate sensitivity toward others and to understand their worldview, their struggles, and their strengths. People in the health and fitness industry must show their clients compassion in addition to providing challenges to improve their health and well-being.

Clients can detect sincerity in the people they depend on for improving their quality of life. They also can detect phoniness and a lack of professionalism and genuineness. Anyone who is employed to improve the physical and mental health of another person and receives payment for this service has a professional and ethical obligation to provide the best care possible. Demonstrating genuine compassion toward the people who depend on the expertise of professionals is essential to building motivation.

This point has been raised previously, but it is worth repeating: Always let your clients tell you their story. People often have a lot to say, and communicating what is on their mind is part of the human spirit. Sometimes storytelling is about sharing the joy and rewards of life, and sometimes it serves a social purpose because it allows us to connect with each other in personal ways. As Loehr (2007) explains, storytelling allows us to explain why things happen to us. He claims that "stories impose meaning on the chaos; they organize and give context to our sensory experiences. . . . Facts are meaningless until you create a story around them" (pp. 4-5). Effective fitness coaches can listen to the stories of others, but sometimes they may also help clients change their stories from "This is why I cannot" to "This is why I can."

Cribben (1981) differentiates successful leaders from effective ones. Leaders, including sport and fitness coaches, who often win or experience positive outcomes may be considered successful. However, only coaches whose team members feel fulfilled and have other positive feelings related to being part of the team in addition to experiencing desirable outcomes may be considered effective. Therefore, winning is only part of the story; it is just one of several desirable outcomes.

The implication for working with clients in the fitness industry is that motivation is multidimensional. Motivational feelings and experiences should not be restricted to whether or not clients meet particular goals;

As indicated earlier, setting goals is both an art and a science. The art component concerns helping the client feel comfortable in setting and trying to reach his goals, while the science component addresses guidelines for effective goal setting so that the goals are motivational, not tasks that induce anxiety, fear of failure, and lack of enjoyment related to exercise and improved fitness and health. Fitness professionals should consider these strategies in applying goal-setting research.

Sample Strategies to Overcome Perceived Barriers to Starting an Exercise Program

Sample Barrier

The client doesn't have enough time to exercise.

Sample Strategies

- Use time management skills to create one hour of exercise time at least three days per week.
- Have a coworker handle the exerciser's responsibilities during lunch on Tuesday and Thursday and take over the coworker's responsibilities on Monday and Wednesday.
- Organize a group exercise program (for a corporate rate) for coworkers located in the workplace, outdoors, or at a nearby fitness club.

Sample Barrier

The client lacks an exercise partner or group.

Sample Strategies

- Attend exercise classes at a local fitness club.
- Ask neighbors, family members, or coworkers to exercise together at appointed times.

- Ask a personal trainer (fitness coach) to help find an exercise partner.
- Learn to exercise alone by developing exercise routines at times and places that feel safe and comfortable.

Other Sample Barriers

_____

_____

_____

Sample Strategies

_____

_____

_____

Sample Strategies to Overcome Perceived Barriers to Exercise Adherence

- Obtain test data on several fitness pretests and compare with test scores after two (or three) months to detect improvement.
- Obtain test data on other health-related measures such as lipids profile (cholesterol), waist circumference, and percent body fat.
- See a mental health professional to be tested for psychological measures such as chronic depression, chronic anxiety, and attitude toward exercise scales that might impede adherence to an exercise program.
- Obtain counseling from a qualified mental health professional to address personal issues.
- Obtain consultation from a registered dietitian or fitness coach who will provide behavior guidelines for further health and fitness improvement.

- Exercise with at least one family member at least one day per week, but more often if at all possible, to reinforce the need to exercise regularly—perhaps just before dinner, first thing in the morning, during lunch, or some other time.

Rate and discuss the effectiveness of strategies for exercise participation and adherence. What were your barriers? Why did these barriers exist? What caused them?

How effective was your strategy in dealing with each barrier? How will you handle these barriers in the future so that exercise becomes part of your lifestyle?

_____

_____

_____

also important are clients' attitudes toward physical activity, their willingness to develop and maintain healthy habits, and the sense of joy and exhilaration they feel during their journey. Why dismiss opportunities for satisfaction just because the final outcome did not match the client's initial goals and expectations? Did the client enjoy the activity? Did she discover the capability to reach challenging goals she never thought possible? Does she now possess twice the energy she had before starting this exercise program? Does she have new friends and feel better about herself since starting the program? The performer's effort and improvement are examples of other reasons to celebrate success that need not concern a particular performance outcome.

Many people do not feel confident in their ability to begin and maintain an exercise program. Perhaps they have started but quit programs in the past; perhaps they do not believe their current fitness level, body weight, or medical condition will allow them to engage in exercise and experience its benefits. To paraphrase the poet Longfellow, we should judge them by what they are capable of doing, not by what they have already done. Fitness

coaches must have realistic but high expectations of their clients' ability to meet performance demands in exercise settings. Coaches with higher expectations of their subordinates elicit better performance, and they also offer more—and better—instruction (Horn and Lox, 2010). The self-fulfilling prophecy, also called the *Pygmalion effect*, posits that we tend to perform at levels consistent with the expectations of others. Fitness clients will respond better to relatively higher expectations. Expect more and you get more back.

At the heart of intrinsic motivation is a mental state that reflects a sense of enjoyment, pleasure, and even fun in performing the activity. Fitness coaches need to nurture a positive attitude, including fun, to produce a motivational climate that causes the client to want to return. One reason so many postcardiac exercise rehabilitation programs are so popular is the social element; patients enjoy showing up to exercise because they have the opportunity to interact with others with similar medical conditions, and they have established friendships. There is a time for hard work for improved fitness, and there is a time for enjoyment, laughter, and new friendships.

SUMMARY

When conducted properly, goal setting is highly motivational to most people who want to improve their physical performance. Setting goals helps focus the performer's effort and provides a means to monitor progress or performance success. Goal setting is not for everyone, however. A personal disposition called *goal orientation* reflects the performer's attraction to setting goals and the extent to which setting goals is motivational and desirable. A low goal orientation represents a preference to not set goals, perhaps due to the anxiety of failing to meet a predetermined goal. Still, goal setting in exercise settings, particularly among people who are less fit, is usually highly desirable because meeting goals gives a sense of achievement and competence, both of which enhance long-term motivation to make exercise a lifestyle habit.

There are numerous guidelines for effective goal setting. Goals should be challenging yet realistic; set in positive, not negative terms (what the performer will do rather than will not do); observable and measureable; and both short term and long term. Goals should also be set for overcoming exercise barriers, that is, the reasons people give for not starting or for dropping out of exercise programs. Fitness coaches should consider goal-setting contracts that compel the exerciser to meet predetermined goals and to use strategies for meeting those goals. Finally, effective goal setting can only occur in the presence of effective fitness coaches. Some of the characteristics of effective fitness coaches include showing clients compassion, empathy, and a desire to see them become healthy and meet their goals. Exercise and fitness coaches also have to appear physically fit and well groomed to be perceived as professional, knowledgeable, and credible; they must practice what they preach.

STUDENT ACTIVITY

Construct an Exercise Contract With Your Client

The contract's content will include

- the date the contract was generated,
- starting and ending points of expected (contracted) behaviors,
- expected behaviors and the level or quality of those behaviors,
- criteria for assessing those behaviors (e.g., what a correctly performed exercise looks like), and
- who evaluates contract content and whether contract goals have been met.

Should there be a penalty for failing to fulfill the contract? While no harsh consequences should result from failure to live up to the contract, at times a minor penalty (e.g., making a charity donation, avoiding desserts for one week) might create a lighthearted but sincere sense of urgency and accountability in meeting contract demands.

You are now working with an exercise novice and are planning this person's goals. Remember the principles of effective goal setting: specific, performance-based (as opposed to outcome-based, but outcomes are OK as long as they accompany more specific and detailed performance goals), challenging but realistic, observable, measurable, and short term as well as long term.

Here are some examples of contract goals:

- I will walk for at least 20 minutes in my neighborhood after dinner.
- I will ride my stationary bicycle or walk on my treadmill at home for 30 minutes during the evening news.
- I will attempt to elevate my heart rate during my walk–jog interval training session to at least 60% of my predicted maximum (computed by subtracting the exerciser's age from 220 and multiplying by .60, that is, 60% of predicted maximum). I will record my heart rate digitally.

Create goals for the client, remembering to consider the client's current fitness level; movement restrictions; illnesses, injuries, or disabilities; and body weight (e.g., walking on a treadmill may be difficult and uncomfortable for someone who is unfit and overweight). Also, avoid setting too many goals. Goals can create anxiety from a fear of failure if they are too numerous and too demanding. You want exercise novices to feel success and achievement, not disappointment and anger about not meeting demanding goals.

Finally, include space for writing a brief progress report to share with the client. Progress reports should incorporate the client's views and perceptions of his progress as well as reasons for making progress or explanations of why progress was slow or nonexistent.

FORM 10.1   EXERCISE CONTRACT GOALS

Today's date: _____

Contract Goal 1: _____

Goal Strategies _____

_____

_____

Client Responsibilities _____

_____

_____

Assessment Times and Dates _____

_____

_____

Progress Report Notes _____

_____

_____

Contract Goal 2: _____

Goal Strategies _____

_____

_____

Client Responsibilities _____

_____

_____

Assessment Times and Dates _____

_____

_____

Progress Report Notes _____

_____

_____

From M. Anshel, 2014, *Applied Health Fitness Psychology.* (Champaign, IL: Human Kinetics).

REFERENCES

American College of Sports Medicine (ACSM). (2010). *ACSM's guidelines for exercise testing and prescription* (8th ed.). Baltimore: Lippincott, Williams, and Wilkins.

Anshel, M.H. (2012). *Sport psychology: From theory to practice* (5th ed.). San Francisco: Benjamin-Cummings.

Anshel, M.H., Weinberg, R.S., and Jackson, A. (1992). Effect of goal difficulty and task complexity on intrinsic motivation and motor performance. *Journal of Sport Behavior, 15,* 159-176.

Berger, B.G., and McInman, A. (1993). Exercise and the quality of life. In R.N. Singer, M. Murphey, and L. Keith Tennant (Eds.), *Handbook of research on sport psychology* (pp. 729-760). New York: Macmillan.

Burton, D. (1992). The Jekyll-Hyde nature of goals: Reconceptualizing goal setting in sport. In T.S. Horn (Ed.), *Advances in sport psychology* (pp. 267-297). Champaign, IL: Human Kinetics.

Burton, D., and Naylor, S. (2002). The Jekyll/Hyde nature of goals: Revisiting and updating goal-setting in sport. In T.S. Horn (Ed.), *Advances in sport psychology* (2nd ed., pp. 459-499). Champaign, IL: Human Kinetics.

Cook, J. (1993). *Book of positive quotations.* Minneapolis MN: Fairview Press.

Cribben, J.J. (1981). *Leadership: Strategies for organizational effectiveness.* New York: AMACOM.

Duda, J.L., and Whitehead, J. (1998). Measurement of goal perspectives in the physical domain. In J.L. Duda (Ed.), *Advances in sport and exercise psychology measurement* (pp. 21-48). Morgantown, WV: Fitness Information Technology.

Horn, T.S., and Lox, C.L. (2010). The self-fulfilling prophecy theory: When coaches' expectations become reality. In J.M. Williams (Ed.), *Applied sport psychology: Personal growth to peak performance* (6th ed., pp. 81-105). New York: McGraw-Hill.

Howley, E.T., and Franks, B.D. (2007). *Fitness professional's handbook* (5th ed.). Champaign, IL: Human Kinetics.

Kingston, K.M., and Hardy, L. (1997). Effects of different types of goals on processes that support performance. *Sport Psychologist, 11,* 277-293.

Klein, H.J., Wesson, M.J., Hollenbeck, J.R., and Alge, B.J. (1999). Goal commitment and the goal-setting process: Conceptual clarification and empirical synthesis. *Journal of Applied Psychology, 84,* 885-896.

Kyllo, L.B., and Landers, D.M. (1995). Goal setting in sport and exercise: A research synthesis to resolve the controversy. *Journal of Sport and Exercise Psychology, 17,* 117-137.

Loehr, J. (2007). *The power of story.* New York: The Free Press.

Mackinnon, L.T., Ritchie, C.B., Hooper, S.L., and Abernethy, P.J. (2003). *Exercise management: Concepts and professional practice.* Champaign, IL: Human Kinetics.

Nicholls, J. (1984). Achievement motivation: Conceptions of ability, subjective experience, task choice, and performance. *Psychological Review, 91,* 328-346.

Orlick, T., and Partington, J. (1986). *Psyched: Inner views of winning.* Ottawa: Coaching Association of Canada.

Wills, T.A., and Shinar, O. (2000). Measuring perceived and received social support. In S. Cohen, L.G. Underwood, and B.H. Gottlieb (Eds.), *Social support measurement and intervention* (pp. 86-135). New York: Oxford University Press.

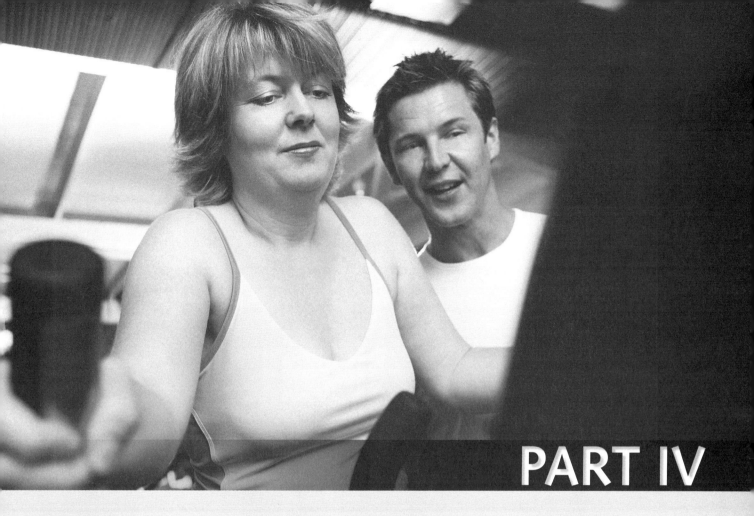

PART IV

PROFESSIONAL CONSIDERATIONS

The final segment of the book, part IV, is dedicated to professional aspects of applied health fitness psychology. It begins with chapter 11, which discusses an area where many health care professionals will find employment and where an important community need is apparent—working with special populations.

One widespread and life-threatening concern is eating disorders, particularly anorexia nervosa and bulimia nervosa. Chapter 12 addresses these and other dysfunctional eating behaviors, including emotional eating—that

is, consuming food due to boredom, stress, or some other emotional reason.

The final chapter is devoted to helping students determine how to become a professional in health fitness psychology. There is an array of professional organizations, each with its own code of ethics, categories of memberships, and criteria for each membership. Professional organizations allow members to remain current with new advances in professional practice and acknowledge areas that need future research and advancement.

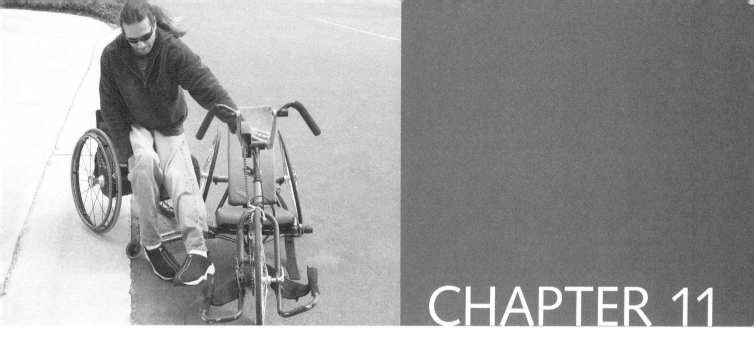

CHAPTER 11

Fitness Consulting With Special Populations

> 66 *Character cannot be developed in ease and quiet. Only through experience of trial* 99
> *and suffering can the soul be strengthened, vision cleared, ambition inspired, and*
> *success achieved.*
>
> Helen Keller, author and activist

CHAPTER OBJECTIVES

After reading this chapter, you should be able to:

- determine the unique needs of various special populations that separate them from the so-called normal population when engaging in regular physical activity,

- describe the psychological barriers that inhibit exercise and other healthy habits for each special population described in this chapter,

- identify the personal and situational factors that promote exercise and other healthy habits for each special population reviewed in this chapter, and

- generate cognitive and behavioral strategies and programs that create a favorable environment in which to initiate and maintain an exercise habit.

Most students who intend to work in the health promotion and fitness industry associate their profession with healthy, able-bodied people who want to improve their fitness, physical appearance, energy, and work productivity while losing weight and maintaining a healthy lifestyle. And, for most people in the health behavior industry, that probably describes their clients. However, there is another category of clients who also require the services of health specialists, but they have special needs that must not be neglected. This chapter addresses this segment of the population.

OLDER ADULTS

Because the baby boomers are reaching retirement age and because people are living longer than ever before, there is going to be a proliferation of older adults in the United States and elsewhere. Keeping this age group physically active is going to have an enormous economic benefit to society—health care costs keep rising due in great part to lack of physical activity and the resultant obesity epidemic. There are, however, special considerations in helping older adults develop a long-term exercise habit.

It is important to note that the geriatric literature differentiates among three categories of older adults: *young-old*, ranging in age from 65 to 74, *old*, aged 75 to 84 years, and *old-old*, aged 85 years and older (Morris, 2004). As medical advances continue to increase the average life span, it is possible these age categories can also change. The main point to remember is that the young-old have more physical capacity for various types and intensities of physical activity than their older counterparts (ACSM, 2010).

An active lifestyle, including exercise, has many advantages for older adults. Numerous studies have shown, for example, that aerobic forms of exercise (i.e., exercise that substantially increases heart rate) slow the aging process, both mentally and physically. Cognitive functioning (e.g., improved short-term memory, reduced chance of dementia) will be better maintained with advanced age (Dorgo, Robinson, and Bader, 2009). Not surprisingly, there is great variation among older adults in

how rapidly they age and the effects of aging on the organism. Though some of these differences are genetically determined, an inevitable deterioration of our anatomy and physiology begins in our mid- to late 20s, and the decline in physiological processes accelerates in our early 70s (Mackinnon, Ritchie, Hooper, and Abernethy, 2003). We can, however, have a strong influence on the rate of aging and our ability to function normally as we become older based on one decision—the decision to engage in regular exercise. Research findings are unequivocal that maintaining a habit of aerobic and resistance exercise will slow the cognitive and physiological aging processes.

ACSM's Guidelines for Exercise Testing and Prescription (2010) provides evidence-based recommendations for exercise programs for older adults. These guidelines are similar to those for younger people; however, two unique characteristics are to provide activities that do not stress the lower limbs and cause discomfort or injury to the low back and lower limbs and to move in a relatively slow and deliberate manner. Tissue that surrounds joints and the general musculature of older people is weaker due to the aging process. For this reason, resistance training is also needed for older adults. Resistance exercises should be carried out using the maximum range of motion without pain or discomfort.

Engagement in regular physical activity decreases with age. Most physicians and other health care workers prescribe exercise to improve and maintain overall function; however, one primary barrier to starting and maintaining an exercise program is the lack of knowledge or experience to exercise alone. Most inactive people, especially older adults, require consultation and supervision from an exercise specialist or an experienced peer.

One strategy that promotes exercise among older adults is called *peer mentoring*. Peer mentors are nonprofessionals who receive quality preparation and therefore provide a unique service to others with similar characteristics (Dorgo et al., 2009). If adequately prepared, older peer mentors are capable of providing basic counseling to their peers that will promote regular physical activity.

Dorgo et al. (2009) examined the effect of peer mentoring among older adults versus the effect of mentoring by qualified kinesiology students on changes in perceived physical, mental, and social function. They found that after a 14-week physical fitness intervention, perceived physical, mental, and social functioning improved significantly for the peer-mentored group, but not for the student-mentored group. Older adults who participated in a physical fitness program with peer support perceived

- overall improvement in physical and mental well-being,
- better social functioning,
- enhanced ability to carry out physical and emotional roles,
- improved general health, and
- increased vitality.

Thus, peer mentoring for older adults was superior to mentoring by young professionals and may lead to increased adherence. The researchers concluded that peer support can improve adherence to structured exercise programs for older adults.

ACSM (2010) recommends the use of weightlifting machines, which allow the lifter greater control and require less skill compared with free weights. Again, with both aerobic and resistance training, exercises should be conducted in a slow and controlled manner.

INJURY REHABILITATION PATIENTS

One of the most important strategies for rehabilitation from injury is various types of physical activity, including exercise. Physical activity is prescribed as a highly important component of injury rehabilitation. Two issues are unique to the rehabilitation process: the psychological factors that help explain injury and the individual needs of patients or clients that must be addressed to ensure an effective rehabilitation program, also called *rehabilitation compliance*.

Three challenges to health care workers in providing injury rehabilitation services to clients and patients are

1. to address the causes of the individual's mental and physical condition,
2. to understand the psychological barriers to successful rehabilitation, and
3. to provide rehabilitation services that overcome those barriers and meet patient needs in returning to preinjury performance levels.

Causes of the Patient Condition

Brewer and Tripp (2005) reviewed the relevant literature on the prevention and rehabilitation of athletic injuries. They reported, for instance,

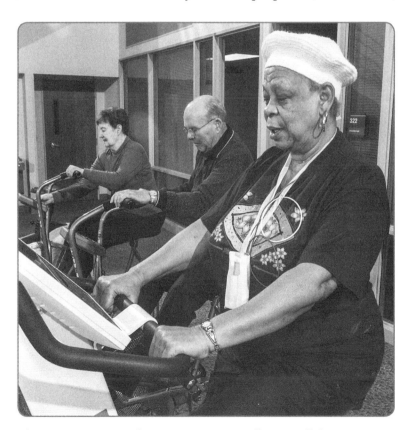

Clients recovering from an injury or illness will have unique psychological needs that the fitness professional should understand in order to improve rehabilitation compliance.

that 30 of 35 studies reviewed showed a strong relationship between stress and occurrence of athletic injury. The relationship between the stress response and injury grows stronger if incorporating the athlete's personality (e.g., sensation seeking, trait anxiety), history of stressors (e.g., chronic life stress), coping resources (e.g., effective psychological and behavioral coping skills, presence of social support), and use of cognitive and behavioral interventions (e.g., visualization, relaxation, regular exercise).

Taken together, these factors suggest that a patient's susceptibility to and recovery from injury is partly a function of personal and situational factors that must be taken into account in the rehabilitation process. For example, highly anxious people who suffer from chronic life stress and have little social support may require far more individualized attention from the rehabilitation therapist or coach; planned interactions with other rehabilitation patients, which is common among cardiac rehabilitation patients, for instance; and motivational statements that reflect improvement and approval. Other patients may prefer a therapist strategy in which they go it alone and are more tenacious, independent, and self-controlling after receiving initial instruction on rehabilitation strategies.

Psychological Barriers to Rehabilitation

The literature is unequivocal in supporting exercise, particularly of light to moderate intensity, as an effective strategy to promote psychological and physical quality of life (Gillison et al., 2009). Not everyone responds to exercise the same way, however. There are personal and situational reasons why some people experience a faster and more effective injury rehabilitation program than others. These reasons are referred to as *psychological barriers*, and the rehabilitation coach needs to examine these factors in order to plan an effective program.

Psychological (personal) barriers to injury rehabilitation can relate to the patients' personality (e.g., self-esteem, neuroticism or stability, trait anxiety), thinking style or ori-entation (e.g., level of optimism, confidence, mental toughness, attentional style, helplessness, competitiveness), emotional reaction to an injury (e.g., anger, confusion, depression, anxiety, fear, frustration), and use of effective coping strategies (e.g., social support, positive self-talk, cognitive reappraisal, monitoring, rationalization, self-deprecating humor, positive expectations) (Anshel, 2006; Brewer and Tripp, 2005; Fisher, 1999; Heyman, 1987).

Only mental health practitioners are trained to administer and interpret psychological inventories that measure many of these conditions. Rehabilitation practitioners, however, can refer the patient to a therapist to obtain this information, review the patient's file in which this information may already be provided, or just be aware of these conditions and adapt the rehabilitation program based on specific patient characteristics. For example, several conditions warrant more sensitive approaches, reassurance, positive feedback, and both emotional and physical support.

Effective Injury Rehabilitation Services

A discussion of the best ways to provide exercise rehabilitation programs is not as simple as a mere list of steps. There is no magical formula because so many physical, psychological, and emotional factors influence the patient's readiness to begin and adhere to an exercise rehabilitation program. One of the factors that complicates a successful rehabilitation program is the dynamic relationship between physical health and mental health in this population. Gillison and colleagues (2009) explain:

> Psychological factors give some insight into why improvements in physical health may not be occurring. For example, lack of change on quality of life measures may indicate that patients do not perceive the benefits of exercise interventions to be meaningful, which may serve to explain their poor adherence to treatment. . . . It seems likely that poor emotional functioning may significantly inhibit the perception of physical benefits. (p. 1708)

Gillison et al. (2009) suggest that quality of life be a primary consideration before generating a patient's rehabilitation program. If patients lack social support (e.g., friends, family, peers) and physical support (e.g., transportation to the exercise venue, proper nutrition, funds for proper exercise apparel), are not highly motivated, and do not have a positive mood state about the physical and emotional demands and challenges of the rehabilitation program, they are unlikely to adhere to the program. The intrinsic motivation needed to set and meet challenging goals and to persist in the program until goals are achieved will be lacking. Health care coaches need to monitor the patient's psychological status concomitantly with physical progress. In fact, psychological and physical outcomes may occur independently. Specifically, desirable psychological outcomes (e.g., improved confidence and self-efficacy) may occur in the absence of improved physical status, and clients may improve physical status while deteriorating psychologically (e.g., chronic depression and anxiety, unpleasant mood state, lack of self-motivation).

Another consideration is the timing of a patient's exercise therapy. Gillison et al. (2009) suggest that introducing an exercise intervention may not be optimal when the patient is battling a chronic illness. This is because exercise adherence is considerably worse when a patient's mood state is negative, which is common when experiencing ill health. Sometimes, however, the patient's health care provider will prescribe a low-intensity exercise program relatively soon after a medical procedure as an integral part of the recovery process. It is suggested, therefore, that the patient's psychological and physical status be monitored simultaneously. Having a better quality of life may increase the patient's ability to engage in exercise behavior. As Gillison et al. conclude, "Identifying whether patients have a sufficiently positive level of quality of life at the outset of an intervention to be able to bring to [the exercise intervention] the [level of] energy and commitment it needs may increase the efficiency and acceptability of interventions" (p. 1708).

CARDIAC AND PULMONARY REHABILITATION PATIENTS

Cardiac rehabilitation refers to programs that help patients with cardiovascular disease (CVD) return to their previous lifestyle, including a resumption of normal physical activity, after experiencing some type of cardiac episode. The mission of these programs is to provide a multidimensional intervention that includes counseling, educating, and supporting patients to make changes in their self-destructive lifestyle and to replace unhealthy habits with healthier routines.

CVD patients form a particularly common segment of the rehabilitation population. Due to the proliferation of heart disease in most Western cultures, cardiac rehabilitation programs are ubiquitous. Often they are associated with hospitals, universities, local fitness clubs, and community recreation centers. They are almost always supervised by a cardiologist who is not usually on-site but who oversees the program, prescribes the program to patients, and provides program staff with individualized exercise protocols for each patient.

CVD comprises several types of heart disease, including myocardial infarction (i.e., heart attack), angina, cardiopulmonary disease, coronary artery bypass surgery, angioplasty, myocardial ischemia, and heart transplant. Candidates for cardiac rehabilitation include patients who have complex conditions requiring multiple medications, who have a pacemaker or valve replacement, or who are recovering from an acute cardiac event (Mackinnon et al., 2003).

In addition to deterioration of cardiac function, CVD has a deleterious effect on mental health. One common type of psychopathology among cardiac patients is depression (Biddle and Mutrie, 2001). Sources of depression include fear of dying, significant lifestyle changes, frequent intake of medication, reduced physical capacity (e.g., easily out of breath, need to monitor bodily processes such as heart rate and blood pressure that were formerly taken for granted), guilt associated with feeling burdensome to family members for making necessary demands on their time, dependency on others for transportation and other activities of daily living, and the financial demands of health care. Depression, anxiety about lifestyle changes and survival, pessimism, and negative mood states need to be replaced by optimism, confidence, and psychological well-being—an important role of program staff (Biddle and Mutrie, 2001; Hayman, 2009).

Coaching the CVD Patient

Providing an exercise program to the CVD patient has several unique aspects. Because the root causes of CVD are multidimensional (e.g., poor diet, sedentary lifestyle, excessive stress, smoking, type A behavior pattern), an effective exercise coach possesses fundamental knowledge of these causes and attempts to work with clients to change as many of their unhealthy habits as possible, albeit slowly. In particular, health coaching attempts to reduce the patient's risk factors (e.g., lack of exercise, smoking, high stress) that lead to CVD. In other words, recovery from CVD entails changing the client's lifestyle. Helping people change their habits is no easy task. On an upbeat note, however, researchers have found that as risk-factor control increases (i.e., patient's unhealthy habits are reduced or eliminated), CVD mortality decreases.

Cardiac rehabilitation clinics are usually supervised or staffed by a person whose degree (often at the master's level) is in exercise science and includes practical work experience or an internship in a cardiac rehabilitation program. Some have had experience assisting cardiologists in administering exercise stress tests. Some clinics also feature registered dietitians and licensed health psychologists. Staff members provide exercise advice and programs for both inpatients (before discharge from hospital) and outpatients (after discharge).

Mackinnon et al. (2003) describe a typical working day in a hospital-based exercise cardiac rehabilitation clinic. Daily routines of cardiac rehabilitation staff members include performing intake procedures for new patients, leading exercise classes, reviewing each patient's exercise prescription, ensuring patients complete the prescribed program, contacting patients who have not attended their planned program, monitoring exercise intensity (e.g., amount of weight resistance during training) and progress, measuring and continually monitoring preexercise and exercise heart rate and blood pressure, assessing percent body fat and muscular flexibility, providing fitness testing, referring patients to the hospital's registered dietitian or psychologist, and completing paperwork on patient progress for subsequent review by the patient's cardiologist or general physician. Most days end with a meeting with the hospital's social worker or counselor to discuss new patients and to review the progress of patients who have been referred for counseling.

It is clear that cardiac patients have suffered a major setback in health and quality of life. Despite persisting in lifelong habits that have contributed to their CVD, they have experienced a life-changing event that requires coming face to face with their mortality over a relatively short time. There are new pressures and burdens to rethink the way they have lived and to allow long-term relationships to develop with medical practitioners, mental health professionals, and rehabilitation experts. They have lost part of their independence, and they must now retain the support of others to do even menial tasks they used to take for granted.

Exercise Strategies for Postcardiac Patients

First and foremost when engaging in any form of physical activity with CVD patients is to follow the exercise prescription of their primary care provider (ACSM, 2009, 2010). Second, the patient's mental health status must be considered before prescribing an exercise program. Chronic anxiety and depression are common reactions to a cardiac event and will affect the patient's motivation to engage in and maintain an exercise rehabilitation program (Lewin et al., 1992; Oldridge, 1995).

A patient with clinical anxiety, depression, or some other psychopathology will not be fully engaged in the exercise rehabilitation process. As the literature clearly indicates, it is not uncommon for CVD patients to experience mental and physical fatigue and general lethargy (i.e., lack of energy), which often lead to exercise noncompliance.

The exercise coach plays an important role in providing a sense of confidence, optimism, and normality in patients' recovery and rehabilitation. It is immensely gratifying for coaches to be on the receiving end of their patients' gratitude and appreciation for providing these lifesaving services. Strategies that are particularly helpful with CVD patients include the following:

- Extensive use of social support is valuable, including group exercise environments that nurture friendships and warm personal interactions.

- Monitoring patient progress is essential in order to reveal progress and improvement in selective measures; therefore, comparing pretest scores with subsequent test results provides valuable incentive to maintain exercise compliance.

- Taking patient attendance at rehabilitation sessions is important to monitor patient commitment and compliance.

- A self-monitoring checklist is advised to provide instruction, guidelines, and the development of routines, all of which promote exercise compliance.

- Remaining in regular contact with the patient's medical care provider is essential (e.g., providing updated test data, monitoring exercise compliance).

- Involvement with a mental health professional is especially important in this population given the frequent onset of anxiety, depression, and other psychological barriers to program compliance and mental health.

Hayman (2009) provides additional recommendations on ways to promote patient compliance with exercise rehabilitation programs.

PREGNANT WOMEN

A pregnant woman should obtain a medical clearance from her physician before beginning an exercise program, regardless of her current fitness and health status. In the early years, there was considerable debate about prescribing exercise for pregnant women. In the 1970s and earlier, the thinking was that considerable exertion, especially during intense cardiorespiratory work, was undesirable for the fetus. In more recent years, this worry has been dispelled. Exercise during pregnancy improves general well-being, reduces physical discomfort, and has psychological benefits (Symons Downs and Hausenblas, 2003). Cardiorespiratory exercise and resistance training in particular are recommended for a pregnant woman, as long as her physician approves (given her health status and medical history) and the level of intensity is commensurate with her current fitness level and health status.

As indicated earlier, exercise for pregnant women also has psychological benefits. Researchers have found that exercise reduces the onset of depression and anxiety, improves mood state, reduces chronic stress, and provides a higher quality of life (American College of Obstetricians and Gynecologists [ACOG], 2003; Thompson, 2007).

What is the final verdict about exercising during pregnancy? Perhaps the first step is to convince pregnant women that exercise is beneficial to their pregnancy. This was confirmed in a study by Symons Downs and Hausenblas (2003), who found that positive attitudes toward exercise and believing it is beneficial to their condition are the best predictors of exercise during pregnancy. From her literature review, Thompson (2007) concluded that due to the enormous demands that pregnancy places on a woman's body, it appears that "for healthy pregnant women, exercise is safe and beneficial during this critical time" (p. 290). Pregnant women with cardiovascular, pulmonary, or metabolic disease, however, as well as those who are obese, should seek physician guidance concerning exercise and the type and intensity of physical activity in which they should engage.

PEOPLE WITH DIABETES

Diabetes mellitus (categorized as type 1 and type 2) is a disease in which the body does not produce or properly respond to insulin, the hormone needed to convert sugar, starch, and other food into energy (ACSM, 2010). These food substances are converted to glucose, an energy fuel source, during the process of digestion. The diabetic patient experiences a lack of insulin and thus glucose cannot enter body cells to be used as an energy source. Without sufficient insulin, glucose will accumulate in the bloodstream, causing high blood sugar, a condition called *hyperglycemia*. If left untreated, hyperglycemia may lead to CVD, blindness, limb amputations, and damage to the liver, kidneys, and nerves (feelings of numbness, among other symptoms).

Although an exercise program is essential for diabetic patients, they first require a medical examination, especially if they are older than 40 or have had the disease for more than 20 years. Members of the health promotion industry should know that, according to medical practitioners, exercise should be avoided if the patient's blood sugar (i.e., blood glucose) is below 70 or above 240 mg/dl or if ketones are present in the urine. See ACSM (2009, 2010) for specific exercise guidelines and special considerations for people with diabetes.

Although it is known that physical activity is beneficial for patients with diabetes, few studies have examined sustained walking in this population. One longitudinal study—conducted over two and a half years—by Duru et al. (2008) examined the factors associated with sustained walking among 5,935 managed care patients with diabetes who walked at least 20 minutes per day at baseline. The researchers wanted to determine the likelihood of sustained walking, defined as walking at least 20 minutes per day, at follow-up two and a half years later. They found that the most important factor that predicted walking behavior was the absence of pain. Not surprisingly, obese patients were far less likely to sustain walking than overweight or normal-weight patients, and patients older than 65

years were less likely to sustain walking than patients younger than 65. Characteristics of the patients' neighborhoods were not related to walking behavior in this study.

Thus, exercise and rehabilitation staff should initiate walking habits as soon as possible, when patients are younger rather than waiting for the retirement years, and they should combine walking and other forms of physical activity with weight-loss programs. They also need to reduce or eliminate the patient's physical discomfort not only through medication but also by offering activity alternatives that are not too uncomfortable, such as water aerobics, exercises that improve flexibility and reduce stress (e.g., Pilates, yoga), and certain resistance training exercises.

PEOPLE WITH PHYSICAL AND MENTAL DISABILITIES

Few people are in greater need of exercise than those with physical impairments. This group is described by the American College of Sports Medicine (2009) as persons who are confined to a wheelchair, deaf, blind, missing a limb, have only one of a set of organs, or persons who may have behavioral, emotional, and psychological disorders that limit a major life activity. *Disabled* or *people with disabilities* are the terms that are most accepted and used by advocacy groups and sport organizations. These groups include the USA Deaf Sports Federation (USADSF), United States Association of Blind Athletes (USABA), United States Cerebral Palsy Athletic Association (USCPAA), Disabled Sports USA, Dwarf Athletic Association of America (DAAA), Special Olympics, and Wheelchair and Ambulatory Sports, USA (WASUSA). The Mental Health America and the American Association on Intellectual and Developmental Disabilities are two of many national organizations in the U.S. that promote health and welfare for the mentally and intellectually disabled. There are also many state organizations; one example in Tennessee is called Pacesetters and promotes this mission on their website: "To empower and support people with disabilities and their families to lead enriched and fulfilled lives" (see www.pacesetterstn.com). Services provided include exercise, social events, handicrafts, and other forms of recreation. Organizations that offer similar services are common in most states and countries.

On an optimistic note, fitness professionals will find that working with people with disabilities is highly satisfying for several reasons. In addition to making a valuable contribution to their lives, these clients tend to be highly self-motivated to engage in regular physical activity and are most appreciative of the opportunities and coaching they receive (Shapiro, 2003). In addition, most disabled people are unfit and overweight (McDermott et al., 2012), at least partly due to physical restrictions in movement capability and low energy, but also partly due to psychopathologies such as clinical depression, low self-esteem, feelings of helplessness, and a general lack of motivation. The literature is replete with studies examining the effectiveness of interventions on improved fitness and other health indicators among people with intellectual disabilities (e.g., Carmeli, Zinger-Vaknin, Morad, and Merrick, 2005; McDermott et al., 2012), traumatic brain injury (e.g., Self, Driver, Stevens, and Warren, 2013), and mental retardation (e.g., Urv, Zigman, and Silverman, 2003). If given the chance to participate in exercise programs, people with disabilities will significantly improve both physical and mental well-being.

From a psychological perspective, Bawden (2006) contends that people with disabilities are "mentally strong" because "they need to be mentally tough to cope with their disability in life itself" (p. 668). This psychological characteristic of mental toughness and a can-do attitude separates this group from other special populations such as older adults and rehabilitation patients, who are more dependent on their coach and in greater need of social support, positive reinforcement, and coping with not meeting performance expectations. Although people with disabilities are as susceptible as anyone else to depression

and other mental illnesses that may impede rehabilitation and a high quality of life, exercise coaches and therapists should recognize their resilience and avoid being condescending. This is especially the case with disabled athletes.

According to Bawden (2006), the primary goal of coaching people with disabilities is "focusing on factors that they can control and understanding those that they can't" (p. 669). People with disabilities must deal with numerous uncontrollable factors, such as "leg spasms, the need to go to the toilet, help from others to gain access to venues, pressure sores, disabled access, transport issues, [and] accommodation issues" (p. 669).

Bawden (2006) offers these guidelines for working with people with physical disabilities:

- Create an appropriate environment in which to conduct an intervention (e.g., easy accessibility to the facility, proper ventilation).

- Be prepared to refer the client to a specialist, such as a licensed psychologist or medical practitioner, if there are concerns.

- Get to know the client's support network of family, friends, and other supporting personnel (e.g., a speech therapist for clients with impaired speech or hearing).

- Use appropriate communication strategies, such as speaking with the client in a respectful rather than patronizing manner and speaking to the person directly, not to the person's interpreter or family member, if the patient is in the room.

- Build trust and ensure confidentiality.

- Don't be afraid to ask the client for more information or clarification. Coaches should know their own strengths and weaknesses and try to improve their skills in providing better services to this population.

McDermott et al. (2012) and Self et al. (2013) offer additional guidelines for working with people with mental and intellectual disabilities. In general, people with intellectual disabilities have inadequate exposure to physical activity and proper nutrition. The result is a relatively high degree of obesity in this population. Therefore, these strategies are of particular importance for this group:

- Feel a sense of purpose and compassion when working with disabled persons, knowing that this work makes a significant contribution to their lives.

- Create opportunities for increased physical activity, including formal exercise programs, participation in various types of sports, and recreational pursuits (e.g., biking, hiking, camping).

- Ensure that leaders of health-related programs (e.g., exercise, nutrition, stress management, sleep quality) are experts in their respective fields; the mentally disabled deserve the same high-quality instruction and mentoring as nondisabled clients.

- Purchase and make available proper sport and exercise equipment that fits the needs of mentally disabled persons so that activities can be performed easily and successfully. For example, equipment should be of appropriate weight and height and be designed for simple movement and mechanics.

- Inform the family members of people with disabilities that they have a role in promoting healthy habits. Examples include engaging in a variety of physical activities, making conscious efforts to reduce stress, maintaining positive emotions prior to bedtime (for improved sleep quality), and including disabled family members in as many family events as possible.

- If food preparation and consumption are components of your program, meals should be nutritious and, if possible, staff should eat with their disabled clients. Often, relationships between people with disabilities and program and administrative staff are nurtured, and trust is developed, when enjoyable activities such as meal time are shared. However, food should never be used as a reward (e.g., "If you finish your exercise routine you can have a piece of cake").

- Address people with mental disabilities with the same respect and integrity shown nondisabled individuals; remember that adult clients are mature adults, not young children.

- Never use exercise or deny opportunities for physical activity as a form of punishment.

- Always try to end your physical activity session with statements and experiences that are positive and encouraging, but also sincere (e.g., "I am seeing improvement in your throwing form, George" or "It's obvious you are getting fitter and jogging further, Jane. Well done").

Identify Your Attitudes and Motives

Asken (1991) suggests that people who want to work with this special population should clearly understand their personal thoughts and motivators. In particular, health workers need to examine their attitudes about disability in general and about the disabled in particular. In addition, the health worker needs to read about the psychology of people with disabilities and be comfortable with experiences unique to this population, including prosthetics, amputated stumps, and adapted self-care related to bowel and bladder incontinence. The consultant must be prepared for and comfortable dealing with these factors.

Four Areas of Specialized Knowledge

Fitness coaches and other professionals should have four areas of specialized knowledge before working with people with disabilities. The first area is to understand the background of psychological trauma associated with disability. As Asken (1991) describes, "The most compelling characteristic of the physically disabled that separates him or her from the able-bodied is the history of having encountered a physically or psychologically traumatic experience resulting in loss of function and the disability" (p. 373).

The second factor is to understand the unique physical responses and medical problems that people with disabilities must confront. Life-threatening medical conditions, for instance, may occur due to bladder dysfunction, lack of proper circulation, or an impaired nervous system resulting in lower maximal heart rates. People who use wheelchairs require increased upper-body strength if they have arm function.

The third factor is the complexity of motivation for a disabled person to continue the road to rehabilitation and improved function. Understandably, feelings of helplessness and hopelessness are not uncommon in this population. Reasons to have hope for meeting performance goals and improved functioning are uneven among the disabled. The coach's primary mission in the beginning is to provide a sense of direction, purpose, and optimism that associates the rehabilitation program with a better quality of life. This is one reason competitive sport is so popular among people with disabilities; it provides value and focus to the rehabilitation process.

The fourth area concerns the benefits of exercise for mental functioning. Exercise helps patients overcome, or at least minimize, the debilitating effects of mental disorders that are common among this population. Similar to the distraction hypothesis (Bahrke and Morgan, 1978) that explains the psychological

benefits of exercise, the disabled individual is focusing on exercise tasks and not on less pleasant aspects of life. As reviewed in chapter 5, increased fitness level usually generates improved mental health.

PEOPLE WITH CHRONIC CONDITIONS

Coaching special populations primarily includes people who have long-term medical conditions. (For examples of conditions, see the Common Chronic Conditions That Improve Through Exercise and Physical Activity highlight box.) Exercise training for people with chronic conditions requires a different regimen than for healthy people. Symptoms of the condition will likely be present throughout the person's life. The exercise coach must select exercises that are compatible with the client's needs, including the psychological characteristics that accompany the illness (Schmitz, 2012). Recurring physical symptoms, for instance, can create mental barriers that result in irregular attendance at exercise sessions. Adherence, therefore, is an important area of concern when working with clients with chronic conditions. A primary goal of exercise and fitness coaches is to create conditions that will motivate people with chronic conditions to develop healthier habits and to make lifestyle changes.

COMMON CHRONIC CONDITIONS THAT IMPROVE THROUGH EXERCISE AND PHYSICAL ACTIVITY

Fibromyalgia	Depression or anxiety
Arthritis	Eating disorders
Alcoholism or drug abuse	Parkinson's disease
Diabetes (types 1 and 2)	Emphysema
Osteoporosis	Organ transplant
Hemophilia	Lupus
Multiple sclerosis	AIDS
Chronic fatigue syndrome	Post-traumatic stress disorder (PTSD)
Traumatic brain injury	

People with chronic conditions need special care and sensitivity. They are not elite athletes. Fitness professionals need to keep the exercises simple to learn and easy to do, model them before asking the client to perform them, and have the client perform them somewhat slowly. People in this population are especially appreciative of having an exercise partner or other social support, and they should not be left on their own if at all possible (Rollnick, Mason, and Butler, 1999). The fitness coach may find them to be high maintenance, meaning that they require persistent attention, ongoing encouragement, lots of performance feedback, and frequent communication as they slowly become comfortable with each exercise technique. Specific strategies to help people with chronic conditions adopt new habits, including exercise, are similar to those for their healthy counterparts, but it is even more important for this population to maintain exercise adherence and adopt healthy lifestyle changes (Gillison et al., 2009; Hayman, 2009). Understandably, in this population there is somewhat more dependence on caregivers.

Social Support

These clients will need to exercise with their coach for several reasons. For one, the coach can model the exercise technique and provide ongoing instruction and encouragement. In addition, the client will develop a trusting relationship with the coach, which is motivational for taking risks in performing new exercises and exercising at higher intensity. Finally, the coach can monitor client attendance and performance improvement, thereby reacting to favorable and unfavorable changes in these areas.

Other forms of social support include the client's physician or other personal care provider. This person should become aware of the exercise program and lend full verbal support to the patient's attempts to initiate and maintain the program. The care provider may also administer medical tests during the year to detect changes in scores. Numbers from tests tend to increase self-motivation to change behavior (Loehr and Schwartz, 2003).

Another form of social support is the client's family and friends. Clients with chronic conditions are better off exercising with another person or with a group of people who are experiencing the same or similar maladies. Exercising with others allows the person to meet social needs as well as become distracted from the exertion that occurs with exercise training.

One person who has been neglected in the search for sources of social support is the client's religious leader. Numerous studies have shown that religious leaders can provide great value and meaning to maintaining a healthy lifestyle (Koenig, 2007). Religious leaders have enormous credibility in their communities when they cite scriptural passages that have inspirational value. People of faith can be encouraged to maintain a healthy lifestyle and to maintain the spiritual dimension in their lives. Exercise reflects their values of faith and of respecting the body as a temple. See chapter 7 for more information.

Building New Habits

Changing habits is a challenging task. The most efficient way to build a new exercise habit is to schedule the exercise sessions for the week and have preexercise rituals in place that facilitate the preparation and execution of an exercise session. Clothing should be prepared in advance, transportation should be planned, and when the client enters an exercise facility, a series of routines should be preplanned and carried out. The time of day to exercise should be compatible with the client's optimal mental and physical readiness, and the exercise environment should be compatible with client needs (e.g., exercising at a time when there are relatively few or relatively many exercisers).

Goals

Several studies have shown that performance goals enhance most forms of physical activity, including sport and exercise. Goals have strong motivational value and also help performers focus their effort toward achieving a particular outcome. Goals should be based on exercise pretests and an exercise prescription. They may reflect movement speed (e.g., "I will complete 1 mile in 10 minutes or less"), number of repetitions (e.g., "I will lift that weight five times"), amount of resistance (e.g., "I will be able to lift 150 pounds, an increase of 50 pounds from my current resistance, within six weeks"), or distance (e.g., "I will run half a mile longer in 30 days").

Another advantage of goal setting is that it provides information about improved performance and competence. Meeting a goal represents improved performance and competence, which is an important component of intrinsic motivation. This creates a sense of satisfaction, which in turn provides feelings of achievement. Taken together, the person now experiences exercise as a source of not only better health but also personal satisfaction and growth. Exercise is then viewed as pleasant and enjoyable.

CANCER PATIENTS

Cancer, a leading cause of death in most developed countries, consists of a complex group of diseases that stem from the progressive and uncontrolled growth of a single cell. There are numerous personal and environmental factors that partially explain the causes of cancer. Evidence is mounting that physically active people have a lower incidence of cancer than their sedentary counterparts. In addition, there is strong evidence that exercise protects against breast cancer in women and prostate cancer in men. There is more moderate support for linking exercise and lower incidence of several other cancers. Regular physical activity is recommended for most cancer patients to improve functional capacity, mental health (including reduced depression), and quality of life.

Moderate exercise counteracts the loss of functional capacity that is common among cancer patients undergoing chemotherapy. This is the primary way exercise causes desirable changes in the well-being of cancer patients (Dimeo et al., 1997). More than 80% of patients undergoing cancer treatment or recovering from surgery experience fatigue and nausea as a side effect of treatment. Anemia is also a common side effect of che-

motherapy, and it reduces aerobic capacity, leading to premature fatigue during aerobic exercise (Sanft and Irwin, 2012).

The most common exercise prescription for cancer patients is to engage in moderate, not high, exercise intensity. As a general guideline, the National Cancer Institute (2010) recommends 30 minutes of walking three to five times per week. In the beginning of an exercise regimen, however, cancer patients should start slowly, walking five times per week for 3 minutes per day in the first week, then three times per week for 10 minutes per day in the fourth week, and so on, slowly working toward a more intense regimen.

Exercise is not always recommended for cancer patients. For example, cancer patients should avoid exercise

- when there is evidence of infection (fever above 37.5 °C or 99.5 °F);
- when there is a low platelet count and cardiac function is not normal;
- when they experience severe fatigue, weakness, or nausea;
- 24 hours before or after chemotherapy; and
- if the cancer has spread (metastasized) to the bone, thereby weakening bone tissue and requiring avoidance of resistance training or high-impact aerobics.

The patient's physician should always be consulted concerning the patient's medical condition, limitations in physical activity, level of readiness for engaging in various forms of physical activity, and individualized exercise prescription. Readers are directed to *ACSM's Guide to Exercise and Cancer Survivorship* (Irwin, 2012) for more detailed information for working with cancer patients.

CULTURAL DIFFERENCES

There are two primary reasons it is important to acknowledge the role of culture in the road to improving health behavior. First, it is important to understand the reasons some cultures are more physically active than others and the types of physical activity they often prefer. Some cultures more than others consider physical activity an important part of their lifestyle. The first reason to study cultural differences in fitness psychology, therefore, is a descriptive one that reflects cultural norms, that is, patterns of behavior or beliefs generally held by members of a particular group. The second reason is an applied one—cultural considerations help determine the nature of programs and the instructional and motivational strategies that will promote the replacement of unhealthy behavior patterns with more desirable ones.

Do cultural norms influence rates of physical activity? In one study, O'Brien Cousins (2000) compared cultural norms for physical activity among older adults living in the United States and Canada with a similar age group living in China. The North Americans viewed physical activity as inappropriate, without benefit, and dangerous, while the Chinese considered physical activity to play an important role in their life and were far more active. Physical activity in China is considered healthy and is performed in large groups each morning (China National Sports Council, 1997). Hong and Lu (1999) report that China provides older adults with more than 200,000 physical activity associations that promote exercise options such as swimming, dancing, and tai chi.

Another culture that strongly encourages physical activity is Scandinavia, which is composed of Sweden, Denmark, Finland, and Norway. Not only are Scandinavians far more active than most other cultures, but studies have shown that Scandinavian university students hold negative stereotypes toward nonexercisers and consider them to be lazy and have low self-control (Lindwall and Martin Ginis, 2006). Exercise and other forms of physical activity are common—even among older adults—and desirable. Perhaps not surprisingly, the life span in these countries is longer than in the United States and Canada, and older adults are more mobile, even bicycling into their 80s.

What are the implications of cultural differences for professionals in the health behavior change profession? Perhaps the main issue here is that people have individualized needs, preferences, and limitations with respect to maintaining an active lifestyle and healthy habits. Individual differences exist, for instance, in preferred type of physical activity—some people enjoy exercise such as walking, jogging, yoga, and Pilates, while others prefer competitive sport. Availability of facilities, equipment, and recreational sport leagues are factors that will influence this decision. Culture also may play a role in determining whether to engage in a physical activity program and the type of program that seems most comfortable and effective.

Finally, another personal factor that will influence participation in physical activity is whether clients feel they need to speak to a mental health professional for any of the following three reasons:

1. To help explain and overcome certain feelings (e.g., self-doubt, low confidence) or emotions (e.g., anxiety) or perceived lack of control or energy that prevent making permanent changes in health behaviors

2. To address feelings of inadequacy, anxiety, depression, lack of confidence, high self-consciousness, or other issues that make it difficult to exercise in public or group settings

3. To help explain their history of quitting programs that improve health and well-being or their inability to adhere to programs and new habits over the long term

What are the barriers to successfully changing health behaviors, what are the sources of these barriers, and what can be done to overcome them? Is there a history of starting new health-related programs and then quitting? What types of mental and behavioral strategies and interventions can a person use to facilitate permanent changes in unhealthy habits, and who can provide support to help ensure these new habits remain integrated into the person's lifestyle? Is there a need to maintain consistent interactions with a mental health professional to keep the client on track and engaged in the behavior change process?

FROM RESEARCH TO REAL WORLD

Each special population has unique attributes, needs, and barriers to initiating and adhering to healthy habits. Health and fitness workers must address each of these unique needs in order to enact long-term behavioral change.

Age Differences

There are differences among young-old, old, and old-old age groups for people in advanced years of life. Although the human organism and its many physiological processes begin to slowly deteriorate in the mid- to late 20s, the level of physical and mental incapacitation does not become apparent until the 70s. Aerobic and resistance exercise will slow the rate at which the body deteriorates (Hong and Lu, 1999).

Rehabilitation

There are three primary challenges to health care workers in providing rehabilitation services to clients and patients:

- Determine the causes of the mental and physical condition.

- Understand the psychological barriers to successful rehabilitation.

- Provide rehabilitation services that overcome those barriers in helping clients return to their previous performance level (Duru et al., 2008; Lewin et al., 1992).

Pregnancy

The enormous physical demands of pregnancy require caution before engaging in vigorous exercise. The conclusions from many studies, however, indicate that it is safe for healthy pregnant women to engage in regular exercise. However, pregnant women with cardiovascular, pulmonary, or metabolic disease, as well as those who are obese, should seek physician guidance to determine the type and intensity of physical activity to engage in (Symons Downs and Hausenblas, 2003).

Chronic Conditions

Clients with chronic conditions include people whose medical conditions are long term. Exercises must be compatible with the client's physical needs (e.g., use of a walker or wheelchair) and with the psychological characteristics that accompany the illness or disability (e.g., embarrassment, guilt, low confidence or self-esteem). Conditions should be created that motivate the person to make lifestyle changes (Fisher, 1999; Hayman, 2009).

Cancer Recovery

Regular physical activity is recommended for most cancer patients to improve functional capacity, the patient's mental status (including depression), and quality of life. The primary way exercise causes desirable changes in well-being is by counteracting the loss of functional capacity that is common among cancer patients undergoing chemotherapy (Dimeo et al., 1997; National Cancer Institute, 2010).

It is imperative that we acknowledge the dangers of a sedentary lifestyle and a culture that reflects habits that are leading to weight gain, premature onset of diseases, lack of energy, poor quality of life, and a shortened life span. Physical activity has to be perceived as the cultural norm and as a common lifestyle choice.

SUMMARY

There is a category of clients who require special skills and training—people who have what are commonly called *special needs*. This chapter addresses this segment of the population, which includes older adults, people who need rehabilitation from injury and disease, cancer patients, pregnant women, and people with physical and mental disabilities. All of these conditions involve special needs and recovery strategies, particularly given their long-term time frame for rehabilitation and the psychological issues that accompany them (e.g., anxiety, depression, denial, hopelessness).

Clients with chronic conditions are especially in need of social support and strategies that promote adherence to new habits that aid

recovery. Conditions and their symptoms may appear throughout the patient's life. A primary goal of exercise coaches is to create conditions that will motivate the person with a chronic condition to develop healthier habits and make lifestyle changes. Medical specialists; exercise, nutrition, and physical rehabilitation coaches; mental health professionals; family members; and friends all play a part in the rehabilitation process that improves recovery and quality of life.

STUDENT ACTIVITY

Developing a Psychological Plan for Special Populations

Perhaps not surprisingly, if exercise is challenging to many people who do not have physical limitations, imagine how difficult and even threatening it must be to people with special needs. This student activity concerns developing a mental plan to improve a person's psychological readiness to maintain the incentive and energy to remain physically active. Exercise for special populations is always in response to the approval of and guidelines set by the client's physician or other licensed medical practitioner. If a person who represents any of the several populations reviewed in this chapter is available, obtain permission from that person and the person's medical practitioner to engage in an 8- to 10-week program of increased physical activity. If you do not already possess fitness coaching skills, try to solicit the assistance of a certified personal trainer or physical therapist who can recommend types of exercises your client can perform. Your job is not to conduct the fitness program with this client but rather to develop a mental plan.

General Objectives of the Mental Plan

- To help the client avoid negative thinking
- To foster positive thinking (such as confidence, optimism, self-control, and mental toughness)
- To promote more consistent performance

Specific Objectives of the Preexercise Phase

- To strengthen feelings of preparation and readiness
- To avoid the intrusion of self-defeating thoughts that produce anxiety
- To improve the client's preexercise emotional state, accompanied by a positive attitude about the exercise experience

Issues to Address With Clients

- *Maintain a positive, uplifting attitude.* The client should enter the exercise area in a positive mood and in anticipation of enjoyment and achieving fitness goals.

He should feel confident and enthusiastic to be there and anticipate a pleasant experience. Remind the client that his body—and his medical condition—are in dire need of physical activity.

- *Use positive self-talk.* As the client enters the facility and begins exercise preparation, he should use self-talk statements such as "I feel good," "I'm ready," "My body needs this," and other positive affirmations that provide an uplifting mood. Prayer is acceptable for highly spiritual clients if they wish.

- *Dress properly.* The client should not wear street clothes for engaging in vigorous physical activity. She should dress for action, including high-quality footwear and apparel that fits the situation and is within her comfort zone.

- *Develop an exercise plan.* Describe the sequence of activities to engage in during the exercise session from start to finish. Your client should know what you are going to do even before entering the exercise facility.

- *Be familiar with the facilities and equipment.* Where should the client begin and what should he do from the time he enters the facility until the time he departs? Having a workout plan will prevent clients from feeling self-conscious and out of place.

- *Provide physical and social support.* Clients with special needs are almost always dependent on another person—social support—to help them handle exercise equipment, enter and exit facilities, use the locker room and restroom, and perform exercise tasks.

- *Develop the set of routines.* What must the client do throughout the exercise session, from start to finish? Clients need to know the full set of exercises; drink water regularly before, during, and after the workout; and feel comfortable ending the session when they are fatigued or have had enough for the day. Some clients, particularly diabetics, may need to consume certain foods to maintain insulin levels.

- *Provide instruction for each exercise.* All clients, but particularly people with special needs, must be instructed on performing the exercises correctly in order to avoid expending too much energy and to obtain the optimal benefits of each exercise.

- *Use cognitive strategies.* Clients should use strategies such as association, dissociation, psyching up, positive self-talk, and attentional focusing when performing the exercises.

- *Use behavioral strategies.* Use strategies such as goal setting and music when possible and if desirable. Some people enjoy setting goals or exercising to music more than others.

Finally, develop a checklist that incorporates these guidelines and work with your client on developing these areas of preparation and execution of exercise sessions. Send clients text messages, e-mails, and other forms of electronic communication as reminders about their exercise sessions. Finally, provide clients with data based on tests that reflect fitness, lipids profile (e.g., cholesterol, triglycerides), and other measures that you anticipate would favorably change over time. Compare pretest data (obtained at the start of the program) with posttest data, which might occur at least 10 to 12 weeks later. Improved scores are highly motivating.

REFERENCES

American College of Obstetricians and Gynecologists (ACOG). (2003). Exercise during pregnancy and the postpartum period. *Clinical Obstetrics and Gynecology, 46,* 496-499.

American College of Sports Medicine (ACSM). (2009). *ACSM exercise management for persons with chronic diseases and disabilities.* (3rd ed.) Champaign, IL: Human Kinetics.

American College of Sports Medicine (ACSM). (2010). *ACSM's guidelines for exercise testing and prescription* (8th ed.). Philadelphia: Williams and Wilkins.

Anshel, M.H. (2006). *Applied exercise psychology: A practitioner's guide to improving client health and fitness.* New York: Springer Publishing Company.

Asken, M.J. (1991). The challenge of the physically challenged: Delivering sport psychology services to physically disabled athletes. *Sport Psychologist, 5,* 370-381.

Bahrke, M.S., and Morgan, W.P. (1978). Anxiety reduction following exercise and meditation. *Cognitive Therapy and Research, 4,* 323-333.

Bawden, M. (2006). Providing sport psychology support for athletes with disabilities. In J. Dosil (Ed.), *The sport psychologist's handbook: A guide for sport-specific performance enhancement* (pp. 665-683). New York: Wiley.

Biddle, S.J.H., and Mutrie, N. (2001). *Psychology of physical activity: Determinants, well-being and interventions.* New York: Routledge.

Brewer, B.W., and Tripp, D.A. (2005). Psychological applications in the prevention and rehabilitation of sport injuries. In D. Hackfort, J.L. Duda, and R. Lidor (Eds.), *Handbook of research in applied sport and exercise psychology: International perspectives* (pp. 319-332). Morgantown, WV: Fitness Information Technology.

Carmeli, E., Zinger-Vaknin, T., Morad, M., and Merrick, J. (2005). Can physical training have an effect on well-being in adults with mild intellectual disability? *Mechanisms of Ageing and Development, 126,* 299-304.

China National Sports Council. (1997). *Report on China mass sports survey.* Beijing: Author.

Dimeo, F., Fetscher, S., Lange, W., Mertelsmann, R., and Keul, J. (1997). Effects of aerobic exercise on the physical performance and incidence of treatment-related complications after high-dose chemotherapy. *Blood, 90,* 3390-3394.

Dorgo, S., Robinson, K.M., and Bader, J. (2009). The effectiveness of a peer-mentored older adult fitness program on perceived physical, mental, and social function. *Journal of the American Academy of Nurse Practitioners, 12,* 116-122.

Duru, O.K., Gerzoff, R.B., Brown, A.F., Karter, A.J., Kim, C., Kountz, D., Narayan, K.M., Schneider, S.H., Tseng, C.W., Waitzfelder, B., and Mangione, C.M. (2008). Predictors of sustained walking among diabetes patients in managed care: The Translating Research into Action for Diabetes (TRIAD) study. *Journal of General Internal Medicine, 8,* 1194-1199.

Fisher, A.C. (1999). Counseling for improved rehabilitation adherence. In R. Ray and D.M. Wiese (Eds.), *Counseling in sports medicine* (pp. 275-292). Champaign, IL: Human Kinetics.

Gillison, F.B., Skevington, S.M., Sato, A., Standage, M., and Evangelidou, S. (2009). The effects of exercise interventions on quality of life in clinical and healthy populations: A meta-analysis. *Social Science and Medicine, 68,* 1700-1710.

Hayman, L. (2009). Lifestyle change and adherence issues among patients with heart disease. In S.A. Shumaker, J.K. Ockene, and K.A. Riekert (Eds.), *The handbook of health behavior change* (3rd ed., pp. 677-692). New York: Springer.

Heyman, S.R. (1987). Counseling and psychotherapy with athletes: Special considerations. In J.R. May and M.J. Asken (Eds.), *Sport psychology: The psychological health of the athlete* (pp. 135-156). New York: PMA.

Hong, Y., and Lu, Y. (1999). Physical activity and health among older adults in China. *Journal of Aging and Physical Activity, 7,* 247-250.

Irwin, M.L. (2012). *ACSM's guide to exercise and cancer survivorship.* Champaign, IL: Human Kinetics.

Koenig, H.G. (2007). *Spirituality in patient care: Why, how, when, and what* (2nd ed.). Philadelphia: Templeton Foundation Press.

Lewin, B., Robertson, I.H., Cay, E.L., Irving, J.B., and Campbell, M. (1992). Effects of self-help post-myocardial-infarction rehabilitation on psychological adjustment and use of health services. *Lancet, 339,* 1036-1040.

Lindwall, M., and Martin Ginis, K.A. (2006). Moving towards a favorable image: The self-presentational benefits of exercise and physical activity. *Scandinavian Journal of Psychology, 47,* 209-217.

Loehr, J., and Schwartz, T. (2003). *The power of full engagement.* New York: Free Press.

Mackinnon, L.T., Ritchie, C.B., Hooper, S.L., and Abernethy, P.J. (2003). *Exercise management: Con-*

cepts and professional practice. Champaign, IL: Human Kinetics.

McDermott, S., Whitner, W., Thomas-Koger, M., Mann, J.R., Clarkson, J., Barnes, T.L., Bao, H., and Meriwether, R.A. (2012). An efficacy trial of "Steps to Your Health," a health promotion programme for adults with intellectual disability. *Health Education Journal, 71,* 278-290.

Morris, V. (2004). *How to care for aging parents.* New York: Workman.

National Cancer Institute. (2010, June 29). Guidelines urge exercise for cancer patients, survivors. *NCI Cancer Bulletin, 7* (13).

O'Brien Cousins, S. (2000). My heart couldn't take it: Older women's beliefs about exercise benefits and risks. *Journal of Gerontology, 55B,* 283-294.

Oldridge, N.B. (1995). Patient compliance. In M. Pollack and D.H. Schmidt (Eds.), *Heart disease and rehabilitation* (pp. 393-404). Champaign, IL: Human Kinetics.

Rollnick, S., Mason, P., and Butler, C. (1999). *Health behavior change: A guide for practitioners.* New York: Churchill Livingstone.

Sanft, T., and Irwin, M.L. (2012). Side effects and persistent effects of cancer surgery and treatment. In M.L. Irwin (Ed.), *ACSM's guide to exercise and cancer survivorship* (pp. 15-28). Champaign, IL: Human Kinetics.

Schmitz, K. (2012). Exercise prescription and programming adaptations: Based on surgery, treatment, and side effects. In M.L. Irwin (Ed.), *ACSM's guide to exercise and cancer survivorship* (pp. 87-112). Champaign, IL: Human Kinetics.

Self, M., Driver, S., Stevens, L., and Warren, A.M. (2013). Physical activity experiences of individuals living with a traumatic brain injury: A qualitative research exploration. *Adaptive Physical Activity Quarterly, 30,* 20-39.

Shapiro, D.R. (2003). Participation motives of Special Olympic athletes. *Adapted Physical Education Quarterly, 20,* 150-165.

Symons Downs, D., and Hausenblas, H.A. (2003). Exercising for two: Examining pregnant women's second trimester exercise intention and behavior using the framework of the theory of planned behavior. *Women's Health Issues, 13,* 222-228.

Thompson, D.L. (2007). Exercise and women's health. In E.T. Howley and B.D. Franks (Eds.), *Fitness professional's handbook* (5th ed., pp. 289-295). Champaign, IL: Human Kinetics.

Urv, T.K., Zigman, W.B., and Silverman, W. (2003). Maladaptive behaviors related to adaptive decline in aging adults with mental retardation. *American Journal of Mental Retardation, 108,* 327-339.

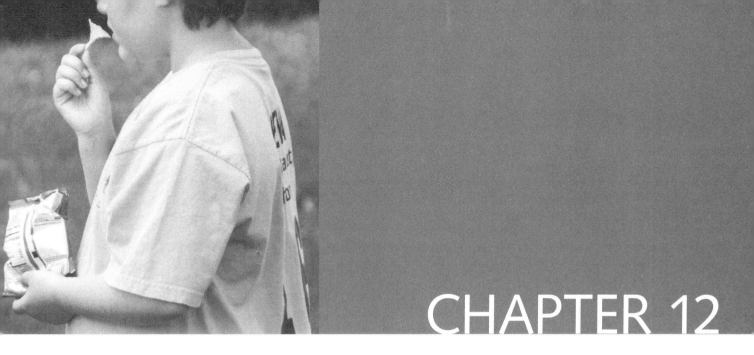

Dysfunctional Eating Behaviors

66 *Champions aren't made in the gyms. Champions are made from something they have* 99 *deep inside them—a desire, a dream, a vision.*

Muhammad Ali, former world heavyweight boxing champion

CHAPTER OBJECTIVES

After reading this chapter, you should be able to:

- describe the sources of poor eating habits, some of which reflect mental health disorders and require counseling;
- understand the differences between disordered eating and eating disorders; and
- provide strategies for eating more responsibly and strategically to improve energy, physical performance, and weight control.

A book on changing health-related behaviors must include a chapter on eating habits and the role of health and fitness professionals in helping clients replace poor eating habits with ways to eat strategically to improve energy and to maintain healthy body weight. Improving mental and physical health, general well-being, energy, and performance requires proper nutrition. Eating a healthy diet, however, is not always simply about making good choices and eating strategically to improve energy and maintain a proper body weight. Two factors get in the way of eating wisely—culture and emotion. For many of us, eating to satisfy hunger has little to do with what we eat. Instead, we seem to consume food to meet cultural expectations, in which eating a large volume of food is a fundamental component of socializing and relaxing. Eating in response to certain emotions, such as stress, boredom, and happiness, is also common, as is passive eating while performing another task such as watching television, a movie, or a sporting event. It appears that much of the time we eat for all the wrong reasons rather than to satisfy our hunger.

Our culture suffers from an array of eating pathologies (i.e., mental illnesses) associated with making poor food choices and lacking awareness of healthy eating habits (Lamarche and Gammage, 2012). Most people need to improve the ability to burn calories rather than being preoccupied, perhaps obsessed, with food intake that results in excessive calories, which are stored rather than used as energy. Nutrition and weight management is a science, and health professionals require knowledge of that science to understand and communicate the causes of improper eating behavior (i.e., types of eating disorders and disordered eating) and to help clients engage in eating and exercise behavior that is consistent with that science.

The purposes of this chapter, therefore, are to describe the sources of poor eating habits, some of which reflect mental health disorders and require counseling, and to provide strategies that consultants and their clients can use in eating more responsibly and strategically for improving energy, performance, and weight control. We begin with an overview of eating disorders and disordered eating, followed by

---

WEIGHT MANAGEMENT: POSITION OF THE AMERICAN DIETETIC ASSOCIATION

The American Dietetic Association (ADA, which changed its name in 2012 to the Academy of Nutrition and Dietetics) defines *obesity* as "a condition characterized by excess accumulation of adipose tissue (i.e., fat stores)" (ADA, 2009, p. 330). The way to maintain a healthy body weight is to manage fat stores. As the ADA states, "Fat stores can only be changed by a whole body energy imbalance brought on by a change in energy intake, energy output, efficiency of energy use, or a combination of any of these components" (p. 330). Although many overweight people rationalize their condition as genetic ("My whole family is overweight, so I can't do anything about it"), the ADA claims "there have been only a limited number of obesity cases identified as being directly caused by a single gene mutation" (p. 330).

The ADA goals of weight management, endorsed by ACSM (ADA, 2009), are not mere reflections of the numbers on a scale but rather an attempt to help people develop healthy lifestyle habits and to set realistic expectations about the time and effort required to manage their weight. The ADA proposes four goals of weight management interventions:

1. Prevention or cessation of weight gain
2. Varying degrees of improvement in physical and emotional health
3. Small, maintainable weight losses or more extensive weight losses achieved through modified eating and exercise behaviors
4. Improvements in eating, exercise, and other behaviors

the most common form of disordered eating, called *emotional eating*, and we finish with a discussion of ways to manage obesity. At the heart of obesity and poor eating habits is the all-too-common failure to manage body weight, primarily due to the combination of consuming too many calories and not getting enough daily physical activity.

This is not new information, but what we need are novel approaches to help people overcome their food addictions, obsessions with food, emotional eating, and other habits that lead to obesity and reduced quality of life. Replacing negative habits with new routines is required. Thus, it is necessary for health and fitness professionals to be familiar with the conditions and concepts related to eating and dietary problems in order to develop strategies for behavior change. Specific recommendations for maintaining a healthy weight and treating eating disorders from a behavioral perspective—not psychotherapy—will be described later.

DISORDERED EATING AND EATING DISORDERS

There are differences between disordered eating and eating disorders, both of which may reflect habits of food consumption driven by psychological factors and reactions to life situations. *Disordered eating* includes a wide range of abnormal eating, such as chronic restrained eating, compulsive eating, habitual dieting, and irregular or chaotic eating patterns (Thompson and Sherman, 2010). Often physical hunger and satiety (fullness) are ignored. Disordered eating has negative effects on overall emotional, social, and physical health. It may cause the individual to feel tired and depressed, decrease mental functioning and concentration, and can lead to malnutrition with risk to bone health, physical growth and brain development. Disordered eating is considered by psychologists as subclinical, and while less life-threatening than a clinical eating disorder, is still dangerous to maintaining proper health (Brewer and Petrie, 2002). Brewer and Petrie assert that female athletes

with disordered eating also may develop amenorrhea and osteoporosis, which may lead to increased bone fractures and permanent bone loss.

Clinical eating disorders, on the other hand, are recognized by psychologists and medical practitioners as life-threatening medical conditions. These include anorexia nervosa, binge eating disorder, bulimia nervosa, and eating disorders not otherwise specified. Eating disorders are typically caused by psychological factors, and all forms of eating disorders and disordered eating should be treated by a licensed mental health professional, not solely by a fitness or nutrition coach.

Disordered eating lies on a continuum ranging from psychopathological and life-threatening (clinical) eating disorders to preoccupation with weight and restrictive eating (O'Dea, 2002; Wein and Micheli, 2002). A disordered eating pattern is a habitual reaction to life situations, such as feeling stress, wanting to appear thin for a particular event, or trying to obtain the approval of another person. Disordered eating is not in itself usually life threatening, but it may lead to transient weight changes, nutritional problems, and serious medical conditions. Disordered eating is usually accompanied by frequent thoughts of food, eating, and one's physical appearance. Disordered eating is typically subclinical and not life-threatening. Emotional eating and other food intake habits unrelated to hunger (e.g., eating when bored, passive eating while distracted with another task) are examples. An eating disorder, on the other hand, is a clinical (i.e., potentially life-threatening) condition that warrants immediate treatment by a licensed mental health professional. About 10% of individuals with anorexia nervosa, for instance, die as a result of this eating disorder. Hospitalization is often needed.

Researchers (Hamilton, Brooks-Gunn, and Warren, 1985; also see Williams, 2006, for a review) contend that the incidence of eating disorders is estimated to be higher in models, dancers, and athletes than in the general population. For example, the prevalence of anorexia nervosa is higher for ballerinas compared with the general American population of adolescent females (Anshel, 2004; Brooks-Gunn, Warren, and Hamilton, 1987). Dance students are seven times more likely than high school students to develop anorexia nervosa (Clough and Wilson, 1993). Brooks-Gunn et al. (1987) reported that one-third of a sample of professional dancers had a disordered eating pattern, while Hergenroeder, Fiorotto, and Klish (1991) found that 43% of dancers at the Houston Ballet Academy were diagnosed with anorexia nervosa. Although these studies are not new, similar patterns of disordered eating remain in more recent research (Beals and Houtkooper, 2006).

Not surprisingly, only licensed clinical psychologists and psychiatrists should counsel people with eating disorders, because these patients often require hospitalization and drug treatment (APA, 2000). Health care consultants who are not licensed to prescribe medication, however, can usually work with clients with disordered eating.

As indicated earlier, the condition of *disordered eating* is often and wrongly used interchangeably with the condition of *eating disorders*. In summary, there are several differences between eating disorders and disordered eating:

- Each condition is treated differently.
- A certain degree of mental illness is associated with each.
- Disordered eating requires patient education and may diminish without treatment, whereas eating disorders require specific medical and mental health treatment, without which the problem will persist and perhaps worsen.

An eating disorder is a potentially life-threatening mental illness, or mental disorder, with multiple determinants and risk factors (APA, 2000; Thompson and Sherman, 2010). People with eating disorders have compulsive thoughts of food, eating, and their bodies. Eating disorders often lead to serious medical problems, and 2% to 10% of people diagnosed with an eating disorder die from this mental illness (Garner et al., 1990; Williams, 2006). The onset of eating disorders generally occurs in adolescence or young adulthood and is largely confined to women (O'Dea, 2002; Striegel-Moore and Smolak, 2001).

Two of the more common eating disorders are anorexia nervosa and bulimia nervosa. As described by Herzog and Delinsky (2001), anorexia nervosa concerns self-starvation; the person refuses to consume sufficient calories to maintain a weight above 85% of expected body weight. People with this condition have a fear of gaining weight or becoming fat despite having a thin or underweight appearance. They perceive their bodies to be larger than their actual size, and females experience amenorrhea (i.e., absence of menstruation). Bulimia nervosa, on the other hand, also called *binge–purge syndrome*, is the tendency to consume an excessive amount of food (binge) and then attempt to quickly vomit the food before digestion. People with this condition place undue importance on their body size, shape, and weight in defining their self-identity.

More than 90% of anorexia nervosa and bulimia nervosa sufferers are adolescent or young adult females, and approximately 5% of women suffer from a partial or subclinical form of either anorexia nervosa or bulimia nervosa (Sundgot-Borgen and Torstveit, 2004). Females in Western cultures are at much greater risk for developing eating disorders than males due to intense social pressures to conform to the current cultural ideals of feminine beauty (O'Dea, 2002).

One possible reason for these gender differences is that body shape and weight become critical determinants of self-esteem in females more than males, particularly in adolescence. This is because interpersonal success is seen as closely linked to physical attractiveness in women (Brownell, Rodin, and Wilmore, 1992; Thompson and Sherman, 2010). According to Johnson, Steinberg, and Lewis (1988), thinness among women has increasingly been seen as a highly valued personal achievement, demonstrating self-control, autonomy, and success. Thus, the pursuit of thinness is commonly perceived as an action or goal via which young women in particular can obtain favorable social responses, thereby enhancing self-esteem.

IRRATIONAL THOUGHTS ON EATING

Often, the thoughts of a person with an eating disorder are not accurate and are based solely on emotion or incorrect reasoning. These individuals have an inner voice that consists of irrational thoughts. Here are some common irrational thoughts of disordered eaters.

Thought: Some foods are bad and I am bad if I eat them.

Fact: Foods are not good or bad; they are highly nutritious or low on the nutrition scale. What I eat does not make me bad or good.

Thought: Because I am overweight, my body is disgusting and embarrasses me.

Fact: I don't judge others by their weight, so why do I judge myself so harshly about my weight?

Thoughts: Food will make me fat. Food is my friend (my enemy). Ignoring my body's signals will make me fat.

Fact: Food is used for fuel and energy. I can turn to other people and to myself, not to food, for love and comfort.

According to Burke (2007), struggling to live up to perfectionistic or unrealistic standards is characteristic of anorexia nervosa. The combination of sociocultural pressures and pressures inherent in the dance profession identify dancers as a vulnerable subgroup of women who are at high risk of eating disorders. The pressure for thinness combined with expectations of high performance such as dance produce the ideal social climate for eating disorders, particularly in vulnerable adolescents (Garner and Garfinkel, 1980). Whether these pressures lead to emotional disturbance and eating disorders is uncertain. However, as mentioned previously, dance students are far more likely to develop eating disorders than nondancers of the same age (O'Dea, 2002).

Although dancers and other people with eating disorders share similar weight and dieting concerns, dancers tend to lack the associated psychopathology (i.e., mental illness) of most eating-disordered patients (ADA, 2005). The pursuit of thinness is not always associated with psychopathology. A related problem associated with eating disorders and far more common in Western cultures is called *emotional eating*.

EMOTIONAL EATING

Emotional eating is a form of disordered eating; it is not associated with mental illness and eating disorders. Sometimes people eat primarily to satisfy an emotional need. Emotional eating, then, is eating for reasons other than hunger (Pinaguy et al., 2003). Instead of the physical symptom of hunger initiating the eating, an emotion triggers it. There is a difference between normal eaters and emotional eaters. Normal eating serves to fuel the body. Normal eaters perceive food as what it is— energy that fuels the body. Emotional eaters, on the other hand, are compulsive about their eating habits. They eat mindlessly as something to do, similar to watching television or staring into space. This eating lacks purpose and is not about satisfying hunger (Burke and Deakin, 2006). Here are some of the various types of eating (Adriaanse, de Ridder, and Evers, 2011; Koball et al., 2012).

- *Restrictive eating* involves seeing food as the enemy. Food is restricted and monitored. Restrictive eaters fear feeling full; feeling full is frightening and shameful.

- *Compulsive eating* involves not paying attention to feeling full. Compulsive eaters eat quickly and often overeat.

- *Emotional overeating* means seeing food as comfort and eating to reward yourself with something nice or to feel better. Emotional overeaters often want to feel more than full— they want to feel overly full, which they find comforting.

In their reviews of related literature, Adriaanse et al. (2011) and Koball et al. (2012) list the following implications of emotional eating:

- After people have identified the beliefs that underlie their behaviors and replaced them with more rational beliefs, behavior change is possible.
- If hunger is not frightening or shameful, it can be allowed to develop and be recognized as a useful signal.
- When someone is thinking rationally about food, dietary choices improve. Food is selected because it's the main source of fuel and energy.
- It is normal to stop eating when full when fullness is recognized without fear, shame, or needing to fill an emotional void.

Rules of Normal Eating

Rules related to normal eating are not rigid. There is no right way to eat; however, there is a right reason to eat and a right way to think about food. Typically, normal eaters

- eat when they are hungry;
- choose foods that will satisfy them;
- stay in touch with their bodies by monitoring weight gain, weight loss, and general feelings;
- are self-aware of their eating habits; and
- stop eating when they are full.

There are several differences between emotional hunger and physical hunger, according to the University of Texas Counseling and Mental Health Center website (http://cmhc.utexas.edu/contact.php):

- Emotional hunger comes on suddenly; physical hunger occurs gradually.
- With emotional hunger, the person is eating to fill a void that is not related to an empty stomach. Specific foods are craved, such as pizza or ice cream, and only those foods will meet the person's needs. Eating in response to actual hunger means the person is open to a variety of food options.
- Emotional hunger feels like it needs to be satisfied instantly with the food that is craved; physical hunger can wait.

- Even when full, the person continues to eat to satisfy an emotional need and is more likely to keep eating. When eating in response to hunger, the person is more likely to stop when full.
- Finally, emotional eating can leave behind feelings of guilt ("Why did I eat that?" or "I shouldn't have eaten that"); eating when physically hungry does not.

Comfort Foods

One of the distinguishing characteristics of emotional hunger is that the person is focused on a particular food, likely a comfort food. Comfort foods are consumed when a person eats in order to obtain or maintain a feeling; they are typically consumed in response to negative moods, such as anxiety or depression, or to maintain positive moods, such as happiness or enthusiasm. The most popular comfort food for both sexes is ice cream. Additional comfort foods, however, differ. In general, according to Wansink (2006), women prefer chocolate and cookies, while men prefer pizza, steak, and casserole. Additionally, what you reach for when eating to satisfy an emotion depends on the emotion. Wansink

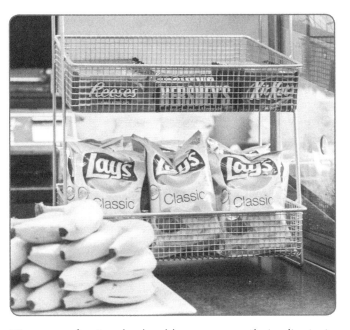

Fitness professionals should encourage their clients to understand the reasons why they choose a bag of chips over a piece of fruit and how to make better choices.

contends that the type of comfort foods people are drawn toward varies depending on their mood. People in happy moods often reach for foods such as pizza or steak, while unhappy people prefer ice cream and cookies. Bored people tend to go for a bag of potato chips. Again, emotional eating feeds a feeling, not a growling stomach.

Overcoming Emotional Eating

Persons who eat emotionally lack the control over their actions that normal eaters practice. In addition to obtaining professional counseling, there are ways to gain greater self-control in one's thinking in order to prevent or manage emotional eating.

- *Recognize and control hunger.* For some people, hunger causes anxiety. Others eat before they are hungry, and still others wait too long after they detect hunger and become too hungry to stop eating when full.

- *Choose foods that will satisfy hunger.* Eating is not satisfying when we eat what we think we should instead of what our body wants. The lack of satisfaction results in the temptation to eat more.

- *Don't fear food denial.* Sometimes emotional eaters have unconscious fears that they will be denied their favorite foods. When that fear is lost, it becomes much easier to choose from a wide range of foods.

- *Stay in touch with your body.* It is important to be aware of your eating habits. You are capable of monitoring your sense of fullness and stopping when satiated.

- *Slow down.* Emotional eaters often eat too quickly, worry about what others think of their food choices, and ignore signs of being full. Avoid all of these.

- *Don't take guilt trips.* Enjoy food without feeling guilty. Food consumption is a biological necessity to sustain life. Food does not have to become the enemy.

- *Pay attention to signs of fullness.* When feeling full, stop eating, even if you think you will make someone happy if you clean your plate or eat another serving. Those extra calories have to go somewhere, and much of the time they are stored as fat.

- *Examine thoughts and beliefs about food and eating.* Abnormal eaters should examine their beliefs and thoughts about food, eating, and their bodies. Are those beliefs rational and accurate? If not, from where did these irrational or inaccurate beliefs come? After people are aware of their irrational thoughts, they can challenge them and change them to be more rational. When that happens, the need for emotional eating is reduced or gone. Often, a mental health professional who is familiar with eating disorders will assist in this process.

- *Plan ahead.* In that moment of weakness or boredom, there's nothing easier than grabbing the ice cream from the freezer and chowing down. But what if indulgences like that aren't in the freezer, fridge, or pantry? Stock your kitchen with fruits, veggies, pudding cups, frozen fruit bars, popcorn, and yogurt. Be sure to wash and cut up the produce when you get it home—when you are in a munching mood, who wants to deal with peeling and cutting up a mango?

- *Allow treats.* There's nothing wrong with an occasional treat. In fact, they often make eating healthy the rest of the time a little easier. Whether it's a small bag of chips during your favorite TV show or an ice cream cone on a warm Saturday afternoon, giving yourself permission to eat a treat eliminates the need for secret binge sessions and the guilt felt after splurging on a favorite food.

- *Keep active while watching television.* Keeping your hands and head occupied can keep you from noshing induced by the television haze. There's always knitting or crossword puzzles, and what about holding onto the mail or a new magazine until you sit down for the evening? Need to write any thank-you notes or pay any bills? It doesn't matter what it is; just keep busy.

Guidelines for practitioners will be described later in this chapter. The next section addresses possible thoughts that accompany an eating disorder and would prompt a person to seek the services of a mental health professional.

BODY DISSATISFACTION

One condition that underlies eating disorders is discontent with one's physical characteristics. This is referred to as *body dissatisfaction*. There appear to be two contradictory obsessions in most Western cultures: an obsession with food, manifested by an emotional relationship with food and overeating, and an obsession with maintaining a proper weight and body size. Both issues reflect eating disorders, irrational thinking about food, and feelings of dissatisfaction with our bodies. Mental health professionals consider this to be dysfunctional, overly self-critical thinking.

The collective term referring to body dissatisfaction, discrepancies between actual and perceived body size, and negative affect when comparing one's body with perceived societal norms is called *body image disturbance*. The greatest source of body image disturbance is sociocultural (Heinberg, Thomspon, and Matzon, 2001). In many cultures, females feel pressured to achieve a near-impossible degree of thinness and to avoid weight gain and obesity (Henry, Anshel, and Michael, 2006). Rodin, Silberstein, and Striegel-Moore (1985) correctly predicted that body dissatisfaction may one day become the societal norm, a phenomenon they called *normative discontent*.

Messages from the mass media appear to be partly responsible for this pressure to be thin. Van den Buick (2000), for example, reported that the degree of watching television correlated negatively with ideal body image among adolescents; frequent viewers preferred a thinner ideal body compared with less frequent viewers. Along these lines, Harrison and Cantor (1997) found that the amount of time spent watching television significantly predicted overall body dissatisfaction. The print media are not exempt from influencing body image, either. Harrison and Cantor reported a significant relationship between reading fashion magazines and body dissatisfaction. In addition, Thomsen, Weber, and Brown (2001) found a strong correlation between frequency of reading women's health and fitness magazines and the use of unhealthy weight practices among high school girls.

Perhaps the most potentially harmful by-product of negative body image is increased risk of eating disorders. Body shape and weight become critical determinants of self-esteem in adolescence because interpersonal success is increasingly seen as closely linked to physical attractiveness (Brownell, Rodin, and Wilmore, 1992). As discussed earlier, thinness has increasingly been seen as a highly valued personal achievement, demonstrating self-control, autonomy, and success (Johnson, Steinberg, and Lewis, 1988). Obesity, or poor weight control, on the other hand, can lead to social discrimination and low self-esteem. Thus, the pursuit of thinness is a common goal through which young women can obtain favorable social responses and, consequently, enhance self-esteem. Distorted body image among females, then, is a common cause of eating disorders, and it may predispose people to relentless dieting or to lack of recognition of the effects of dieting. Typical causes of a distorted body image are low self-esteem, perfectionism, and body dissatisfaction (Clough and Wilson, 1993; Reel and Gill, 1996).

Again, one group of people who appear to be particularly vulnerable to body dissatisfaction and distorted body image is dancers. Dancers who fail to meet and maintain a predetermined ideal body composition are rapidly deselected from professional participation. There is a brief window for demonstrating competence in the dance field. Apparently, the point at which it is determined whether a dancer will become successful is age 21, after which time the dancer's chances are greatly reduced (Druss and Silverman, 1979).

Another factor that exacerbates the likelihood of disordered eating among dancers is that, in the absence of strict dieting, exercise alone may not result in the desired weight loss. For example, Cohen, Segal, Witriol, and McArdle (1982) studied 15 professional ballet dancers from the American Ballet Theatre and found that the caloric expenditure for an entire one-hour ballet class averaged only 200 calories for women versus about 500 calories per hour for swimming and skating (Brooks-Gunn, Warren, and Hamilton, 1987). According to Cohen et al. (1982) and Cohen, Potosnak,

Frank, and Baker (1985), these findings suggest that classical ballet is a relatively inefficient method of burning calories. Thus, without a safe and nutritious dietary intervention, dancing cannot burn enough calories to reduce weight and maintain the low weight required for the classical dance physique. The chronic dieting behavior of dancers may be important in the pathogenesis of eating disorders (Garner and Garfinkel, 1980). The demands for thinness and the low caloric expenditure of dance make eating disorders all too common in the dance world (Brooks-Gunn, Burrow, and Warren, 1988).

MULTIDISCIPLINARY APPROACH TO COMBATING EATING DISORDERS

Causes of eating disorders are complex and arise from multiple sources. In addition, treatments must target the exact type of eating disorder being addressed and meet the patient's individual needs. O'Neil and Rieder (2005) recommend the following members of a consulting team to help clients overcome inappropriate eating habits.

• *Registered dietitian:* This professional meets the specific knowledge and educational requirements of the ADA. The title *registered dietitian* is used exclusively to describe a person who has obtained registration and has met educational (e.g., completed an ADA-approved program) and knowledge (e.g., passed a national exam) requirements. This person will deliver an individually tailored dietary prescription for the patient and monitor patient progress and adherence to the prescribed program.

• *Exercise specialist:* This person should be certified to offer fitness testing, prescription, and instruction. There are a variety of certification programs in the United States and other countries, but the most recognized is ACSM, which offers separate tracks in clinical certification and health and fitness certification.

• *Mental health professional:* This is a category that includes several titles and credentials of professionals (e.g., therapist, social worker, counselor, psychologist) who provide psychological services to clients. Psychiatrists are physicians (i.e., MDs) and therefore are not included in this group. The title *psychologist* is reserved for a person who has completed a PhD from a program approved by the APA, including an extensive internship program. As part of the team, mental health professionals offer testing to detect psychopathology (i.e., mental illness) that might impede progress or lead to quitting the program, and they offer counseling services to address any barriers that might prevent the person from adhering to and successfully completing the program.

• *Medical practitioners—physician and nurse:* Inclusion of a medical practitioner is essential to establish the credibility of the program—that it is based on sound medical research—and to have a medical expert to help patients address their medical needs. The medical practitioner should be familiar with conditions related to obesity, including diabetes and medications that are commonly prescribed to combat obesity (e.g., diet pills) and obesity-related conditions.

• *Lifestyle counselor:* This professional helps the client to develop a new set of routines that replace the person's former unhealthy lifestyle. The lifestyle counselor often serves as the anchor for all members of the team and services provided. O'Neil and Rieder (2005) suggest that the person be a certified member of the American Association of Lifestyle Counselors (AALC) or the American Council on Exercise (ACE).

STRATEGIES FOR OBESITY MANAGEMENT

Health and fitness professionals can take numerous approaches to changing unhealthy eating habits. The ADA, with the written endorsement of ACSM, has generated an evidence-based list of ways practitioners can help prevent or manage obesity. There is a noticeable absence of any particular diet or other program that has been marketed and popularized in the mass media. These

---

UNDERSTANDING AN EATING DISORDER NOT OTHERWISE SPECIFIED

Individuals who experience a mix of anorexia and/or bulimia and/or binge-eating symptoms, but who are not categorized into one of the medical categories, have what mental health professionals call an *Eating Disorder Not Otherwise Specified* (ED-NOS). Only professionals who are educated and licensed in mental health diagnoses can detect and treat this condition. For additional information visit www.nedic.ca/knowthefacts/definitions.shtml#disordered.

Individuals with ED-NOS may exhibit all the symptoms of anorexia with these exceptions:

- Women may continue to experience menstruation.
- Men will not typically experience abnormally low sex hormones.
- Both men and women may lose weight but still remain in the normal weight range.

Others may have all the symptoms of bulimia but may

- Not binge and/or purge as often as is required to be categorized as having bulimia
- Purge, or compensate for normal eating by inducing vomiting, using laxatives or over-exercising, but not often enough to be diagnosed with one of the other clinical eating disorders
- Chew food repeatedly and often spit it out rather than swallow it
- Binge-eat regularly and compensate for it through the use of laxatives or by vomiting, etc.
- Remain within a normal weight range despite disordered eating

---

suggestions instead come from the abundant scientific literature. There is some redundancy with the earlier list of ways to regulate emotional eating.

Brewer and Petrie (2002) offer the following guidelines for preventing and treating eating disorders, with strong implications for athletes and dancers whose cultures emphasize weight loss and body size:

- Deemphasize weight as an important factor (i.e., avoid dieting)
- Eliminate weighing athletes in front of one another (unless medically necessary)
- Eliminate unhealthy but often accepted cultural standards that hasten eating disorders, such as "cutting weight" in wrestling or fat loss in gymnastics
- Treat each athlete as an individual and develop individualized training regimens that are based on health, not weight
- Control the competitiveness that exists on sport teams regarding weight loss or changes in body size

According to a report by the National Institutes of Health (NIH, 1998),

an increase in physical activity is an important component of weight loss therapy, although it will not lead to substantially greater weight loss over 6 months. Most weight loss occurs because of decreased caloric intake. Sustained physical activity is most helpful in the prevention of weight regain. In addition, it has a benefit in reducing cardiovascular and diabetes risks beyond that produced by weight reduction alone. For most obese patients, exercise should be initiated slowly, and the intensity should be increased gradually. The exercise can be done all at one time or intermittently over the day. Initial activities may be walking or swimming at a slow pace. The patient can start by walking 30 minutes for 3 days a week and can build to 45 minutes of more intense walking at least 5 days a week. With this regimen, an additional expenditure of 100 to 200 calories per day can be achieved.

All adults should set a long-term goal to accumulate at least 30 minutes or more of moderate-intensity physical activity on most, and preferably all, days of the week. This regimen can be adapted to other forms of physical activity, but walking is particularly attractive because of its safety and accessibility. Patients should be encouraged to increase "everyday" activities such as taking the stairs instead of the elevator. With time, depending on progress and functional capacity, the patient may engage in more strenuous activities. Competitive sports, such as tennis and volleyball, can provide an enjoyable form of exercise for many, but care must be taken to avoid injury. Reducing sedentary time is another strategy to increase activity by undertaking frequent, less strenuous activities. (pp. ix-xx)

Regulation of Food Intake

Results of repeated studies indicate that the most important factor in weight control is what's called a *negative energy balance*. This means that to avoid weight gain, a person must reduce energy intake, preferably by 500 to 1,000 calories per day, in order to achieve a 1- to 2-pound (.5-1 kg) weight loss per week (ADA, 2009; NIH, 1998). Specific ways to reach this goal include changing diet composition, increasing meal frequency (i.e., eating more frequently), timing meals a certain way (e.g., eating breakfast), and eating smaller portions.

Diet Composition

The ADA (2009) claims that "a low-fat, reduced-energy diet is the best studied weight-loss dietary strategy and is most frequently recommended by governing health authorities" (p. 333). A low-fat, low-energy diet in combination with increased physical activity and lifestyle counseling is an effective way to lose weight. Although some people feel that a variation in food intake should include reduced carbohydrate, the ADA concluded the following based on their review of research: "Consumption of a low-carbohydrate diet is associated with a greater weight and fat loss than traditional reduced-calorie diets during the first 6 months, but these differences are not significant after 1 year" (p. 334).

Portion Control

While the restaurant industry is trying to place more and more food on your plate with the expectation that you can actually eat all of it, the ADA (2009) strongly asserts that these enormous portions are highly destructive to weight control: "Effectively reducing portion sizes appears to be an important weight gain prevention strategy for everybody (regardless of weight) as marketplace food and drink portions now exceed standard serving sizes by a factor of at least twofold" (p. 334). The term *portion distortion* is used to describe the perception that large portions are appropriate amounts to eat at a single occasion. The ADA claims that the distortion "is reinforced by packaging, dinnerware, and serving utensils that have also increased in size" (p. 334).

Eating Frequency

Perhaps the most important strategy related to eating frequency is eating breakfast. For a variety of reasons, many people avoid eating a full breakfast or anything at all in the morning. Bad idea! Nutrient intake, such as calcium and fiber intake, may be compromised if breakfast is not consumed. The result is often poor choices made from available foods, including from vending machines, office candy jars, and fast-food restaurants, that are "energy dense but nutrition poor" (ADA, 2009, p. 335). Breakfast also improves appetite control (i.e., people who skip breakfast often overeat at lunch), dietary quality, and metabolism (i.e., eating breakfast increases metabolism, which burns more calories per minute at rest).

With respect to the number of meals consumed per day, the jury is still out. Several studies have shown that eating several small meals per day (i.e., about every three to four hours) helps prevent weight gain. Frequently consumed meals consisting of small portions will help maintain energy, increase metabolism, and reduce the likelihood of fat storage, which results when too much glucose is ingested in a short time (Whitnesy and Rady-Rolfes, 2004).

Meal Replacements

The ADA (2009) makes the following recommendation regarding meal replacements: "For people who have difficulty with self selection and/or portion control, meal replacements (e.g., liquid meals, meal bars, or calorie-controlled packaged meals) may be used as part of the diet component of a comprehensive weight management program. Substituting one or two daily meals or snacks with meal replacements is a successful weight loss and weight maintenance strategy" (p. 335).

Very-Low-Energy Diets

This type of diet is the only food source during an active weight-loss period. Usually in liquid form, it supplies about 800 calories or less per day, but it is enriched with protein and provides 100% of the daily value of essential vitamins and minerals. The purpose of this type of diet is to lose a lot of weight quickly while maintaining nutrition and lean body mass. The ADA (2009) recommends medical monitoring for people on these diets. People with a BMI under 30 should not use low-energy diets due to medical risks. As is the case with virtually all diets, long-term adherence to a very-low-energy diet is poor. Such diets lack a normal eating pattern and are inconsistent with typical food preferences. There is also a high likelihood of weight regain with this type of diet. Low-energy diets are usually prescribed for people before bariatric (i.e., stomach-reducing) surgery to reduce overall surgical risk in patients with severe obesity.

Physical Activity

Physical activity, of which exercise is just one option, forms the other side of the energy–weight control equation: calories burned, or out (as opposed to calories consumed, or in). According to the ADA (2009), an energy deficit of 500 to 1,000 calories is necessary to achieve a 1- to 2-pound (.5-1 kg) weight loss per week.

For most adults, many of whom lead a sedentary lifestyle, exercise alone without reduced caloric intake is a difficult approach to reach this objective. In a review of past studies that examined the separate roles of exercise and dietary changes on reducing weight, the ADA concluded that "the magnitude of weight changed due to physical activity is additive to that associated with a dietary intervention achieving energy restriction. . . . An individual may burn an additional 1,000 kcal per week by exercising 30 minutes 5 days a week" (p. 336). In other words, engaging in regular physical activity is almost required if a person wants to lose weight. Dietary restrictions alone are rarely sufficient to reach this goal. The ADA also provides guidelines, endorsed by ACSM, for engaging in regular physical activity to maintain a healthy body weight and increase fitness (see the next section).

WEIGHT MAINTENANCE

The ADA and ACSM (2009) recommend three categories of physical activity for weight maintenance. The first category is to reduce the risk of chronic disease in adulthood by engaging in at least 30 minutes of moderate to intense physical activity on a minimum of three days per week, preferably every other day (e.g., Monday, Wednesday, Friday; Tuesday, Thursday, Saturday) on most days of the week. The second category is to help manage body weight and prevent weight gain in adulthood by engaging in 60 minutes of moderate- to vigorous-intensity activity on a minimum of three days a week. The third category is to prevent weight regain after weight loss by engaging in 60 to 90 minutes of daily physical activity at moderate intensity "while not exceeding energy requirements" (p. 336), which means to avoid overeating.

In addition to recommending daily doses of physical activity, the ADA (2009) has also proposed weekly exercise periods. These include 150 minutes of moderate-intensity aerobic physical activity per week for significant health benefits and 300 minutes of moderate-intensity physical activity per week for more extensive health benefits.

Here are 10 guidelines from Otten, Hellwig, and Meyers (2006) for eating to maintain optimal energy and reduce the likelihood of becoming obese.

1. *Eat every two to three hours.* This is important in order to maintain an elevated metabolism (number of calories burned per minute to sustain life). This does not require eating a full meal every two to three hours, but you do need to eat a total of six to eight small meals and snacks that conform to the other rules in this list.

2. *Eat complete, lean protein each time you eat.* Eat food that comes from an animal with each meal, or if you're a vegetarian, you need to eat nonanimal sources of complete protein.

3. *Eat vegetables every time you eat.* In addition to a complete, lean protein source, you need to eat vegetables every time you eat (every two to three hours, ideally). You can include an occasional piece of fruit as well; however, do not skip the veggies.

4. *Eat carbohydrate.* Eat fruits and veggies whenever you want. You can eat carbohydrate that is not a fruit or a vegetable (e.g., simple sugar, rice, pasta, potatoes, bread); however, it is preferable to save these types of carbohydrate until after exercising. Heavily processed grains are dietary staples in North America, but they lead to heart disease, diabetes, and cancer. You can reward yourself for an intense workout with a good carbohydrate meal right after exercising because your body best tolerates these types of carbohydrate after exercise. For the rest of the day, eat lean protein and a selection of fruits and veggies.

5. *Eat healthy fat.* There are three types of fat—saturated, monounsaturated, and polyunsaturated. Forget about the old maxim that eating fat makes you fat. Eating all three kinds of fat in healthy balance (about equal parts of each) can dramatically improve your health and even help you lose fat. Saturated fat usually comes from animal products, and butter or coconut oil can be used for cooking. Monounsaturated fat should come from mixed nuts, olives, and olive oil. Finally, polyunsaturated fat should come from flaxseed oil, fish oil, and mixed nuts.

6. *Forget consuming calorie-containing drinks, even fruit juice.* All drinks should come from non-calorie-containing beverages. Try to omit fruit juice, alcoholic drinks, and sodas. The best choices are water and green tea. Researchers have found that sipping soft drinks all day will add at least 10 pounds (5 kg) of body weight a year.

7. *Focus on whole foods.* Most dietary intake should come from whole foods. There are a few times when supplement drinks and shakes are useful; however, most of the time, whole, largely unprocessed foods are best for nutrition and weight control.

8. *Break the rules by 10%.* Optimal progress does not require 100% nutritional discipline. The difference between 90% adherence and 100% adherence to your nutrition program is negligible when maintaining healthy nutrition and weight control. So, 10% of the time you can allow yourself fun foods and drinks that break the rules. For example, if you're eating 6 meals per day for 7 days of the week, that's 42 meals, and 10% of 42 is about 4. Therefore, you're allowed to break the rules during 4 meals each week.

9. *Develop food preparation strategies.* The most challenging part about eating well is making sure you can follow the previous eight rules consistently. This is where preparation becomes important. Even knowing what to eat may not result in eating properly if the right foods are not available; you will fail to eat correctly without planning ahead.

10. *Balance daily food choices with healthy variety.* People who are busy or have low incomes will not spend much time preparing gourmet meals. A list of tasty, easy-to-make foods will be needed. However, once a day or a few times a week we all need to eat something that's different and tasty to stave off boredom and stagnation.

*The information presented here is not intended as medical advice or as a substitute for medical counseling. The information should be used in conjunction with the guidance and care of your physician. Consult your physician before beginning any meal program as you would with any exercise and nutrition program. If you choose not to obtain the consent of your physician or work with your physician while following the recommendations in the program, you are agreeing to accept full responsibility for your actions.

SUMMARY

Much of what has been reported in this chapter requires support from mental health professionals such as licensed psychologists, licensed professional counselors, or social workers, people who have been certified to provide counseling by the state in which they have a professional practice. There are other areas, however, that require a coach, or consultant, who need not be licensed in the area of mental health (Dunford, 2006). For example, registered dietitians and fitness coaches both play an important role—dietitians help clients regulate food intake and fitness coaches help them plan and carry out action plans that incorporate proper physical activity choices, schedules, and content. Exercise and nutrition are firmly grounded in scientific research that validates the correct ways to maintain a healthy lifestyle. This literature must be known and applied when certified fitness coaches and registered dietitians work with clients. People who want to improve their fitness, develop healthy dietary habits, and learn other desirable lifestyle strategies would do well to invest both time and financial resources in the opportunity to work with experts in these areas—at least until they gain the proper skills and information.

STUDENT ACTIVITY

Managing Emotional Eating

Do you eat for emotional reasons rather than in response to physical hunger? Does someone you know eat impulsively, particularly high-fat or salty foods? Perform the actions in the following list or help a family member or friend do them (Wansink, 2006) in attempting to control emotional eating.

- Recognize emotional eating and learn what triggers this behavior in you.
- Make a list of things to do when you get the urge to eat and you're not hungry, and carry the list with you. When you feel overwhelmed, you can put off the desire to eat by replacing eating with another enjoyable activity.
- Try taking a walk, calling a friend, playing cards, cleaning, doing laundry, taking a nap, or doing something productive to take your mind off the craving.
- When you get the urge to eat when you're not hungry and you can't distract yourself, find a comfort food that's healthy instead of junk food. Comfort foods do not need to be unhealthy.
- For some, leaving comfort foods behind when dieting can be emotionally difficult. The key to controlling the intake of comfort foods is moderation, not elimination. Try dividing comfort foods into smaller portions; for instance, if you have a large bag of chips, divide it into smaller containers or baggies. Then the temptation to eat more than one serving can be avoided.
- Your memory of a particular food peaks after about four bites. Therefore, if you only have those few bites, you'll remember it as just as good of an experience and consume far fewer calories than if you polished off the whole serving. So have a few bites of cheesecake and then call it quits and put the rest away for another time. You'll get the same amount of pleasure at a lower cost and fewer calories.
- Last, remember that emotional eating is something that most people do when they're bored, happy, or sad. It might be a bag of chips or a steak, but whatever the food choice, learning how to control your eating and using moderation are key.

After three weeks of staying in intermittent contact with your client or monitoring your own thought and behavior patterns, did food consumption change? Did you (or your client) change the way you thought about food? How often did you detect emotional eating? Did self-awareness of this eating pattern result in changed food consumption?

REFERENCES

Adriaanse, M.A., de Ridder, D.T.D., and Evers, C. (2011). Emotional eating: Eating when emotional or emotional about eating? *Psychology and Health, 26,* 23-39.

American Dietetic Association (ADA). (2005). Practice paper of the American Dietetic Association: Dietary supplements. *Journal of the American Dietetic Association, 105,* 460-470.

American Dietetic Association (ADA). (2009). Position of the American Dietetic Association: Weight management. *Journal of the American Dietetic Association, 109,* 330-346.

American Psychiatric Association (APA). (2000). *Diagnostic and Statistical Manual of Mental Disorders (DSM-IV-R)* (4th ed. rev.). Washington, DC: Author.

Anshel, M.H. (2004). Sources of disordered eating patterns between ballet dancers and non-dancers. *Journal of Sport Behavior, 27,* 114-124.

Beals, K., and Houtkooper, L. (2006). Disordered eating in athletes. In L. Burke and V. Deakin (Eds.), *Clinical Sports Nutrition* (pp. 201-226). New York: McGraw-Hill.

Brewer, B.W., and Petrie, T.A. (2002). Psychopathology in sport and exercise. In J.L. Van Raalte and B.W. Brewer, *Exploring sport and exercise psychology* (2nd ed., pp. 307-323). Washington, DC: American Psychological Association.

Brooks-Gunn, J., Burrow, C., and Warren, M. (1988). Attitudes toward eating and body weight in different groups of female adolescent athletes. *International Journal of Eating Disorders, 7,* 749-757.

Brooks-Gunn, J., Warren, M., and Hamilton, L. (1987). The relation of eating problems and amenorrhea in ballet dancers. *Medicine and Science in Sport and Exercise, 19,* 41-44.

Brownell, K., Rodin, J., and Wilmore, J. (1992). *Eating, body weight and performance in athletes: Disorders of modern society.* Philadelphia, London: Lea and Febiger.

Burke, L. (2007). *Practical sports nutrition.* Champaign, IL: Human Kinetics.

Burke, L., and Deakin, V. (2006). *Clinical sports nutrition.* New York: McGraw-Hill.

Clough, M., and Wilson, B. (1993). The relationship between eating disorder characteristics and perfectionism among 22 dance students 17-21 years. *Sport Health, 11,* 5-8.

Cohen, J., Potosnak, L., Frank, O., and Baker, H. (1985). A nutritional and hematologic assessment of elite ballet dancers. *Physician and Sportsmedicine, 13,* 43-52.

Cohen, J., Segal, K., Witriol, I., and McArdle, W. (1982). Cardiorespiratory responses to ballet exercise and the $\dot{V}O_2$ max of elite ballet dancers. *Medicine and Science in Sports and Exercise, 14,* 212-217.

Druss, R., and Silverman, J. (1979). Body image and perfectionism of ballerinas: Comparison and contrast with anorexia nervosa. *General Hospital Psychiatry, 1,* 115-121.

Dunford, M. (2006). *Sports nutrition: A practice manual for professionals* (4th ed.). Chicago: American Dietetic Association.

Garner, D., and Garfinkel, P. (1980). Socio-cultural factors in the development of anorexia nervosa. *Psychological Medicine, 10,* 647-656.

Garner, D., Olmsted, M., Davis, R., Rockert, W., Goldbloom, D., and Eagle, M. (1990). The association between bulimic symptoms and reported psychopathology. *International Journal of Eating Disorders, 9,* 1-15.

Hamilton, L., Brooks-Gunn, J., and Warren, M. (1985). Sociocultural influences on eating disorders in professional female ballet dancers. *International Journal of Eating Disorders, 4,* 465-477.

Harrison, K. and Cantor, J. (1997). The relationship between media consumption and eating disorders. *Journal of Communication, 7,* 40-67.

Heinberg, L.J., Thompson, J.K., and Matzon, J.L. (2001). Body image dissatisfaction as a motivator for healthy lifestyle change: Is some distress beneficial? In R.J. Stiegel-Moore and L. Smolak (Eds.), *Eating disorders: Innovative directions in research and practice* (pp. 215-232). Washington, DC: American Psychological Association.

Henry, R., Anshel, M.H., and Michael, T. (2006). Effects of aerobic and circuit training on fitness and body image among women. *Journal of Sport Behavior, 29,* 281-303.

Hergenroeder, A., Fiorotto, M., and Klish, W. (1991). Body composition in ballet dancers measured by total body electrical conductivity. *Medicine and Science in Sports and Exercise, 23,* 528-533.

Herzog, D.B., and Delinsky, S.S. (2001). Classification of eating disorders. In R.H. Striegel-Moore and L. Smolak (Eds.), *Eating disorders: Innovative directions in research and practice* (pp. 31-50). Washington, DC: American Psychological Association.

Johnson, A., Steinberg, R., and Lewis, W. (1988). Bulimia. In K. Clark, R. Parr, and W. Castelli (Eds.),

Evaluation and management of eating disorders, anorexia, bulimia and obesity (pp. 187-227). Champaign, IL: Life Enhancement.

Koball, A.M., Meers, M.R., Storfer-Isser, A., Domoff, S.E., and Musher-Eizenman, D.R. (2012). Eating when bored: Revision of the Emotional Eating Scale with a focus on boredom. *Health Psychology, 31*, 521-524.

Lamarche, L., and Gammage, K.L. (2012). Predicting exercise and eating behaviors from appearance evaluation and two types of investment. *Sport, Exercise, and Performance Psychology, 1*, 145-157.

National Institutes of Health (NIH). (1998, September). Clinical guidelines on the identification, evaluation, and treatment of overweight and obesity in adults: The Evidence Report. NIH Publication No. 98-4083. Washington, DC: National Heart, Lung, and Blood Institute.

O'Dea, J. (2002). Can body image education programs be harmful to adolescent females? *Eating Disorders: Journal of Treatment and Prevention, 10*, 1-13.

O'Neil, P.M., and Rieder, S. (2005). The multidisciplinary team in the management of obesity. In D.J. Goldstein (Ed.), *The management of eating disorders and obesity* (2nd ed., pp. 355-366). Totowa, NJ: Humana Press.

Otten, J., Hellwig, J., and Meyers, L. (Eds.). 2006). *Dietary reference intakes: The essential guide to nutrient requirements.* Washington, DC: National Academies Press.

Pinaguy, S., Chabrol, H., Simon, C., Louvet, J.-P., and Barbe, P. (2003). Emotional eating, alexithymia, and binge-eating disorder in obese women. *Obesity Research, 11*, 195-201.

Reel, J.J., and Gill, D.L. (1996). Psychosocial factors related to eating disorders among high school and college female cheerleaders. *Sport Psychologist, 10*, 195-206.

Rodin, J., Silberstein, L.R., and Striegel-Moore, R.H. (1985). Women and weight: A normative discontent. In T.B. Sonderegger (Ed.), *Psychology and gender: Nebraska Symposium on motivation* (pp. 267-307). Lincoln, NE: University of Nebraska Press.

Striegel-Moore, R.H., and Smolak, L. (2001). Conclusion: Imagining the future. *Eating disorders: Innovative directions in research and practice* (pp. 271-278). Washington, DC: American Psychological Association.

Sundgot-Borgen, J., and Torstveit, M.K. (2004). Prevalence of eating disorders in elite athletes is higher than in the general population. *Clinical Journal of Sport Medicine, 14*, 25-32.

Thompson, R.A., and Sherman, R.T. (2010). *Eating disorders in sport.* New York: Routledge.

Thomsen, S.R., Weber, M.M., and Brown, L.B. (2001). The relationship between health and fitness magazine reading and eating-disordered weight-loss methods among high school girls. *American Journal of Health Education, 32*, 133-138.

Van den Buick, J. (2000). Is television bad for your health? Behavior and body image of the adolescent "couch potato." *Journal of Youth and Adolescence, 29*, 273-281.

Wansink, B. (2006). *Mindless eating—why we eat more than we think.* New York: Bantam-Dell.

Wein, D., and Micheli, L. (2002). Nutrition, eating disorders, and the female athlete triad. In D.L. Mostofsky and L.D. Zaichkowsky (Eds.), *Medical and psychological aspects of sport and exercise* (pp. 91-111). Morgantown, WV: Fitness Information Technology.

Whitnesy, E., and Rady-Rolfes, S. (2004). *Understanding nutrition* (10th ed.). New York: Thompson/Wadsworth.

Williams, M. (2006). *Nutrition for health, fitness, and sport* (5th ed.). New York: McGraw-Hill.

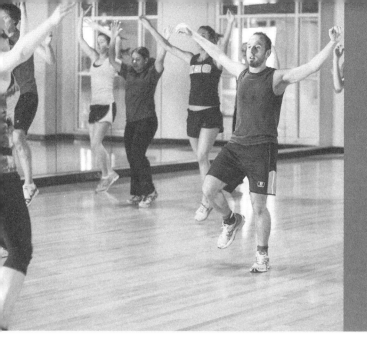

CHAPTER 13

Professional Organizations and Ethics

66 *There is no passion to be found playing small, in settling for a life that is less than* 99
the one you are capable of living.

Nelson Mandela, 11th president of South Africa

CHAPTER OBJECTIVES

After reading this chapter, you should be able to:

- identify the names, mission, and websites of the many organizations related to health fitness psychology;

- explain the meaning, purpose, and content of an organization's code of ethics;

- list the ethical issues that are common in most professional organizations;

- identify the ways in which health fitness psychology is affiliated with the fields of sport science and psychology;

- define *credentialing* and differentiate among the subprocesses of credentialing called *licensure*, *certification*, and *registry*; and

- describe employment opportunities that reflect training and education in health fitness psychology.

This chapter describes the means by which fields of study and practice related to health fitness psychology are recognized and represented by a group of uniquely educated and skilled professionals. Professional organizations exist to provide structure, growth, and state-of-the-art knowledge through conferences and publications. The document that provides guidance and governance for a profession in working settings is called the *code of ethics*. An ethics code provides integrity and structure to the values and standards of a profession, and it fosters public trust by establishing high standards (Whelan, Meyers, and Elkins, 2002). Although no code of conduct or set of ethical guidelines can account for all possible situations or ethical dilemmas, an ethical code is intended to regulate the conduct of organization members (Pauline et al., 2006). Professional organizations represent well-defined areas of expertise, research, and practice. Codes of ethics allow organizations to grow and to represent a field of professional expertise.

Professional organizations related to health fitness psychology represent psychology, such as the American Psychological Association (APA); sport and exercise psychology, such as the Association for Applied Sport Psychology (AASP), European Federation of Sport Psychology (FEPSAC), and British Association of Sport and Exercise Science (BASES); sports medicine, such as the American College of Sports Medicine (ACSM); behavioral medicine, such as the Society of Behavioral Medicine (SBM); and health, such as the American College Health Association (ACHA). Each of these organizations has subspecialty memberships or interest groups in the area of exercise or fitness.

Thus, the field of applied health fitness psychology is represented by five professional areas: psychology, sport and exercise psychology, sports medicine, behavioral medicine, and health. Each of these areas is represented by organizations that promote each field of expertise. Ways to promote and recognize the skills of organization members is the process called *credentialing*. Credentialing ensures that members of a profession meet predetermined and published standards. The processes that regulate these procedures are called *licensure*, *certification*, and *registry* and will be described later.

PROFESSIONAL ORGANIZATIONS

Professional organizations have the enormously important role of defining and promoting the growth, development, and recognition of an area of expertise that requires education and professional experience. Perhaps the organization that is recognized by health professionals throughout the world as the leading authority on health and fitness from both physiological and psychological perspectives is the American College of Sports Medicine (ACSM; www.acsm.org). Perhaps this is why ACSM is among the organizations that are relatively active in applied health fitness psychology. The main objective of ACSM is to support and promote health and fitness through research, education, and practice. ACSM is viewed as a superb resource for mental health professionals concerning issues related to exercise, fitness, and health.

In 2003, ACSM created a code of ethics that includes its primary mission of generating and disseminating knowledge about all aspects of the exerciser (ACSM, 2010). There are four components of the code:

1. Striving to improve and disseminate to the public knowledge and skill about the benefits of their professional expertise

2. Maintaining high professional and scientific standards and not collaborating with people who violate these standards

3. Safeguarding the public and ACSM against members who are deficient in ethical conduct

4. Improving the health and well-being of individuals, the community, and society

The American Psychological Association (APA; www.apa.org) forms another substantial professional body that represents the academic qualifications and professional standards for health fitness psychology. Divisions 38 (Health Psychology), 47 (Exercise and Sport Psychology), and 13 (Society of Consulting Psychology) are particularly relevant to the field.

Fitness psychology is also compatible with the growth of information technology. Discussing professional issues, accessing recent articles and events, finding job placements, and seeking professional advice or assistance have become increasingly popular and simplified in recent years with online services that are accessible nationally and internationally. In addition to CD-ROM library search programs (e.g., PsychLit, Sportsdisc), Listservs such as sportpsy@listserv.temple.edu provide opportunities to interact through e-mail with other students, practitioners, researchers, and educators sharing information or debating various issues.

The link between health fitness psychology and psychology is also strong in Canada (www.scapps.org), Europe (e.g., Britain, France, Germany, Ireland, Greece, Portugal, Italy), Australia, New Zealand, and Asia (e.g., China, India, Philippines, South Korea, Thailand, Singapore) as well as in international organizations (e.g., International Society of Sport Psychology, www.issponline.org; Society of Behavioral Medicine, www.sbm.org). Many countries have sport and exercise psychology organizations, conferences, and publications (written in their national language, although abstracts are usually published in English) that serve practitioners and researchers. These organizations give members an opportunity to communicate their research experiences, exchange ideas, hear and interact with established practitioners whose work in sport and exercise behavior is well known, discuss and perhaps generate guidelines or policies about controversial issues, and bring back new and exciting ideas to their programs, classes, and state or regional organizations.

Another advocate of exercise and wellness since 1920 is the American College Health Association (ACHA; www.acha.org), which is associated with college health professionals throughout the United States and internationally, forming a powerful, collaborative network. According to its mission statement, ACHA provides advocacy, education, communications, products, and services as well as promotes research and culturally competent practices to enhance the ability of members to advance the health of all students and the campus community. Improved fitness forms one of the primary objectives of this organization.

The *American Journal of Health Promotion* (www.healthpromotionjournal.com), a peer-reviewed publication devoted exclusively to health promotion since 1986, provides a forum through its annual Art and Science of Health Promotion Conference for the diverse disciplines that contribute to health promotion. According to the website of the conference (www.healthpromotionconference.org), one of its goals is to reduce the gap between health promotion research and practice by delivering the most current and relevant research in the field while addressing its practical application.

The Association for Applied Sport Psychology (AASP; www.appliedsportpsych.org), founded in 1986, promotes the ethical practice, science, and advocacy of sport and exercise psychology. AASP is an international, multidisciplinary, professional organization that offers certification to qualified professionals in sport, exercise, and health psychology. The *health and exercise psychology* component of this organization focuses on the application of psychological principles to promote and maintain health-enhancing behaviors over the life span (e.g., play, leisure, physical activity, structured exercise) and the psychological and emotional consequences of those behaviors. Researchers in this area also investigate the role of exercise in disease remediation, injury rehabilitation, and stress reduction.

The North American Society for Psychology of Sport and Physical Activity (NASPSPA; www.naspspa.org) develops and advances the scientific study and practice of motor behavior (development, learning, and control) and sport and exercise psychology. The association also facilitates the dissemination of information and improves the quality of research and teaching in these disciplines.

Various other organizations in the United States have direct and indirect links to the mission of improving fitness and developing an exercise habit. These organizations include the American College of Lifestyle Medicine, American College of Preventive Medicine, Wellness Council of America, and American School Health Association.

Table 13.1 summarizes the main organizations that promote the combination of health, fitness, and psychology.

There is a clear political and philosophical battle for territory and ownership in representing the field, but ACSM is gaining recognition and credibility as the primary organization that oversees the field of exercise psychology. It has clearly taken the lead in promoting educational requirements and developing policy in recognizing exercise psychology as a reputable field of training, research, and practice.

Arguments in favor of one field having a greater identification with exercise psychology over another field are beyond the scope of this section. There are two fields of study, or academic disciplines, that have valid claims on maintaining a strong influence on the development of exercise psychology. One area is sport science, which includes physical education, exercise science, health and human performance, kinesiology, human movement, and others. The second discipline is psychology.

Neither field is going to be the sole representative of exercise psychology. There is much to be said for the fact that both disciplines bring to the field complementary needs and skills. Examining how each discipline contributes to the growth and development of health fitness psychology reveals the importance of bringing together both disciplines in an effort to provide the best quality of education, research, and practice of the field, and it reveals how exercise science and psychology have their own unique features that are needed by athletes, exercisers, dancers, actors, rehabilitation patients, law enforcement officers, and others who want to improve some aspect of human performance. Neither discipline has a monopoly on the truth, but following is an attempt to accurately represent the best interests of each.

Affiliation With Sport Science

Exercise psychology is being taken seriously by the academic community, but there remains controversy, sometimes contentiousness, concerning which academic discipline should

Table 13.1 Professional Organizations That Promote Health Fitness Psychology

Organization	Purpose
American College of Sports Medicine (ACSM)	World's largest sports medicine and exercise science organization
Association for Applied Sport Psychology (AASP)	Promotes research and practice in examining personal and situational factors that influence sport performance, and to a lesser degree, exercise
American Psychological Association (APA)	Promotes understanding (through research and practice) of the psychological factors that influence health and human performance
European Federation of Sport Psychology (FEPSAC)	Comprises European organizations that promote sport and exercise, such as the British Association of Sport and Exercise Sciences (BASES) and the German Association of Sport Psychology (ASP)
Society of Behavioral Medicine (SBM)	Examines relationships among the psychobehavioral factors that influence health, illness, behavior, and performance
International Society of Sport Psychology (ISSP)	Promotes factors that lead to excellent performance in exercise and sport
North American Society for Psychology of Sport and Physical Activity (NASPSPA)	Promotes theoretical and applied research and practice of concepts that improve understanding of the relationship between mental processes and performance outcomes

govern the education, training, and practice of fitness psychology students, researchers, and practitioners. Exercise psychology has also received increased attention in recent years by professional organizations. The APA, AASP, and ACSM all have active missions and programs in the area of exercise psychology. As indicated earlier, exercise psychology focuses on cognitive, psychophysiological, and situational factors that influence exercise behavior (see Anshel, 2006; Buckworth and Dishman, 2002; Lox, Martin Ginis, and Petruzzello, 2010; and Watson, Zizzi, and Etzel, 2006, for reviews of this emerging field).

Examples of topics studied in this area include effects of physical activity on the exerciser's emotions (e.g., arousal, anxiety, mood state) and certain psychological dispositions (e.g., confidence, depression, self-esteem), reasons why some people engage in exercise programs while others do not, positive and negative addiction to exercise, factors that influence an exerciser's perceived exertion, the effect of exercise on preventing or treating mental illness (e.g., depression, irrational thinking, low self-esteem), the effects of cognitive strategies (i.e., mental skills) on exercise performance (e.g., association, dissociation, psyching up, positive self-talk), the influence of cognitive and behavioral interventions on exercise adherence, and other topics.

A perusal of the *Directory of Graduate Programs in Applied Sport Psychology* (Sachs, Burke, and Schweighardt, 2011) clearly indicates that sport and exercise science (e.g., departments of physical education, kinesiology, human movement, or health and human performance) is the primary area from which exercise psychology programs are offered, almost always in conjunction with sport psychology. It is the rare psychology department that includes a course or specialization in exercise or sport psychology. This is understandable, given the strict requirements of psychology departments in order to have a program approved by the APA. In most states, psychologists can be licensed only if they graduate with a PhD from an APA-approved program. Often, there is simply no opportunity to complete

additional courses (i.e., electives) beyond those needed for licensure or meeting other program requirements. The result is that few graduate students in psychology ever complete a course in sport or exercise psychology, and full programs that specialize in this content area are rare.

Not surprisingly, sport and exercise psychology courses consist primarily of graduate students from departments of exercise and sport science (rather than psychology departments) who complete internships and practica to develop skills in exercise and sport psychology. Further testimony to the origins of sport psychology comes from the sport psychology literature, which widely acknowledges the father of sport psychology, Dr. Coleman Griffith, a professor of physical education (Anshel, 2012). It is apparent, then, that exercise science and physical education educators and researchers are the founders of this field.

Members of the exercise science field recognize the importance of providing appropriate interventions based on the development and mastery of requisite skills and knowledge. They contend that the practice of exercise psychology clearly warrants a level of sophistication that goes beyond traditional training in psychology.

Affiliation With Psychology

Health psychology has been an active part of the academic community and a field within the discipline of psychology for many years. The APA, which has over 50 divisions, or specialization areas, admitted Division 38, Health Psychology, in 1978, and started publishing the journal *Health Psychology* in 1982 (Matarazzo, 1982).

Anshel (2012) provides four points that justify the field of psychology as the primary caretaker of exercise and sport psychology. First, the legal title of *psychologist*, as in using the title *exercise psychologist* or *performance psychologist*, is governed by the field of psychology. Second, the status of licensure that allows clinicians, counselors, and therapists to receive third-party payments (i.e., paid by the client's health insurance) is also governed by psychology. Third, education and training in counseling or clinical psychology consist of developing the skills needed to administer and interpret psychological tests that are available only to licensed mental health professionals, who are trained specifically for this purpose. And, fourth, only psychologists may conduct various forms of psychotherapy with their clients. Just a few of the psychological issues that occur in applied health fitness psychology include emotional eating, social physique anxiety (i.e., feeling anxious about one's physical appearance), chronic depression or anxiety, sleeplessness, and irrational thinking (e.g., "I do not deserve to be fit, healthy, or more attractive").

The decision to pursue graduate training in sport and exercise psychology should be primarily determined by one's professional aspirations. If the student plans on an academic career, then the sport and exercise sciences are more likely to have courses in sport and exercise psychology and therefore require an academically trained person to teach and supervise graduate students in this area. If, however, private practice is the goal, then the student should follow the road to licensure as a psychologist, obtaining the academic credentials needed to enter a graduate program in psychology. People with an academic background in the exercise or sport sciences will not be eligible to enter a graduate program in psychology unless they complete several prerequisite courses in psychology.

The sport and exercise science professional will be financially compensated not by third-party payments but by clients' personal payments. This means two things, according to Anshel (2012). First, payment for services rendered by the licensed mental health professional will be partly supported by a third party,

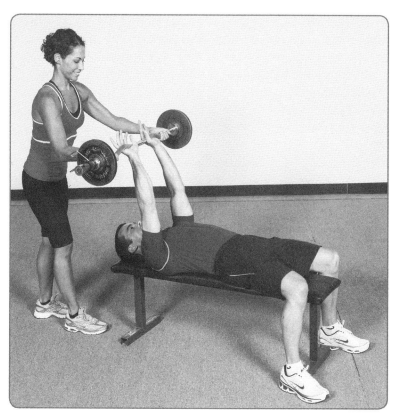

Nonlicensed consultants should not engage in any form of client psychological counseling or psychotherapy but instead restrict their techniques to enhancing exercise performance.

the client's insurance policy, whereas service provided by a nonlicensed professional will require the client to pay the full consultation fee out of pocket. Second, licensure means that the psychologist can be covered by an insurance policy—a requirement to guard against possible lawsuits. Practice insurance is almost always required in order to engage in any form of counseling, although each state and country has its own guidelines, policies, and laws. In addition, nonlicensed consultants may not engage in any form of counseling or psychotherapy because they do not have the proper educational background and legal recognition. The content of their services is restricted to performance enhancement techniques.

CREDENTIALING

Every area of professional practice and expertise requires certain skills and standards that must be published, disseminated to the public, and demonstrated. The process that ensures that members of a profession meet predetermined and published standards is called *credentialing*. Subcomponents of credentialing are licensure, certification, and registry processes.

Licensure is a restrictive legal process designed to regulate the behavior of an organization's members. *Certification* is a nonlegal classification carried out by an organization and is typical of most professional organizations. *Registry* is another nonlegal certification classification indicating recognition of professional status and an expected level of competence.

BASES, a British organization, includes a credentialing process called *accreditation* for providing services as a sport psychology consultant. According to its website (www.bases.org.uk), the BASES credentialing program includes supervised experience, the purpose of which is to provide sport and exercise scientists with the guidance, environment, and opportunities to facilitate the development of the competencies expected for accreditation. For a young practitioner, supervised experience is a key stepping-stone to a career in sport and exercise science.

In addition, as cited on its website, all BASES members must adhere to a strict code of conduct. Violation of this code can result in sanctions, including removal of accreditation. The code of conduct ensures a minimum level of service to individuals or groups who make use of the services offered by sport and exercise scientists. BASES accreditation is awarded to those practitioners who are deemed by the association to have the minimum knowledge, skills, and understanding necessary to practice as a sport and exercise scientist. Members may achieve accreditation as a result of work in applied sport or exercise science support, research, or pedagogy. In all cases the process and the judgment of knowledge, skills, and professional practice will apply, although how these are expressed will differ.

Credentialing in Australia is handled through the Australian Psychological Society (APS). According to its website (www.psychology.org.au), the APS College of Sport and Exercise Psychologists is a professional association of psychologists who are inter-

ested in how participation in sport, exercise, and physical activity may enhance personal development and well-being throughout the life span. The APS College of Sport and Exercise Psychologists develops and safeguards the standards of practice and supervised experience. It sets the quality of service in sport and exercise psychology, and it advises and makes recommendations regarding the education and training of sport and exercise psychologists. In addition, it acts as a focal point for consumer and other general inquiries relating to sport and exercise.

The APS website offers specializations in the following areas: performance enhancement and mental skills development; anxiety and stress management; concentration and mental preparation; overtraining and burnout; team building and leadership; communication skills and conflict resolution; health and wellness coaching; weight management; debriefing and program evaluation; recovery and restoration; injury rehabilitation; psychological assessment; video analysis of sport emotions and performances; balancing of sport, study, employment, and family life; career transitions (for example, layoffs and retirement); and coping with grief and loss.

Licensure

Licensure bestows a particular status that includes an achieved level of education, successful passing of at least two examinations, government and legal recognition, insurance reimbursement to practitioners, and entitlement to use the title *psychologist*. In the most basic terms, people must be licensed to advertise, market, and use the title of *psychologist* in the state (and country) in which they practice. Countries, states, and provinces vary in their requirements for licensure; however, one standard that remains consistent is receiving a doctorate from the psychology department of a university that has a clinical or counseling program that has been approved by the APA. The specific components of an APA-approved program are beyond the scope of this chapter; however, doctoral students who seek this credential must complete extensive coursework and field supervision by a licensed psychologist and must pass two examinations, the Examination for Professional Practice in Psychology (EPPP) and the jurisprudence exam concerned with ethics and the law. Additionally, each state has its own criteria for achieving licensure (e.g., required number of hours of field supervision and internship).

There is one important exception to the policies that surround licensure. Employees (e.g., professors, instructors, coaches) of an educational institution (e.g., university, college, secondary education) who engage in exercise psychology coaching exclusively within the confines of the institution's athletic program and do not advertise their services to the public in the community may also use the title of *fitness psychologist*.

In sum, the title *psychologist* is legally protected. Only licensed psychologists may refer to themselves as a *sport psychologist, health psychologist, fitness psychologist*, or *exercise psychologist*. This statutory process is understandable given the client's reliance on expertise in addressing mental health issues and the potential harm and legal liability that can occur in the absence of mastery over treatment interventions and quality care.

Licensed clinical psychologists may use the title *health psychologist* when they have attained a particular level of education and expertise. They practice psychology in health-related settings, such as hospitals and rehabilitation centers, and address the influence of thought patterns, emotions, and other psychological factors on health or illness. There is also a graduate degree, professional practice, and credential called *licensed professional counselor (LPC)* that requires licensure and may receive insurance payments.

If the title *psychologist* is legally protected, what titles are available for nonpsychologists? Are the titles *coach* or *consultant* available? What are the ethical boundaries of practice in the emerging field of health fitness psychology? Does a health psychologist require specific knowledge and expertise in the area of exercise science? Should this person be able to provide fitness tests and prescribe exercise programs to clients?

The answers to these questions form a gray area—an absence of certainty, final decisions, and consistency in all geographical areas. In addition to the EPPP examination and the jurisprudence exam concerned with ethics and the law, each state has its own rules and its own licensure board to arbitrate who may become or remain licensed, so there are exceptions to these criteria. For instance, the LPC is a licensed mental health professional who may also obtain third-party payments and reimbursements from insurance companies and from the government. However, only earning a doctoral degree (PhD) will allow a person to use the title *psychologist*, including *exercise psychologist*, whereas the LPC only requires a master's degree.

Some professionals in exercise science prefer to avoid the title *psychologist* due to the public perception that people who see a psychologist have mental problems (sometimes viewed as a sign of weakness or personal problems). Visiting a psychologist is threatening for many people. Alternative titles include *coach, consultant*, and *trainer*. Specific examples include *fitness coach, personal trainer, mental skills coach, performance coach* or *consultant, life skills coach*, and *performance counselor*. There are many mental health issues, however, that require the education and training of a licensed psychologist or LPC.

Many people who represent themselves as health, fitness, or exercise psychologists have never taken a course in exercise science, read a book on the psychology of fitness or exercise, or mastered the relevant literature. On the other hand, there are people with expertise in exercise science who market themselves as exercise psychologists but lack the credential of licensure and are not able to conduct mental health counseling, also called *psychotherapy*. Is carrying out mental health counseling when not properly credentialed an unethical act or a misrepresentation of the person's skills? Providing services for which one is not properly trained may result in litigation, either by a professional organization or by the client.

TITLING ETHICS

Who, if anyone, should own health fitness psychology? Is the answer dependent on the open market? Is it the person who delivers the most effective service? What professional organizations best represent this area of study and practice? The answers to these questions are unknown, because health fitness psychology is a relatively new and emerging area of study and expertise. What is known, however, is that a variety of organizations (e.g., AASP, APA, SBM) all have the strengths, knowledge, expertise, marketing skills, credentials, and motivation to make a valuable contribution to the health and well-being of others and to change the culture that maintains unhealthy behavior patterns.

Still, as in all areas of academic and practice, ethics are imperative. For example, earlier we discussed the title *psychologist*. The rule is clear: If practitioners are not legally recognized as psychologists, they may not use this title to describe the service they provide. Does this mean that psychologists who possess expertise and knowledge in sport psychology may refer to themselves as *sport*

psychologists? Yes, under either of two conditions: They are licensed psychologists, or they practice sport psychology in an educational institution such as a college. However, nonpsychologists who work with athletes can use other titles, such as *mental skills coach*, *performance coach*, and *sport psychology consultant*.

Sachs (1993) warns against claiming to have expertise in areas in which the person is untrained and inexperienced. He contends that "just as psychologists trained in marital and family counseling would not ethically note themselves as having expertise in substance abuse counseling (unless, of course, they were trained in this area), psychologists who do not have training in exercise and sport should not be calling themselves 'sport psychologists'" (p. 922). Although many licensed psychologists may be excellent clinicians or counselors, sport psychology may not be within their field of expertise. As Sachs notes, "Clinical or counseling excellence does not necessarily transfer to the exercise [fitness/health] and sport setting" (p. 922).

Certification

This credential reflects the completion of certain criteria in order to represent a level of education, training, and expertise in carrying out a specific service. AASP, for example, offers its members the opportunity to use the title *certified consultant of the Association for Applied Sport Psychology (CC-AASP)* if they have completed specific educational courses and a specific number of hours of supervision by another CC-AASP. Athletes, parents, coaches, or anyone else who wishes to use the services of a CC-AASP may consult a registry of people who have met the criteria to provide an expected level of service to the client. The criteria include attending a minimum number of AASP conferences, completing at least 400 hours of supervised practical experience, and submitting three professional reference letters. In addition, many university programs and mental health professionals in private practice provide internships that allow aspiring consultants to receive supervised experience

working with clients and developing consultation skills. The consultant may or may not be a licensed psychologist, which would be an issue only if the client were seeking psychotherapy due to a psychopathological problem (e.g., suicidal thoughts, low self-esteem, substance abuse or addictive behaviors) that required a licensed psychologist.

Training and experience often dictate what we do and how we do it. Trained psychologists, therefore, rely on their clinical training in providing mental health services and coaching in the area of fitness, and exercise or fitness psychology consultants with a sport science background rely on their mental skills training. The required knowledge, credentials, and skills to provide psychological services to various populations are still being debated by scholars, writers, and practitioners. Current law in the United States posits that any licensed psychologist can claim to be a sport psychologist even though that person may never have taken a course in sport psychology or experienced athletic competition directly.

On the other hand, people trained in the sport sciences but not in educated and trained in psychology can refer to themselves by other titles that exclude the term *psychologist*, such as *sport psychology consultant*, *mental skills coach*, and *sport performance consultant*.

Registry

Part of the credentialing process in most organizations is called *registry*, a nonstatutory (i.e., not governed by law) credentialing procedure that indicates professional recognition. For example, a sport psychologist who has a position with the United States Olympic Team is expected to qualify for the United States Olympic Committee (USOC) Sports Psychology Registry. This entails being a CC-AASP and a member of the APA.

The benefits of registry include restricting membership of a group or organization to people who possess the specific background, experience, and skills that reflect a particular profession or area of expertise. Consumers of a particular service expect that professionals who represent that service possess the requisite skills needed to successfully address and resolve issues. Clients should feel they are obtaining professional consultation with an expert who is properly trained in dealing with and solving problems. Registry regulates the inclusion and exclusion process by ensuring that anyone who represents the field of training and practice possesses the proper competencies. Organizations who have registries include the APA, the American Nurses Association (ANA), ACSM, and the American Medical Association (AMA).

EMPLOYMENT OPPORTUNITIES

Employment opportunities for people with expertise in health fitness psychology often depend on the individual's previous education; qualifications, particularly with respect to credentialing; work experience; and professional aspirations. The person's undergraduate major will help determine the type of employment for which the person is skilled, qualified, and eligible. Someone with aspirations to be a university professor and researcher would need to obtain a doctorate, either in psychology or exercise science (often depending on the person's undergraduate major). A person who prefers to work as a practitioner can become a mental health professional (e.g., licensed psychologist, LPC, therapist), exercise physiologist, or a combination of these. Licensure can include a specialization in health psychology so that the individual is a licensed health psychologist. It is the combination of psychology and exercise science, however, that is currently lacking in the health and fitness area.

A career in fitness psychology requires completed classes in exercise physiology, testing, and prescription. Recreational centers (e.g., YMCA, community centers) and private fitness clubs are two employment options. These jobs usually entail either directly leading exercise classes or supervising others in providing this service. Fitness testing and prescription and the supervision of postcardiac programs (i.e., exercise for patients who have been diagnosed with CVD and require a strictly controlled exercise program) are other program options.

Completing university courses in counseling psychology, health psychology, and sport psychology, preferably at both the undergraduate and graduate levels, would be advisable in order to develop skills in detecting mental illness. This is because mental illness, which should lead to referral to a licensed psychologist, often accompanies dropping out of exercise and reflects self-destructive, unhealthy habits (e.g., overeating, poor sleep, clinical depression and anxiety, low self-esteem). It is safe to assume that fitness professionals need to learn how to detect red flags that suggest a mental health issue and refer that client to a mental health professional.

Other issues that the fitness professional will need to address include exercise motivation, the use of mental skills (also called *cognitive strategies*, discussed in chapter 9) to enhance an exerciser's emotions and performance, and ways to encourage exercise novices and prevent them from dropping out. The ability to render fitness tests and prescribe an individualized exercise program is helpful and establishes a trusting relationship with clients. The exercise specialist should also read books and journals on exercise psychology topics, attend conferences where various topics in this area are studied and communicated through presentations, and interact with fellow professionals in the field.

Mental health professionals or graduate psychology students may also want to enter the field of applied health fitness psychology. They should complete courses in basic and applied exercise physiology (often offered as two separate courses) and exercise testing and prescription, and, if possible, they should complete an internship in an exercise facility under the supervision of two professionals, one who represents exercise physiology and one who represents fitness and health psychology.

People who possess skills in exercise science and mental health consulting offer a specialization that is unique to the community, and many types of professionals, such as medical practitioners, psychologists, rehabilitation therapists, sport coaches, and dietitians, can refer patients or clients to their practice. Given the serious condition of community health, the proliferation of obesity and related type 2 diabetes, and the aging of the population, this area of specialization is needed more than ever before.

PROFESSIONAL ETHICS

Ethics provide the moral component of professional practice, forming a system of principles for a particular code of conduct, particularly related to exercise psychology (Pauline et al., 2006). This code is communicated as a set of guidelines that describe acceptable actions or procedures a person may use to work at a level of expertise that has been predetermined by a professional body, usually a national psychological organization or a state psychology licensure board.

According to Pauline et al. (2006), "An ethics code provides integrity to a profession, professional values and standards, and fosters public trust through the establishment of high standards" (p. 64). As Fisher (2003) points out, a set of ethical guidelines cannot account for all possible situations or ethical dilemmas. Current beliefs and professional standards and practices can change with time, thereby creating changes in ethical codes and standards.

Expanding a field of education, research, and practice, which is one objective of this book in developing a field called *applied health fitness psychology*, requires recognizing certain boundaries of appropriate and ethical behaviors, particularly by practitioners. One ethical concern addressed earlier in the chapter is the use of titles, an issue collectively called *credentialing* (APA, 2002). This section addresses the ethical issues of accountability, performance enhancement, psychological inventories, sensitivity to individual needs, up-to-date knowledge, and referrals.

Accountability

Psychologists are accountable to and must maintain confidentiality with clients. Without client permission, no one obtains information about meeting content, unless—and this is a legal matter—clients express feelings about harming others or themselves (e.g., thoughts of suicide or breaking the law). In that case, the psychologist must notify medical staff, another mental health professional with particular expertise, or law enforcement. Clients must give permission for the consultant or psychologist to reveal meeting-related content to another person, such as the client's physician, fitness coach, insurance company, or family member. Sachs (1993) offers what is probably the safest approach: "Whatever arrangement is entered into must be clearly specified in advance, preferably in writing, and explained and understood by the [client or others]" (p. 923).

Performance Enhancement Techniques

Perhaps among the most debated issues in applied psychology is the extent to which certain techniques are viewed as effective or as evidence-based standard care. The field of applied sport psychology has experienced an abundance of self-proclaimed, exaggerated claims of treatment effectiveness. Some of these claims have been questioned, even from members within the profession (e.g., Landers, 1988; Morgan, 1988; Singer and Anshel, 2006a). Using inventories to measure certain psychological characteristics in exercise settings as a predictor of performance outcomes or exercise adherence is particularly unproven (Watson et al., 2006).

In short, health and fitness psychology practitioners must be prudent about offering conclusive evidence of treatment effectiveness claiming credit for anything about the client's success. In their review of literature, Singer and Anshel (2006a) concluded that "abuses of interventions or claims of beneficial interventions are primarily attributed to those individuals without credentials and formal educational training. Unfortunately, there are many opportunistic entrepreneurs who exaggerate their competencies" (pp. 69-70).

Psychological Inventories

Despite the widespread use of psychological inventories in counseling psychology, researchers (e.g., Schutz and Gessaroli, 1993) and practitioners (e.g., Carlstedt, 2008; Singer and Anshel, 2006b) have questioned the validity and usefulness of scores derived from many of these measures. The use of inventories as part of consulting in exercise settings may include using an inventory without proper knowledge about how to interpret its results or without understanding its intended purpose or the sample for whom it was constructed and validated (Gauvin and Russell, 1993). The client should always retain the right to say to the counselor or coach, "Your interpretation of my score doesn't sound like me. It's off base."

Anshel (2012) suggests answering the following six questions before using an inventory with clients in exercise settings:

1. What are the purpose and goal of using this particular inventory?

2. Is an inventory necessary in this situation?

3. Can the information be obtained from a personal interview instead?

4. Does the inventory have a diagnostic purpose, perhaps to disclose a limitation in some psychological characteristic of the client or to address a particular psychopathology such as depression, chronic anxiety, or neuroticism (Johnsgard, 2004)?

5. How (e.g., in writing, face-to-face meeting) and to whom (e.g., the client, the client's medical care practitioner or mental health professional) will the inventory scores be interpreted and shared?

6. Does the consultant have the credentials—educational, legal, and experiential—to interpret and apply the findings of the inventory in a clinical or consultative setting?

Inventories that are published in research journals must prove they are valid and measure what the researcher intended, a process called *psychometric*, or *statistical*, *validation*. An inventory that is meant for diagnostic purposes (e.g., evidence of low confidence) or predictive purposes (e.g., likelihood of dropping out of the program) will be expected to have greater predictive power and have more extensive statistical proof that it correctly describes, categorizes, or predicts a particular outcome. Consultants should be cautious about the purpose of the inventory and to interpret results correctly. Just because the inventory was published in a scholarly (refereed) journal article does not automatically mean it can provide valid information about a particular client in a counseling or clinical setting. See Sachs (1993) for guidelines for using psychological inventories in exercise and sport settings.

Sensitivity to Individual Needs and Differences

One size does not fit all in the world of applied health fitness psychology. The consultant must take into account the exerciser's personal needs, fitness goals, culture, gender, ethnicity, previous exercise experiences, motives for exercising, attitudes about exercise, preferred versus nonpreferred types of exercise, physical limitations and other health concerns, and expected outcomes (e.g., weight loss, improved fitness, increased energy, ability to play sports). The consultant should be aware of individual differences, try to understand and be sensitive to these differences, and integrate these differences into an effective intervention to improve exercise performance and outcomes. Psychological counseling, or psychotherapy, should not be applied unless the client indicates a clear need for psychological counsel by a mental health professional.

The Need to Update Knowledge

Is it ethical for a doctor to diagnose an illness and then prescribe drugs based on her knowledge from medical school 10 or 20 years ago without consulting recent journals and more current information? A specialist who fails to provide the client with alternative therapies and interventions that reflect state-of-the-art information about the most recent advances in the field may be considered ineffective, or worse, unethical. Applied health fitness psychology is a field of rapidly advancing knowledge. The applied exercise psychology literature consists of studies that test theories and examine the effectiveness of various exercise-related models and interventions related to improving exercise performance and exercise adherence. The applied literature can also generate and validate inventories that describe, explain, or predict exercise performance quality and outcomes.

ASSOCIATION FOR APPLIED SPORT PSYCHOLOGY

The largest organization whose focus is on the development of sport psychology (and, to a lesser extent, exercise psychology) is the Association for Applied Sport Psychology (AASP). According to the AASP ethics code (www.appliedsportpsych. org/about/ethics/code), the purpose of ethical principles and procedures is to ensure "that the profession will regulate itself to do no harm, and to govern itself to ensure the dignity and welfare of individuals we serve and the public . . . and to develop and enforce guidelines that regulate their members' professional conduct. . . . A code of ethical principles and standards guides professionals to act responsibly as they employ the privileges granted by society. A profession's inability to regulate itself violates the public's trust and undermines the profession's potential to be of service to society."

The organization has six principles of ethical conduct (paraphrased here). As the AASP website notes, its ethics code partly reflects the APA ethical principles of psychologists and code of conduct (APA, 1992).

- **Principle A: Competence.** AASP members maintain the highest standards of competence in their work and recognize the boundaries and limitations of their professional competencies and expertise.
- **Principle B: Integrity.** AASP members are honest and fair in promoting integrity in the science, teaching, and practice of their profession. When describing or reporting their qualifications, services, products, fees, research, or teaching, they do not make statements that are false, misleading, or deceptive.
- **Principle C: Professional and scientific responsibility.** AASP members are responsible for safeguarding the public and AASP from members who are deficient in ethical conduct. They uphold professional standards of conduct and accept appropriate responsibility for their behavior.
- **Principle D: Respect for people's rights and dignity.** AASP members respect the rights of individuals to privacy, confidentiality, self-determination, and autonomy, mindful that legal and other obligations may lead to inconsistency and conflict with the exercise of these rights.
- **Principle E: Concern for others' welfare.** AASP members seek to contribute to the welfare of those with whom they interact professionally. When conflicts occur among AASP members' obligations or concerns, they attempt to resolve those conflicts.
- **Principle F: Social responsibility.** AASP members are aware of their professional and scientific responsibilities to the community and to society.

It is also helpful for the health fitness psychology consultant to master fundamental knowledge about ways to properly exercise, improve fitness, and help clients reach their goals and meet their needs. Focusing on mental health alone does not allow the consultant to apply specific strategies (e.g., the motivational effects of goal setting) to attain certain performance outcomes.

Knowing When to Refer

Inherent in consulting ethics is acknowledging the limitations of a consultant's expertise and stating when a client requires the intervention of another consultant or mental health professional whose background and skills might be more effective in addressing the client's needs. Nonpsychologists, for example, should not attempt to determine the causes of and prescribe remedies for a client's apparent depression or chronic anxiety. These are possible psychological disorders that require the input of a licensed psychologist or other mental health professional. Proper ethics dictate that consultants assist the client by acknowledging limitations in their own knowledge and training and by knowing when to refer the client to a colleague with superior expertise.

The evolution of applied health fitness psychology mandates that practitioners become aware of the relevant literature, read current books and journals, join professional organizations and attend annual conferences, join and participate in online groups such as Listservs where current and sometimes controversial issues are discussed, develop a network of professional colleagues to call on for advice or referral, and become innovative and creative in generating new locations of practice. Examples of new locations include rehabilitation and medical centers, clinics, and hospitals; fitness clubs; after-school programs; college campuses; sport teams; private practice in psychology; the arts (e.g., dancers, actors, musicians); and the corporate sector.

FROM RESEARCH TO REAL WORLD

Students and practitioners will find the information in this chapter particularly valuable if they are interested in becoming health care professionals. Gaining knowledge, learning new skills, and becoming an expert and effective professional in the health care industry does not end with a college degree. Learning and improving your skills is a continual process that never ends—and that's a good thing. There is a sense of excitement when developing one's career.

Tasks toward career development include

- attending annual professional conferences where new advances in the field are communicated,
- subscribing to and reading scholarly and applied publications,
- participating in in-service training to improve skills and to learn new ways to improve job effectiveness,
- obtaining credentials that reflect mastery of professional skills and eligibility for organization memberships, and
- being aware of and mastering cutting-edge expertise for carrying out specific treatment strategies and interventions.

Entering a professional field and building a career path starts with following the ethical codes of key organizations that represent the profession. The codes must be read, reviewed, and remembered as an integral part of fulfilling your mission of helping others.

SUMMARY

Professional organizations exist to promote structure, growth, and state-of-the-art knowledge to members primarily through conferences and publications. They represent well-defined areas of expertise, research, and practice. The field of applied health fitness psychology is represented by at least five professional areas: psychology, sport and exercise psychology, sports medicine, behavioral medicine, and health. Each of these areas is represented by organizations that promote that particular field of expertise.

Promoting and recognizing the skills of organization members is the process called *credentialing*, which ensures that members of a profession meet predetermined, published standards through the processes of licensure, certification, and registry. Professional organizations also have codes of ethics, which provide guidance and governance to members in working settings and foster public trust by establishing high standards.

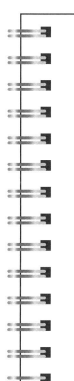

STUDENT ACTIVITY

Digging Deeper Into Professional Organizations

Visit the website of a professional organization related to psychology, health, sports medicine, behavioral medicine, or fitness or exercise psychology and attempt to retrieve the following information about the organization:

- Its mission or vision statement
- Its goals or objectives
- Its code of ethics
- Evidence of its registry
- Categories of memberships (e.g., student, professional)
- Criteria and requisite skills and knowledge for membership

Does the organization include content that concerns you? Seems unfair? Is disorganized? Is not informative or clear? How can this website content be improved to better reflect the goals and standards of this profession?

REFERENCES

American College of Sports Medicine (ACSM). (2010). *ACSM's guidelines for exercise testing and prescription* (8th ed.). Philadelphia: Lippincott, Williams and Wilkins.

American Psychological Association (APA). (1992). Ethical principles of psychologists and code of conduct. *American Psychologist, 47* (12), 1597-1611.

American Psychological Association (2002). Ethical principles of psychologists and code of conduct. *American Psychologist, 57,* 1060-1073.

Anshel, M.H. (2006). *Applied exercise psychology: A practitioner's guide for improving client health and fitness.* New York: Springer.

Anshel, M.H. (2012). *Sport psychology: From theory to practice* (5th ed.). San Francisco: Benjamin-Cummings.

Buckworth, J., and Dishman, R.K. (2002). *Exercise psychology.* Champaign, IL: Human Kinetics.

Carlstedt, R. (2008). Position paper on the state of applied sport psychology. *Journal of the American*

Board of Sport Psychology (www.americanboardofsportpsychology.org).

Fisher, C. (2003). *Decoding the ethics code: A practical guide of psychologists.* Thousand Oaks, CA: Sage.

Gauvin, L., and Russell, S.J. (1993). Sport-specific and culturally adapted measures in sport and exercise psychology research: Issues and strategies. In R.N. Singer, M. Murphey, and L.K. Tennant (Eds.), *Handbook of research on sport psychology* (pp. 891-900). New York: Macmillan.

Johnsgard, K. (2004). *Conquering depression and anxiety through exercise.* Amhert, NY: Prometheus Books.

Landers, D.M. (1988). Sport psychology: A commentary. In J.S. Skinner, C.B. Corbin, D.M. Landers, P.E. Martin, and C.L. Wells (Eds.), *Future directions in exercise and sport sciences* (pp. 475-486). Champaign, IL: Human Kinetics.

Lox, C.L., Martin Ginis, K.A., and Petruzzello, S.J. (2010). *The psychology of exercise: Integrating theory and practice.* Scottsdale, AZ: Holcomb Hathaway.

Matarazzo, R.D. (1982). Behavioral health's challenge to academic, scientific, and professional psychology. *American Psychologist, 37,* 1-14.

Morgan, W.P. (1988). Sport psychology in its own context: A recommendation for the future. In J.S. Skinner, C.B. Corbin, D.M. Landers, P.E. Martine, and C.L. Wells (Eds.), *Future directions in exercise and sport psychology* (pp. 97-110). Champaign, IL: Human Kinetics.

Pauline, J.S., Pauline, G.A., Scott, R., Johnson, S.R., and Kelly, M. (2006). Ethical issues in exercise psychology. *Ethics and Behavior, 16,* 61-76.

Sachs, M.L. (1993). Professional ethics in sport psychology. In R.N. Singer, M. Murphey, and L.K. Tennant (Eds.), *Handbook of research on sport psychology* (pp. 921-932). New York: Macmillan.

Sachs, M.L., Burke, K.L., and Schweighardt, S.L. (Eds.) (2011). *Directory of graduate programs in applied sport psychology* (10th ed.). Morgantown, WV: Fitness Information Technology.

Schutz, R.W., and Gessaroli, M.E. (1993). Use, misuse, and disuse of psychometrics in sport psychology research. In R.N. Singer, M. Murphey, and L.K. Tennant (Eds.), *Handbook of research on sport psychology* (pp. 901-917). New York: Macmillan.

Singer, R.N., and Anshel, M.H. (2006a). An overview of interventions in sport. In J. Dosil (Ed.), *The sport psychologist's handbook: A guide for sport-specific performance enhancement* (pp. 63-88). New York: Wiley.

Singer, R.N., and Anshel, M.H. (2006b). Assessment, evaluation, and counseling in sport. In J. Dosil (Ed.), *The sport psychologist's handbook: A guide for sport-specific performance enhancement* (pp. 89-120). New York: Wiley.

Watson, J.C., Zizzi, S., and Etzel, E.F. (2006). Ethical training in sport psychology programs: Current training standards. *Ethics and Behavior, 16,* 5-14.

Whelan, J.P., Meyers, A.W., and Elkins, T.D. (2002). Ethics in sport and exercise psychology. In J.L. Van Raalte and B.W. Brewer (Eds.), *Exploring sport and exercise psychology* (2nd ed., pp. 503-523). Washington, DC: American Psychological Association.

Epilogue

We live in a culture, in fact, in a *world*, that is focused on immediate gratification. Our vision is short term; we want the fruits of our labors sooner, not later. Too often we are prepared to sacrifice the long-term benefits of maintaining daily rituals, and instead choose less healthy options that bring about short-term gratification. We need to *show* children and students the huge advantages of investing time and energy—making time for wise choices that improve health and well-being—in return for much larger rewards later. Instead of reacting in the easiest way, we need to remember our values and make choices that support those values. For example, many people consider their family the most important thing in their lives, but we are of little value to our families if we are sick, lack energy, and lose enthusiasm for life.

Healthy habits should be viewed as an investment in the future. We are taught to understand the need to put away some of our income for retirement, meaning we have less cash for spending in the short term. We should be making the same parallel case for investing in our future health by acting more responsibly and treating our bodies—our temples—with respect. We need to understand why, as a culture, we engage in self-destructive behaviors, doing things every day that we *know* are not good for us.

Many possible reasons for self-destructive behaviors are discussed in this text, but there remains one possible reason that has gone largely unexplored in the health and fitness literature and may also explain a person's insistence on self-destructive habits: the lack of common sense, also known as stupidity, a concept explored extensively by Dr. James F. Welles (1986). This is an appropriate and important topic because health care professionals need to examine all possible explanations for people's propensity toward self-destructive habits and their refusal to change even though they understand the dire consequences. Why would someone know-

ingly continue harmful behaviors that may lead to poor health and even premature death?

The word *stupid*, which can serve as an adjective or noun, comes from the Latin verb *stupere*, which means being numb or astonished. From a formal perspective, Welles (1986) defines stupidity as a lack of intelligence, understanding, reason, wit, or sense. It may be hereditary, assumed, or reactive (i.e., being stupid with grief or despair). To Welles, stupid describes a person who is slow of mind, perhaps lacking intelligence, care, self-awareness, reason, or common sense. It also represents dullness of feeling or sensation (i.e., senseless, insensitivity) or lacking interest or purpose (exasperating). It can either imply a congenital lack of capacity for reasoning or a temporary state of slow-mindedness.

With respect to the current context of changing health behavior, stupidity takes on a slightly different meaning. Stupidity is not unconscious or unintentional, according to most authors. Stupidity reflects a mentality that is considered to be informed, deliberate, maladaptive, or dysfunctional. Stupidity is often distinguished from ignorance. According to Dr. Robert Sternberg, editor of the book *Why Smart People Can Be So Stupid* (2002), there is a difference between acting and being stupid. Some behaviors are so irresponsible, heedless, thoughtless, negligent, or outrageous that they invite the label. The act of smoking, for instance, is considered stupid regardless of the intent and motives of the smoker. Some people will knowingly, consciously, purposefully, and habitually demonstrate self-destructive behavior patterns because of their refusal to understand and initiate better alternatives that will help prevent highly undesirable outcomes.

Behavior may be inaccurately labeled stupid if the action follows limited or inadequate information and resources. Along these lines, justifiable mistakes should not be labeled stupid. Thus, while stupidity provides one explanation for irrational and unhealthy actions, it is prudent to refrain from labeling actions as stupid unless we know more about a person's knowledge of the consequences of actions. The primary job of health professionals is to provide clients and patients with this knowledge.

A person acting in a stupid manner must *know* she is acting in her own worst interest; stupidity is a choice, not a forced act or accident. Those who are diagnosed with high bad cholesterol, low good cholesterol, and other undesirable scores on a lipid profile are warned by physicians to follow certain dietary and exercise guidelines or face dire consequences. Yet patients who continue the same behavior patterns might be said to be inhibited by their stupidity. They are inhibited in developing clear perceptions and fail to appreciate the need to change features of their lifestyle to improve their health. Stupidity may be the only explanation that accurately reflects the actions of some individuals whose self-destructive behavior patterns border on a death wish.

Stupidity provides one more possible reason some people fail to grasp the seriousness of their unhealthy habits, and why they continue to do things every day that they know are unhealthy. Not surprisingly, they might get sick and do nothing to change the habits that likely cause their ill health. Some individuals even acknowledge that their poor health reflects their lifestyle, yet they fail to commit to changing their behavior.

If certain behaviors can be attributed to stupidity, what can health care professionals do? Referring to a person as stupid, either to that person directly or to another person, is rude, unprofessional, and counterproductive, so identifying the behavior in this way is a bad strategy. With respect to health behavior change, the person engaging in self-destructive behaviors must be informed, with respect and candor, about the costs and consequences of his unhealthy behavior patterns (e.g., financial costs, long-term consequences to health). After this action, however, it is the client's decision whether to change behavior, assuming his unhealthy habit is legal. When one of my students informed me that he refuses to use his

seat belt because one of his friends survived a car accident without wearing it, whereas someone who used a seat belt did not, I could only inform him of the benefits of using seat belts and that it was the law to use it when in a moving vehicle. The decision to wear it was his choice completely. In the end, stupidity is inherent in a society of people who are free to make choices about the way they live. No one, including health professionals, can force behavior change. Making poor choices about unhealthy behavior patterns is not against the law—so far.

What health professionals can do is to provide good information and engage the barriers to regular physical activity head on. Let's review (from chapter 4) some of these barriers and what health professionals can do to prevent and overcome them.

• *Replace negative with positive attitudes toward exercise.* Teachers, coaches, and parents must avoid using exercise as a form of punishment. This common form of punishment runs contrary to the position statement of the National Association for Sport and Physical Education and is a leading cause of negative feelings toward exercise. A student's negative experiences with sport and physical education can lead to long-term unpleasant feelings toward exercise in adulthood. Exercise and other forms of physical activity should be fun. Let's not penalize children whose sport skills are mediocre by having them sit on the sideline or criticize them for their lack of skills. Increase opportunities for sport skill instruction.

• *Prevent exercise burnout.* Can a person burn out from too much exercise? Absolutely, especially if the person is coerced into a training program that is intense and long term. Coaches and physical education teachers can include other forms of physical activity such as performing alternative sport skills or engaging in more playful forms of physical activity (e.g., relay races) to keep exercise fun and prevent burnout.

• *Overcome the perception of no time.* Not enough time is the leading excuse for not exercising in virtually all related studies, but this may be a matter of perception rather than reality. As discussed in chapter 4, all we need is 3 hours per week (on alternate days) of vigorous exercise to meet physiological needs. That's a mere 1.5% of our week. Health professionals have to learn time management strategies in order to help clients and patients determine time management strategies for adhering to a regular exercise schedule. There *is* enough time for an exercise program if the person views it as a necessary component of maintaining health. Not enough time to exercise is among the greatest myths of our culture.

• *Provide strategies for reducing financial costs.* While the expenses associated with starting an exercise program can be prohibitive for some, exercise need not cost much money. It is not necessary to buy a membership to a fitness club, pay for an exercise coach or personal trainer, purchase new exercise apparel (although some items, like high-quality running shoes, will help prevent discomfort and perhaps injury), and pay for transportation to the exercise facility. Exercising at home—using purchased fitness equipment or walking and jogging on the street—is one approach to overcoming expenses, and so is sharing costs for equipment and transportation to attend an exercise facility.

• *Teach proper exercise technique.* There are right and wrong ways to perform various types of exercise. Health professionals, particularly in the fitness industry, should ensure that every person who steps into an exercise facility receives at least elementary coaching on the proper exercise techniques. Incorrect use of equipment can lead to injury and drastically slow progress, both of which are leading causes of quitting an exercise program. This cause of dropping out of programs can easily be remedied.

• *Keep goals realistic and performance based.* Goal setting serves the purposes of increasing motivation, providing direction of effort, determining the standards of successful performance, and feeling rewarded for achieving that success. Goals that are too ambitious, lack concreteness, and are based on outcomes (e.g., losing weight) but not on performance (e.g., completing 10 biceps curls) can inhibit the benefits of goal setting. Unmet goals can lead to perceived failure and dropout. Goals either are unnecessary—depending on the client's preferences—or should be challenging yet realistic. Health professionals need to help clients maintain patience in meeting performance goals.

• *Provide clients with regular feedback on progress.* Progress, also referred to as achievement and perceived competence, is a primary source of exercise motivation. Health professionals should acknowledge all indicators of progress, especially if determined numerically, such as the client's performance speed, distance, number of repetitions, and changes in test scores.

• *Provide social support.* Most people need someone to depend on physically (e.g., exercise coaching, transportation to an exercise venue, exercising together) or emotionally (e.g., motivational statements or messages of encouragement). The process of showing care, comfort, or assistance to another person is collectively called social support, and it is essential for maintaining exercise adherence. Novice exercisers, in particular, might feel lonely or need the companionship and support of others. Coaching is one form of social support. Health professionals need to be sure that each client has her preferred level of support—physically and emotionally—in order to enjoy the exercise experience.

After reading this book, you should feel more prepared to help overcome these barriers and to provide routes to maintaining regular physical activity for your clients who are willing to pursue change. By doing this, you can make an incalculable difference in their lives.

The good news is this: Humans are born with the desire and capacity to survive. What so many clients and patients fail to realize—perhaps reflecting human nature—is that fulfilling dreams require energy, and energy necessitates good health. This is where you as the health care professional become so important. Most clients and patients need assistance, usually referred to as social support, to overcome their self-destructive nature and to reach their goals so that they can be happy and productive members of society. You can provide a wake-up call indicating that clients' behavior patterns are leading them down the path of destruction, poor health, premature disease, a lower quality of life, and a shortened life span. The costs and consequences of actions are enormous, and you—the health care professional—need to play the role of truth teller. Whether your clients and patients are receptive to the truth is their choice. But if they are not, they might not live long enough to walk down the aisle at their children's weddings or to see their children graduate.

It's all about helping clients being receptive to the truth and then helping them making the right choices. As Loehr and Schwartz (2003) explain, "Facing the truth about the gap between who we want to be and who we really are is never easy. Each of us has an infinite capacity for self-deception" (p. 148). We tend to push away or repress information that we find unpleasant, upsetting, or contrary to the way we perceive the world. "Until we can clear away the smoke and mirrors and look honestly at ourselves, we have no starting point for change," Loehr and Schwartz assert.

The truth sets us free. Let the journey begin!

REFERENCES

Loehr, J., and Schwartz, T. (2003). *The power of full engagement: Managing energy, not time, is the key to high performance and personal renewal.* New York: Free Press.

Sternberg, R. (Ed.). (2002). *Why smart people can be so stupid.* New Haven, CT: Yale University Press.

Welles, J.F. (1986) *Understanding Stupidity.* Orient, NY: Mount Pleasant Press. www.stupidity.net/story2.

Index

Note: Page numbers followed by an italicized *f* or *t* refer to the figure or table on that page, respectively.

About the Author

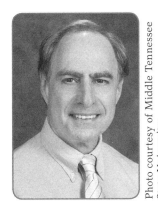

Mark H. Anshel, PhD, is a professor in the department of health and human performance with a joint appointment in the psychology department at Middle Tennessee State University in Murfreesboro. He is the author of more than 135 research publications, four fitness books, and multiple editions of the text *Sport Psychology: From Theory to Practice*. His research since 2007 has concerned the effectiveness of a cognitive-behavioral model on exercise participation and adherence called the Disconnected Values Model. Anshel is recognized as an international leader in providing evidence-based programs and linking research with practice in the areas of exercise and fitness psychology and sport psychology.

Over the course of his career, Anshel has gained hands-on experience consulting with more than 3,000 clients on healthy habits, particularly the use of exercise. His practical career experience began with seven years as a fitness director in community recreation. From 2000 to 2002 Anshel served as a performance coach at the Human Performance Institute in Orlando, Florida, where he provided corporate clients with a cognitive-behavioral program on replacing unhealthy habits with more desirable lifestyle routines. He also served as a performance consultant and researcher related to improving wellness and coping skills with the Murfreesboro Police Department from 2005 to 2011.

In 2009, Anshel was awarded the Distinguished Research Scholar Award from Middle Tennessee State University. Anshel is a fellow of the American Psychological Association (Division 47, Exercise and Sport Psychology). He is the founder and director of the Middle Tennessee State University Employee Health and Wellness Program, which received grant funding of $130,000 over two years. Anshel also served for 10 years on the editorial board of the *Journal of Sport Behavior*.

In his free time, Anshel enjoys jogging, writing on health-related topics, and reading current events and health-related research. He resides in Murfreesboro, Tennessee.

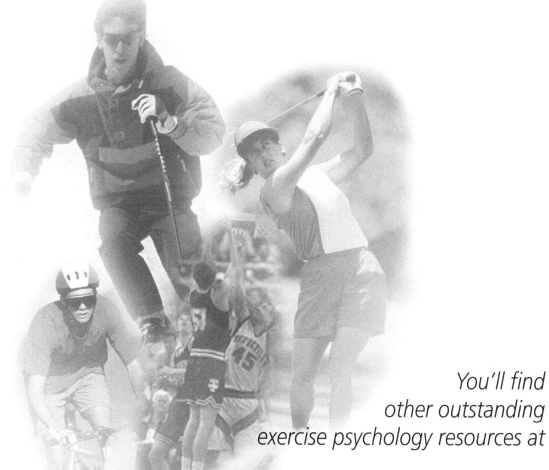